THE NEW PARKINSON'S DISEASE
TREATMENT BOOK

OTHER BOOKS BY THE AUTHOR

The Parkinson's Disease Treatment Book: Partnering with Your Doctor to Get the Most from Your Medications. New York: Oxford University Press; 2005. 532 pp.

Parkinson's Disease Treatment Guide for Physicians. New York: Oxford University Press; 2009. 382pp.

Dementia with Lewy Bodies and Parkinson's Disease Dementia. New York: Oxford University Press; 2014. 250pp.

The New Parkinson's Disease Treatment Book

◆ ◆ ◆

Partnering with Your Doctor to Get the Most from Your Medications

SECOND EDITION

J. ERIC AHLSKOG, PhD, MD

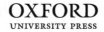
OXFORD
UNIVERSITY PRESS

OXFORD
UNIVERSITY PRESS

Oxford University Press is a department of the University of
Oxford. It furthers the University's objective of excellence in research,
scholarship, and education by publishing worldwide.

Oxford   New York
Auckland   Cape Town   Dar es Salaam   Hong Kong   Karachi
Kuala Lumpur   Madrid   Melbourne   Mexico City   Nairobi
New Delhi   Shanghai   Taipei   Toronto

With offices in
Argentina   Austria   Brazil   Chile   Czech Republic   France   Greece
Guatemala   Hungary   Italy   Japan   Poland   Portugal   Singapore
South Korea   Switzerland   Thailand   Turkey   Ukraine   Vietnam

Oxford is a registered trademark of Oxford University Press
in the UK and certain other countries.

Published in the United States of America by
Oxford University Press
198 Madison Avenue, New York, NY 10016

Library of Congress Cataloging-in-Publication Data
Ahlskog, J. Eric.
[Parkinson's disease treatment book]
The new Parkinson's disease treatment book : partnering with your doctor to get the most
from your medications / J. Eric Ahlskog, Ph.D., M.D. — Second edition.
pages cm
Revision of: Parkinson's disease treatment book. 2005.
Includes index.
ISBN 978-0-19-023186-6
1. Parkinson's disease—Treatment—Popular works.   I.   Title.
RC382.A365 2015
616.8′3306—dc23
2015008118

1 3 5 7 9 8 6 4 2
Printed in the United States of America
on acid-free paper

♦ ♦ ♦

Contents

Part Four
The Cause and Progression of Parkinson's Disease

Part Five
The Movement Problems of Parkinson's Disease: Medication Rationale and Choices

Part Six
Beginning Treatment of Parkinson's Disease: Medication Guidelines

Part Seven
The Early Years on Medications

Part Eight
Later Medication Inconsistency: Motor Fluctuations and Dyskinesias

Part Nine
Other Treatment Problems: Not Just a Movement Disorder

Part Ten
Nutrition, Exercise, Work, and Family

Part Eleven
Surgery and Procedures for Parkinson's Disease: Present and Future

Part Twelve
Parkinson's Disease Information Services

♦ ♦ ♦

Acknowledgments

The practice of medicine starts with medical school and residency, which provide the basis for the real education on the front lines in the clinic and hospital. The first edition of this book, published a decade ago, especially acknowledged the countless patients in my clinic that have taught me so many invaluable lessons. Now, ten years later, I am even more indebted to my patients. I have done my best to listen to them and recognize the treatment principles that have surfaced in their care. Medicine is not a job but a calling; the important responsibility for peoples' health strongly reinforces the lessons learned in their care. I have religiously read the appropriate medical journals and been attentive to new ideas; however, the richest source of knowledge has been taught to me by the people under my care. To them, I dedicate this book.

I also am very indebted to mentors along the way of my medical and scientific career. This includes Professor Mark Rilling at Michigan State University; Professor Bartley Hoebel at Princeton University; and Professor Barry Levin at Dartmouth Medical School. Their support along my career path was crucial and provided me with superb role models.

The medical environment of the Mayo Clinic cannot be overestimated as an influence on my medical career and the care of my patients. Despite the busy patient calendars, adequate time has been available for the most complex of patient problems. I have some very smart and experienced medical colleagues whom I can call upon for advice. As I have gotten older, I find myself giving advice more often than before; however, I still seek advice as often as in years past. It seems that I can always find a colleague who has special expertise in every area of medicine. The resources of the rich Mayo medical environment have been an important source of personal intellectual stimulation. I have had many mentors and role models at Mayo, some of whom have now passed on. Their work lives on in their trainees, including me.

The preparation for a career in medicine started early in childhood, raised as an only child by two loving parents who emphasized the virtues of honesty, humility, respect for others, and, later, hard work and perseverance. They formed the basis for all that I have done since with my life and career. Much of what they taught me was by example; they were immigrants, learning English as a second language. Their childhoods were spent on farms nearly a century ago, with horses instead of tractors, and simple lives with few conveniences. They survived the Great Depression and both World Wars, deferring many things but maintaining optimism for the future. Their marriage was late in life and I was not born until they were middle-aged, my father 50 and my mother 42. They had learned to play the hands they were dealt and were thankful for small blessings. Their life perspectives and the wisdom they accumulated from these challenges were subtly conveyed to me. "Always do the right thing; never lie; never do something that would make you ashamed; money is far less important than your good name"; these were principles that are a good starting point for those destined to become physicians. Later, I understood by their examples the importance of life goals and working hard to attain them. Interestingly, I was never encouraged to have a medical career, but rather to choose life's work that would make them and me proud. I owe much to them, and I frequently think about Dad and Mom, and their examples.

Thanks also very deservedly goes the Joan Bossert, who is the Vice President of the Brain and Behavioral Sciences Division of Oxford University Press. She took on the challenging task of editing my first edition of this book a decade ago. To call it heavy editing would be a gross understatement. I learned much from her deletions and suggestions, and applied these principles to the subsequent books that I have written, including this one. Her writing mentorship has benefitted many readers!

Among the most important contributors to this book and someone who especially deserves my thanks and appreciation is my wife, Faye. She never scolded over the eight months that I spent weekends in front of my computer at the Clinic, churning out the chapters of this book. For all those eight months, she welcomed me home and never complained. I could not have done this without her loving support. To her and to my wonderful sons, Michael, John, and Matthew, I send my love and thank them for their encouragement.

J. Eric Ahlskog, PhD, MD

THE NEW PARKINSON'S DISEASE
TREATMENT BOOK

1

◆ ◆ ◆

Background

This second edition of this book for people with Parkinson's disease follows one decade after publication of the first edition. Since that time, no cure for the disease has been discovered, and there have been no major breakthroughs in treatment of symptoms. However, we are collectively becoming wiser in the symptomatic treatment of Parkinson's disease. With another decade of clinical practice, patients have continued to teach me valuable lessons. The goal of this book is to translate those lessons and the published medical literature into an updated text that informs patients as they work with their clinicians.

For those of you who have read the first edition of this book, you will note that most of the chapters have been rewritten and others have undergone major revisions. In part, this reflects new data and emerging research on Parkinson's disease. However, it also reflects my own ongoing experience in the clinic working with Parkinson's disease patients and their families. Clinicians on the front lines of medicine learn daily from their patients. Some things work, and some do not. What appears useful in the short term may later fail or have adverse consequences.

The revisions of this book also reflect a more narrowed focus. In the first edition, I attempted to cover all reasonable medication strategies, recognizing that other clinicians have differing views; people reading that book will be cared for by some of these clinicians. Hence, that book was very comprehensive.

Medications strategies that I personally did not prescribe or rarely prescribed were discussed, as I knew that some of these would be encountered in other clinics. In this edition, however, I have chosen to be more selective in the treatment strategies presented; these are based on my full-time clinic experience over the past three decades. For example, I have omitted anticholinergic drugs as options for treating Parkinson's disease, as they are more likely to cause side effects than to produce benefits. I have taken a more directed view of precisely which drug among many is my preferred first choice for treating Parkinson's disease— carbidopa/levodopa—and why. Hence, this book is shorter and consistently more to the point.

Since publication of the first edition of this book, I wrote a parallel book for clinicians, *The Parkinson's Disease Treatment Guide for Physicians* (Oxford University Press, 2009), that mirrors the first edition of this book, chapter by chapter. This current second edition for patients maintains the same chapter organization and is in sync with the physician's version.

This book reflects my experience from my own medical practice and does not necessarily represent the views of the Mayo Clinic. Those finding fault with anything written herein have only me and my patients (who have taught me much about Parkinson's disease) to blame.

Why This Book?

Parkinson's disease (PD) is, indeed, a treatable condition. Medical treatment has increased patients' longevity and allowed most people with PD to remain active and productive for many years. The responses to the available drugs are often striking and occasionally border on the miraculous. PD is among the most treatable of all chronic neurological conditions.

The medical treatment of PD, unfortunately, is not always simple. There are multiple medications available, and these can be used in a variety of ways. The choice of drug, the dose, and the timing often are crucial; therapy must be individualized to meet each person's unique requirements. Also, the distinction between the symptoms of PD and medication side effects is a frequent source of confusion, with potential for ineffective or inappropriate treatment. Sometimes, treatable symptoms are not even recognized as part of PD. The difference between optimal and ineffective therapy may be the difference between a nursing home and independent living. The goal of this book is to help each and every person with PD achieve the best treatment.

Numerous texts have been published on the subject of PD, targeting either the patient or the physician. While many of the texts for patients and families have been excellent sources of information, treatment is addressed in only a general sense. Medications are described, but not how and when to use them, nor are the dosages and which medications address which problems.

Rather, these treatment details are deferred for patients to discuss with their doctors. Specific therapeutic guidelines generally have been reserved for texts written for physicians. Yet even many of these physician-directed books are written in general terms. The reason for this relatively superficial discussion is obvious; for any given problem, a variety of treatment strategies may be appropriate. Hence, a general, nonspecific overview avoids offending those with different treatment philosophies.

A different approach has been taken with this book: this is a nuts-and-bolts treatment book addressed to those with PD and their families. It is also meant for the patient's physician, with the intent of making treatment a team approach. After all, physicians, patients, and families are all on the same team. If patients have a good understanding of not only their disease but also of the appropriate drugs, doses, and the rationale for using these, optimal treatment should be facilitated.

Writing a technical book addressing the nuances of medical therapy is challenging; the language of medicine must be translated into words that laypeople understand. On the other hand, the content cannot be watered down; otherwise the purpose of the book would be defeated. But is this level of discussion really necessary? Should the patient cross the threshold into the domain of the physician? Why not let the doctor handle it all? For simple problems, this philosophy of passive reliance on one's physician works well. PD, however, is not a simple problem. Complex problems require complex solutions, and these open the possibility for misunderstanding and miscommunication.

People with PD often misinterpret symptoms or describe them ambiguously. This situation is challenging to the treating clinician, especially given a typically busy practice. The pressures of modern medicine force physicians to maximize efficiency. Hence there is often insufficient time in a busy practice to wade through the complex symptoms of PD. This book is meant to provide the knowledge that people with PD need to assist their physician in this process. Proactive patients and families who are good observers and recognize treatment principles can help maximize therapeutic outcomes. This book is not intended to make patients their own doctors; it is intended to open avenues of informed communication, stimulate discussion, and streamline the decision-making process.

Are the guidelines and recommendations provided in this book the best strategies for treatment of PD? As one might expect, there are often several therapeutic solutions to the same problem. In this text, I have chosen those that have worked best for my patients and have withstood the test of time. They have been distilled from over 30 years of experience of treating people with PD at the Mayo Clinic. This experience has been both in the clinic as a full-time, patient-seeing neurologist and as a clinical-investigator, responsible for PD treatment protocols. One thing I recognized early in my practice was the importance of listening to the people I was treating. They have taught me countless and invaluable lessons about PD that cannot be found in medical textbooks.

In cases where there is more than one reasonable approach, I have tried to present alternative strategies, with the arguments for each. For example, the choice of the initial medication for PD therapy continues to be debated. The arguments for this and other treatment issues can become extremely complex and occasionally supported by misinformation. In this book I have decided to err on the side of being selective and to advise what I believe works best. Moreover, I wanted to avoid paralysis by analysis. This should not be interpreted as disavowing all other treatment strategies.

This book has one more goal: to help the layperson wade through the morass of information about PD in the lay press and on the Internet. It seems that every few months a "new treatment for Parkinson's disease" is acclaimed. With all these "new treatments" it is surprising that anyone still suffers with PD. Many people come to their neurology appointments armed with newspaper clippings and pages downloaded from Internet sites. Some of this information is instructive, but not all is accurate and often it is misleading. Furthermore, some of the more useful and informative websites are a bit sophisticated, and the uninitiated reader may get lost in the medical terms. I hope this book will provide sufficient background so that such information can be understood, judged, and put into the proper perspective.

This book is dedicated to the proposition that PD is not an irreversible sentence to canes, walkers, and disability. Admittedly, lives are changed substantially by PD, and for many, the problems will be limiting. However, even when disability is in the cards, it often can be forestalled for many years by optimal treatment. We have medications available to keep people with PD within the mainstream of life; this book addresses how to take full advantage of such treatments.

How to Use This Book

This book starts with the premise that most readers know little about medical science. It begins with discussions of elementary principles of brain function and of PD, and provides a working medical vocabulary. Medicine has a language all its own, and medical specialty areas have an even more unique lexicon. A clear understanding of words used to describe the nuances of parkinsonism facilitates communication with physicians. If you forget definitions as your read further, you can refer to the glossary at the end of the book.

This book was written to be read from cover to cover; however, there may be certain chapters that do not pertain to you, and these may be skimmed rather than read in detail. Bear in mind that what does not relate to you today may be relevant in the future; hence, it's not a bad idea to at least have a sense of what is discussed in each chapter.

The book begins with introductory chapters that introduce you to the brain and PD, followed by chapters detailing treatment of the movement problems of PD. Parkinson's disease, however, is not simply a problem of tremor and movement. The symptoms go beyond that, and recognition of the broad spectrum of symptoms is critical to optimal treatment. Questions frequently arise: "Is my sciatica due to Parkinson's disease?" "Why am I sleepy all the time?" Pain, insomnia, cramps, shortness of breath, and a wide variety of other problems are typically attributed to other conditions when, in fact, they are due to PD or to the medications used to treat PD. Beginning with Chapter 19, we tackle these non-movement problems and how best to treat them.

Parkinson's disease is a very heterogeneous disorder with marked variability from person to person. Within this book, many potential problems are described, such as difficulty swallowing, urinary incontinence, dementia, and so on. Do not assume that you are destined to develop this full gamut of difficulties. Many of these problems will never become issues for individuals with PD. For example, dementia is present in a minority of people examined in PD clinics; when it develops, it is typically much later in the disease course. Minor swallowing problems or urinary difficulties are frequent, but troublesome difficulties may never occur. Even when many of these problems do develop, they are often treatable. Thus, the extensive list of problems discussed in this book should not be viewed as the likely template for your PD.

The focus of this book is on the medical treatment of PD. However, we are now in an era in which there are increasing surgical options. Currently, brain surgery is not appropriate for most individuals with PD, but it is a consideration for a distinct minority. I have placed this surgical discussion near the end of the book, since brain surgery is currently an appropriate consideration only after medical therapies have been exhausted.

One final comment is in order: the physician must always be the final arbiter of the treatment decisions. I have written this book exactly as I conduct my own medical practice. However, when a patient is with me in the office, I can confirm my clinical impression with firsthand evidence; I can ask clarifying questions, observe behavior, and examine. An objective clinician-observer is necessary to filter and interpret the clinical data to be sure the treatment fits the problem. It is difficult to make objective medical decisions about ourselves. Furthermore, it is easy to jump to inappropriate conclusions after reading something. Hence, your doctor must be a party to all treatment decisions.

But what if your doctor chooses an alternative strategy, different from what you have read in this book? This book is meant to provoke discussion, but not to dogmatically tell each person with PD what he or she must do. Your physician is privy to the details of your unique problem.

This may influence him or her to structure your medical treatment along different lines. Bear in mind that there is often no single correct answer to many problems, and multiple therapeutic strategies often arrive at the same destination. The guidelines in this book work in my practice, but only for those people I can interview and examine. Your doctor must make the ultimate call.

PART ONE

◆ ◆ ◆

Basic Facts about the Brain and Parkinson's Disease

2

♦ ♦ ♦

A Primer on the Brain

A text on Parkinson's disease (PD) should start with a discussion of the brain. After all, this is a brain disorder. As you might imagine, this is not a simple matter; the brain is incredibly complex. Not only is brain structure complicated, but so is human thought and action. How amazing that the human brain can derive complex mathematical equations, compose great novels, and also direct the swing of a baseball bat toward a curving baseball thrown at 90 miles per hour! Although we are not close to understanding how the brain mediates the genius of a mathematician or the artistry of a composer, we do understand many elementary things about brain function. What we have learned has led to breakthroughs in the medical treatment of many neurological conditions.

PD stands as a shining example of how our understanding of brain function provided a rational basis for symptomatic treatment. Over decades, multiple scientists and clinicians each contributed insights, putting pieces of the PD brain puzzle together. From these aggregate efforts, effective symptomatic treatment of PD was predicted and later confirmed in clinical trials. We now are able to treat many PD symptoms based on our knowledge of brain mechanisms. We continue to build upon these scientific principles and, as such, the treatment of PD remains a work in progress.

This chapter outlines elementary principles about the brain and how it is organized. You will be introduced to the medical language of PD, with approximately 25 new terms, which are again defined in the glossary at the end of this book. This will provide the necessary background for subsequent chapters.

Neurons: The Primary Component of the Brain

The brain is very much like the computer on your desk. A computer has small electronic components that are interconnected and integrated in complex circuits. Through multiple series of electrical processing, computers are able to perform complicated tasks.

The primary unit of the brain is the brain cell, or *neuron*. These may be conceived as analogous to components of computer microchips. The normal brain contains approximately 10 billion of these neurons. Each is capable of receiving and sending electrical signals within complex brain circuits. One neuron transmits signals to as many as 10,000 other neurons within these circuits.

What do these neurons look like? Glance at Figure 2.1 and then read on. Neurons are brain cells and share many of the properties of all the other cells within the body. You may recall from your biology classes that all cells have a nucleus. The blueprints for cell function, that is, DNA, are stored and activated within the nucleus. All cells have metabolic machinery for producing the structural building blocks making up the cell. They also have metabolic machinery for producing energy necessary for cell function. As you can see

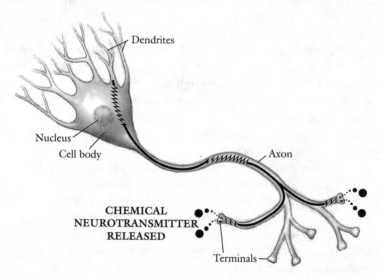

2.1   The elementary component of brain circuits is the neuron. It has a cell body with a nucleus, like other cells throughout the body. However, it is unique in having a long, wire-like extension called the axon; this allows communications with other neurons. The final event in transmission of the signal is release of a neurotransmitter from the terminals of that axon.

from Figure 2.1, at one end of the neuron is the cell body that contains the nucleus and most of the metabolic machinery. This is also the area where most of the signals from other neurons are received.

Electrical circuits need wires; the neuron has a wire-like extension called the *axon*, shown in Figure 2.1. These axons may be quite long, allowing transmission of signals across broad expanses of brain and spinal cord. The signal that starts in the cell body of a neuron (or dendrite) passes down the axon by electrical transmission.

Finally, on the end of the wire-like axon are small bulbs, called *terminals*. It is called a terminal for obvious reasons; it is at the end, or terminus. These terminals contain a specific brain chemical called a *neurotransmitter*. These neurotransmitters are released to signal the next neuron in the circuit. Each type of neuron releases one primary neurotransmitter. The neurons are some-times named by the neurotransmitter they secrete, adding the suffix *-ergic*. For example, neurons that secrete dopamine as the neurotransmitter are called *dopaminergic*; those that release acetylcholine are called *cholinergic*; when glutamate is the neurotransmitter, the neurons are called *glutamatergic*.

A single neuron receives these chemical messages from many other neu-rons. Most of these incoming signals are received either on the *dendrites* (shown in Figure 2.1) or the cell body. These dendrites often form a bushy reception network for these incoming signals.

To recap, when the cell body portion of the neuron is activated by another neuron, an electrical signal is initiated and transmitted to the other end, down the axon. When the electrical signal passes down the axon and reaches the terminals, it induces release of the neurotransmitter. This neurotrans-mitter signals the next cell in the circuit. Hence, signaling from one brain cell to the next is electrical until the very end; the final step involves chemical transmission.

Neurotransmitters and Receptors

The neurotransmitter released by one neuron binds to a specific site on the next brain cell; this is where the chemical signaling occurs to complete the transmission. That second brain cell is not activated by just any neurotrans-mitter. Only the specific neurotransmitter used in that circuit is effective. Why wouldn't any neurotransmitter work? The reason is that there is a specific *receptor* for every neurotransmitter. That receptor is located on the receiving end of neurons. Other chemicals in the area do not activate that receptor; it must be the specific neurotransmitter employed in that brain computer circuit, as shown in Figure 2.2. Once that neurotransmitter binds to the receptor, electrical signals are generated in that next neuron.

One single neuron may receive neurotransmitter input from hundreds or thousands of other neurons. This myriad of neurotransmitter signals may be

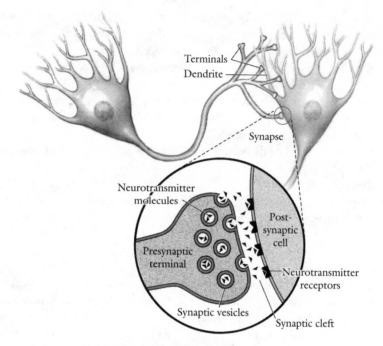

2.2   The terminals of neurons release a neurotransmitter to signal the next neuron in the circuit. The chemical neurotransmitter is expelled into a tiny space, the synapse, and attaches to the receptor. This receptor on the other side of the synapse receives either an activating or inhibitory signal, depending on the specific neurotransmitter.

either *excitatory* or *inhibitory*; that is, some neurotransmitters tend to activate the next neuron, whereas others have a dampening (inhibitory) effect. Thus, the summation of all of these neurotransmitter influences determines whether the next neuron in the circuit will fire or not. If enough of the excitatory receptors are activated on that next neuron, the summation of these will cause passage of the electrical signal down the axon to the terminal. The terminal then releases a finite amount of neurotransmitter and the sequence then continues in the next neuron in the circuit.

These neurotransmitters are contained within multiple discreet packages, called *vesicles*, and stored in the terminal, ready for release. The specific site where terminals release their neurotransmitter to activate the receptor is called the *synapse* (see Figure 2.2). Thus, a synapse includes the *presynaptic* terminal, the *postsynaptic* receptor, and the tiny space in between.

An External View of the Brain

Now that we have a sense of brain components at the microscopic and submicroscopic level, we will take a step back and look at the bigger picture.

Figure 2.3 illustrates two views of the brain, including from the side (revealing the connection with the spinal cord), and sliced through the middle.

- Note the *cortex*, which is the thick region of outermost brain circuitry shown in Figure 2.3. The cortex is most highly developed in humans, less developed in monkeys, and even less developed in lower species. Complex human thought and language are presumed to have their origins largely within the cortex. Some neurological conditions, such as Alzheimer's disease, result in widespread damage to the cortex. Such widespread cortical damage may impair the ability to think, remember, and communicate (dementia).

- At the back of the brain is the *cerebellum*, just above where the neck meets the skull. As Figure 2.3 shows, it is shaped like a tree in full leaf. The cerebellum integrates with other brain regions and modulates coordination. This area is spared in PD but degenerates in some disorders that resemble PD. The incoordination due to cerebellar damage is called *ataxia*. You may recognize such ataxia in people who have consumed too much alcohol; alcoholic beverages tend to impair cerebellar function, causing unsteadiness, hand incoordination, and slurred speech.

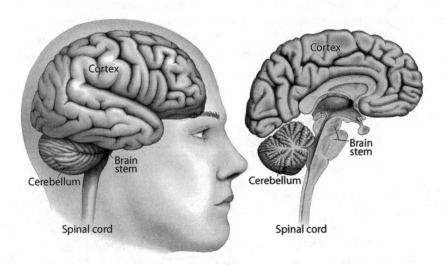

2.3 The external surface of most of the brain is covered by thick layers of interconnected neurons, the cortex; this is where human thought and memory is processed. The cortex is also where complex movement patterns are organized. Beneath the cortex (subcortex), more elementary processing of movement occurs, such as in the basal ganglia. The final common pathway of movement signals travel from cortex and subcortex down through the brainstem and into the spinal cord. The cerebellum is located over the brainstem and modulates the movement signals passing downstream to the spinal cord. The cerebellum is crucial for normal coordination of movement.

- The *brainstem* is located underneath the cerebellum, as shown in Figure 2.3. At the top of the brainstem is the substantia nigra, which we will discuss in detail in subsequent chapters. This area degenerates in Parkinson's disease and is primarily responsible for the slowness, stiffness, and other movement symptoms. Multiple other collections of brain cells are located in the brainstem. Many of these mediate elementary functions such as breathing, eye movement, swallowing, and jaw opening. Also, information passing from the spinal cord to the brain, and vice versa, goes through the brainstem. This is conducted along cable systems containing countless axons. Such nervous system cables are called *tracts*.

- The *spinal cord* is a continuum of the brainstem (Figure 2.3). This is the final common pathway for translating thought and intentions into goal-directed movements of the trunk and limbs. The decision to wave goodbye, throw a ball, or write a sentence originates in the cortex. The thought activates motor programs within and just below the cortex (i.e., cortex and subcortex). The brain computer code for the specific movement(s) is then conducted downstream, via the tracts passing through the brainstem into the spinal cord. Neurons within the spinal cord are then activated in the proper sequences to move muscles appropriately. The spinal cord also sends information in the opposite direction. When we stub our toe, sensors in the skin and joint are stimulated. These sensors send signals up nerves in the leg to the spinal cord. Initial processing of these signals occurs within the spinal cord. Subsequently, passage of these (stubbed toe) signals continues up to the brain. The pain signals activate groups of neurons at several levels of the brain, including brainstem, subcortex, and cortex.

Brain Centers Directly Affected by Parkinson's Disease

Now that we have a sense of the general design of the brain, we can focus on those areas responsible for many of the symptoms of Parkinson's disease (more will be said about this in Chapter 3). Neurons within the brain are organized into well-delimited regions called *nuclei*. Many nuclei can be easily recognized with the naked eye when looking at a brain slice. Early anatomists often named these nuclei based on their appearance. Hence, certain nuclei have very descriptive names, such as the "superior and inferior olives" (shaped like olives) or "red nucleus," named because of its reddish tint.

The most important nucleus that degenerates in those with PD and is responsible for many of the symptoms is the *substantia nigra*. This is located at the top of the brainstem (midbrain region), as shown in Figure 2.4. The

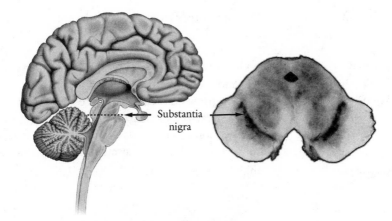

2.4 The substantia nigra provides the dopamine signaling that is crucial for normal movement. It degenerates in Parkinson's disease. The dark pigment of the substantia nigra makes is easy to recognize even in the absence of a microscope. It is located at the front end of the brainstem, in the midbrain.

substantia nigra neurons contain a black pigment; hence the name that translates into "black substance."

The darkly pigmented cell bodies of the substantia nigra send axons to another area of the brain called the *striatum*, as shown in Figure 2.5. The striatum is actually two nuclei, the *putamen* and *caudate*.

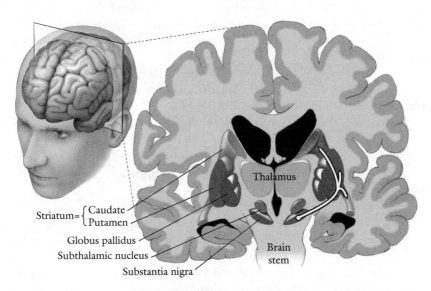

2.5 The substantia nigra neurons send axons to the striatum; these signal the striatum by releasing the neurotransmitter dopamine. The striatum includes two nuclei: caudate and putamen. Also shown are the globus pallidus and subthalamic nucleus; these two nuclei are integral components of the basal ganglia and are targets for deep brain stimulation treatment of PD. The brain ventricles are shown as black spaces in this figure.

Figure 2.5 also illustrates three other brain nuclei relevant to this discussion: the thalamus, globus pallidus, and subthalamic nucleus. They are intimate components of movement control circuits. Although they are not substantially damaged in Parkinson's disease, they are the three primary sites for PD brain surgery, which is addressed in Chapter 33.

We previously mentioned how groups of neurons release a common neurotransmitter, which signals the next set of neurons. The neurotransmitter for the substantia nigra projections to the striatum is *dopamine*; hence they are called dopaminergic neurons. In PD, these substantia nigra cells degenerate; consequently, dopamine levels plummet in the striatum. These dopaminergic substantia nigra cells are crucial to PD, as we discuss further in Chapter 3.

Brain Circuits Relevant to Parkinson's Disease

In a very simplistic sense, the connections of these brain nuclei may be conceptualized similar to an electrical wiring diagram. The brain movement control circuits are much more complex than this, but the major connections (projections of axons) are often thought of as electrical circuits.

The programming of walking and other movements partially occurs within the striatum. Projections from the striatum are primarily to the *globus pallidus*. The globus pallidus is a crucial output nucleus of this system, which processes and relays the signals to other brain nuclei. The globus pallidus is also called the *pallidum*. A major projection from the globus pallidus is to the *thalamus*. The thalamus is at the very center of the brain and contains multiple subdivisions. It is sometimes conceptualized as a relay station to and from the large expanse of cortex. The thalamus has widespread interconnections with all areas of the cortex. These nuclei are illustrated in Figure 2.5.

To reiterate, the striatum is a nodal point for brain movement circuitry. It sends output to the globus pallidus, which projects to the thalamus, and ultimately the thalamus projects to the cortex. Not surprisingly, signals from cortex are transmitted back to the striatum, forming a complete loop; this allows the cortex to provide feedback to the striatum.

Of special relevance to PD, this striatal-pallidal-thalamic-cortical loop is directly modulated by the dopaminergic substantia nigra. The nigral projection to the striatum maintains proper activity in the striatal-pallidal-thalamic-cortical circuit; when this dopaminergic control is lost, motor activity slows or is lost. That is the substrate for many of the symptoms of PD and also for symptomatic treatment.

An important aside relates to the *subthalamic nucleus*, also shown in Figure 2.5. This nucleus has become a target for neurosurgeons treating PD, as will be discussed in Chapter 33. The subthalamic nucleus is another relay station in these subcortical movement control circuits. It receives input from the striatum and projects to the globus pallidus. It is located just below the thalamus (hence, *sub*-thalamic). Its function, however, is distinct from that of the thalamus. This nucleus has an interesting history. For decades, it has been recognized that a stroke within the subthalamic nucleus causes an unusual syndrome, characterized by wild, flailing involuntary movements in the limbs on the opposite side of the body (known as hemiballismus).

General Terms Relating to PD Brain Circuits

Two other anatomic terms need to be defined since they are frequently encountered in reading about PD: basal ganglia and extrapyramidal. The precise anatomic definitions of these terms vary slightly, depending on the author. They refer to the subcortical brain motor control systems that we have been discussing. *Basal ganglia* is an encompassing term for both the striatum (caudate and putamen) and the globus pallidus. Both the substantia nigra and subthalamic nucleus have intimate connections with the striatum and globus pallidus, and they are typically included in the concept of the basal ganglia. Thus, the core nuclei of the basal ganglia are striatum and globus pallidus, plus their interconnected nuclei, the substantia nigra and subthalamic nucleus.

The term *extrapyramidal* is often used interchangeably with *basal ganglia*. It primarily refers to the basal ganglia nuclei plus their connections (which also includes certain connections with the cortex). Clinicians often use this term when referring to symptoms and signs caused by damage to these circuits; for example, they might say, "The patient had an extrapyramidal gait."

The term *extrapyramidal* derives from the need to distinguish this system from the pyramidal circuit. The pyramidal circuit is often referred to as the corticospinal tract and represents an elementary motor control system originating in the cortex. The name *pyramidal* derives from the appearance on a cross-sectional view of the brainstem, where this pathway was noted to be shaped like a pyramid. Hence, the other major motor control system (basal ganglia and connections) was termed extrapyramidal.

3

◆ ◆ ◆

Parkinson's Disease: Changes in the Brain and Beyond

Parkinson's disease (PD) is notoriously a brain disorder that impairs movement; it is characterized by slowness, stiffness, and often tremor. PD, however, affects the nervous system beyond brain motor regions, and the symptoms extend well beyond movement problems. PD affects certain brain regions but spares many others. It has specific microscopic and biochemical signatures. Although people with PD may seem quite varied in their symptoms, there are fundamental nervous system features that pervade this condition. In this chapter we will introduce such basic concepts. To begin, we discuss how PD fits into the larger context of all brain disorders and the relationship to other neurodegenerative diseases.

Neurodegenerative Disease

In general, a variety of insults may damage the brain and cause it to malfunction. This includes such disorders as strokes, tumors, brain infections (encephalitis), and trauma. One such category of brain disorders is *neurodegenerative disease*. Neurodegenerative diseases affect specific groups of brain cells, which slowly die (degenerate). Neurodegenerative disease encompasses a variety of conditions, most of which occur for unknown reasons. Well recognized within this category are Alzheimer's disease and Lou Gehrig's disease (amyotrophic lateral sclerosis, or ALS). PD is a neurodegenerative disease.

The loss of brain cells in these neurodegenerative disorders does not happen quickly; rather, it is a very slow process, progressing over years. The degeneration of these specific brain regions is typically incomplete, and not every neuron dies. Furthermore, the degeneration is confined to limited brain areas; much of the brain is spared. Which neurons degenerate, and which are spared, depends on the specific neurodegenerative disease. For example, in Alzheimer's disease, memory, language, and thinking neurons are selectively lost. In ALS, the neurons activating our muscles degenerate. In Parkinson's disease, most (but not all) of the symptoms are due to degeneration of the substantia nigra, although other neuron systems may be affected much later in the disease course.

What causes neurodegenerative diseases is largely unknown, although clues are now starting to surface. Undoubtedly, there will be a different cause for each class of neurodegenerative disorder. However, we are beginning to appreciate that there are some common themes, and what we learn about one disorder may help us understand the others.

The Substantia Nigra, Dopamine, and Parkinson's Disease

The substantia nigra, which degenerates in PD, is pivotally placed within movement control systems in the brain. The substantia nigra sends axons to and throughout the striatum, where it regulates the firing rates of neurons within movement circuits. We call this the *nigrostriatal pathway*, which is a contraction of the two words, *nigra* and *striatum*. The two components of the striatum, the caudate and putamen, are not equally affected; the putamen is more profoundly depleted of input from the substantia nigra.

Signaling from one neuron to the next is by release of a neurotransmitter, which is dopamine in the nigrostriatal system. Thus, when a substantia nigra neuron is activated, dopamine is released within the striatum; we categorize these neurons as dopaminergic. Researchers have recognized that this dopaminergic nigrostriatal pathway is constantly active, with ongoing dopamine release constantly modulating striatal neurons.

The neurons within the striatum have specific receptors that recognize and respond to dopamine. These dopamine receptors are not activated by other neurotransmitters.

When the substantia nigra cells are lost in PD, dopamine levels plummet within the striatum. When there is no dopamine, striatal cells do not activate properly and the symptoms of PD result. Experimentally, this can be demonstrated in animals. When a monkey or rat is administered a drug that lowers brain dopamine levels, these animals walk and move just like people with PD. Conversely, drugs that restore these animals' brain dopamine levels reverse these symptoms.

Medical treatment of PD capitalizes on the recognition that loss of brain dopamine is primarily responsible for the movement problems of PD. The major drugs used to treat PD symptoms either elevate brain dopamine levels or substitute for the lost dopamine.

What Is a Lewy Body and Why Should I Care?

The first important insight into the underpinnings of PD occurred around a century ago. In 1913, Dr. Frederick Lewy described unique microscopic changes in the brains of people with PD. He noted that brain cells from those with PD contained small, round collections of some type of biological material. These have since been known as *Lewy bodies*. They are found in specific areas of the brain and, notably, within the substantia nigra among people with PD. They are now recognized as the microscopic hallmark of PD. Pathologists look for these when asked to determine after death whether someone truly had PD. Lewy bodies cannot be seen with the naked eye. A microscopic view of a Lewy body is illustrated in Figure 3.1.

In typical PD, Lewy bodies are found in only specific areas of the nervous system, usually associated with loss of neurons (e.g., substantia nigra). Presumably, the process causing PD generates Lewy bodies, and this mechanism ultimately results in cell death of some of these neurons.

Although Lewy bodies often occur in only limited brain regions in typical PD, they become more widespread in individuals with long-standing

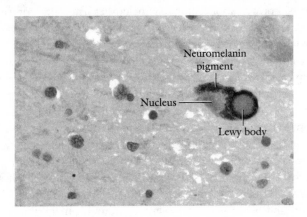

3.1 A substantia nigra neuron is shown, recognizable by the dark pigment. Within this neuron is a Lewy body.

PD, especially the elderly. This results in other symptoms, such as cognitive impairment (dementia). In a related condition called *dementia with Lewy bodies*, Lewy bodies are more diffusely found in both motor and cognitive regions of the brain. People with this disorder experience thinking and memory problems early in the disease course. Dementia with Lewy bodies is discussed in greater detail in Chapters 6 and 23 (see also J.E. Ahlskog's *Dementia with Lewy Bodies and Parkinson's Disease Dementia*, Oxford University Press, 2014).

A Brain Protein: Alpha-Synuclein

Because Lewy bodies mark the areas of degeneration, they are presumed to hold a key to the understanding of PD. What is contained within these Lewy bodies? A variety of component substances have been identified, but one in particular stands out: alpha-synuclein.

The alpha-synuclein story starts with the search for the gene causing parkinsonism in successive generations of several unique Italian-Greek families. Members of these families initially surfaced in the clinic of Dr. Lawrence Golbe, at the Robert Wood Johnson University Hospital in New Brunswick, New Jersey. He recognized the inheritance pattern (autosomal dominant) and appreciated the potential importance to understanding sporadic PD if the causative gene could be identified. It is extremely rare for PD to be passed from generation to generation; otherwise, these Italian-Greek families were typical of PD.

Through several years of extended travel to trace the family trees and collect blood samples, the products of his work led to the discovery of the abnormal gene. The gene coded for a previously unrecognized brain protein, alpha-synuclein.

Little was known about alpha-synuclein at the time of this discovery, although we now know that it is universally found in synaptic terminals throughout the normal brain. Shortly after the discovery of this alpha-synuclein mutation, scientists looked for this mutation among people with typical PD. Despite the investigation of many people with PD, no one, outside of a few European families, was found to carry this genetic abnormality. So why would this be relevant to PD in general? Its importance became apparent when a special stain was developed that marked where alpha-synuclein aggregates within the brain: alpha-synuclein is found in high concentrations in Lewy bodies! Although this is not the abnormal (mutated) alpha-synuclein like that of the Italian-Greek families, the high concentrations in Lewy bodies suggested a role for alpha-synuclein in typical PD. Based on this and other evidence, scientists now speculate that there may be something abnormal about the production or metabolism of alpha-synuclein that predisposes affected individuals to typical PD. More is said about this in Chapter 8, where we address current theories about the cause of PD.

Lewy Bodies in Normal People

Are Lewy bodies found only among people with PD (or Lewy body dementia)? In fact, Lewy bodies are found on postmortem examination in about 15% of neurologically "normal" seniors. This is approximately 10 times the prevalence of PD. Would these normal individuals have developed PD if they had lived longer? Or was the disease-causing process incomplete or aborted? Is PD actually a very common condition, with only a fraction of those predisposed developing it? This is food for thought, and we will discuss this further in Chapter 8.

More about Lewy Bodies

Lewy bodies are indeed the microscopic marker of Parkinson's disease. However, they are only the most visible part of the Lewy neurodegenerative process. They were first recognized because they were the easiest to see when PD brains were studied microscopically. Now with the use of special tissue stains that specifically label alpha-synuclein in the brain, Lewy bodies are easily seen. However, also visualized are much smaller accumulations in axons and dendrites, termed *Lewy neurites*. Small deposits (Lewy dots) are also apparent in affected brain regions of those with PD. Thus, there is a spectrum of microscopic Lewy neurodegenerative changes.

The current consensus is that the tiniest aggregates of this alpha-synuclein (Lewy) process may be the most toxic. Conversely, Lewy bodies, which are huge cellular clumps, may represent the neuron's garbage basket; that is, they are not toxic per se, but rather represent the cell's means of sequestering waste material. Lewy bodies reveal evidence of the Lewy neurodegenerative process, telling us that the affected neurons are trying to defend themselves. Thus, in this book, when we refer to Lewy bodies, it will be as a marker of the Lewy neurodegenerative process.

Why Are Symptoms of Parkinson's Disease Asymmetric (More on One Side Than the Other)?

People with PD typically experience their *initial* symptoms predominantly or exclusively on one side of their body, perhaps in only one limb. Why is this so? Shouldn't the degeneration of PD be uniform? In fact, the loss of the substantia nigra cells is somewhat haphazard. Even with progression, PD remains asymmetric, affecting one side of the body more severely than the other. Why some substantia nigra cells succumb and others survive is unknown.

PD Symptoms Outside the Motor System

Although the problems with movement and tremor have received most of the publicity in PD, non-movement symptoms are also common. Some of these non-movement symptoms have their substrate outside the nigrostriatal dopaminergic system. In other words, the nigrostriatal system is not the only brain circuit to degenerate.

These non-motor symptoms are detailed in later chapters (see Part IX); however, we will briefly consider a few of them here, to put things into their anatomic perspective.

- Depression (feeling blue) is common in PD and often is not simply a psychological reaction to the life changes caused by PD. Depression has a neurochemical basis, and the deficiency of dopamine may play a role. A reduction in other brain neurotransmitters, such as serotonin or norepinephrine, may also be important. Neurons releasing serotonin are located primarily in the midline of the brainstem; these degenerate in PD, although less severely than in the substantia nigra. Neurons containing the neurotransmitter norepinephrine also tend to degenerate in PD; they are also predominantly found in brainstem regions, and deficiencies have been implicated in depression. Most antidepressant medications enhance serotonin or norepinephrine neurotransmission, as will be discussed in Chapter 22.

- A variety of sleep disorders are experienced by those with PD. Dopamine deficiency underlies some but not all of these sleep problems. Sleep centers are located primarily in the brainstem, and degeneration in these areas is probably responsible for certain of these problems.

- With advancing PD, thinking and memory problems occur in some individuals with PD. Although slowness of thinking (bradyphrenia) relates to loss of the dopaminergic nigrostriatal system, more substantial problems (dementia) reflect more widespread degeneration, especially that involving the cortex.

- Problems with bowels, bladder, and low blood pressure are common in PD. These are due to degeneration within the autonomic nervous system, which is the internal nervous circuitry that unconsciously controls bladder, bowels, sweating, heart rate, and blood pressure.

Thus, although movement problems from nigrostriatal dopamine deficiency take center stage in PD, other brain circuits are also affected. These problems tend to be more difficult to treat but are not hopeless, as will be addressed later in this book.

Not All Movement Problems Are Due to Dopamine Deficiency

While most of the movement problems of PD respond to medications that replenish dopamine, some respond incompletely or not at all. Late in the disease course this may become more problematic. Poor balance in advanced PD is a prime example; whereas dopamine replenishment effectively treats other aspects of walking, prominent imbalance rarely responds. If degeneration of the dopaminergic substantia nigra were solely responsible for all PD movement symptoms, we would be able to normalize everyone's walking, movement, and balance. In fact, other brain movement control circuits degenerate to a limited extent.

Other Brain Neurotransmitters

For PD problems that are not due to dopamine deficiency, why not also target other neurotransmitters in the interconnected movement circuits? Unfortunately, this strategy is unworkable. A fundamental problem is that most of the other relevant brain neurotransmitters are more widely distributed throughout the brain. Drugs targeting these neurotransmitters have influence well beyond the intended target, causing unintended adverse effects. Prototypic of this problem are neurons releasing the neurotransmitter glutamate (termed *glutamatergic* neurons). Glutamate neurotransmission is an important component of basal ganglia function; however, glutamate is widely distributed throughout the brain. Drugs that block glutamate (e.g., amantadine) do address certain PD problems, but their role and dose are limited because of the more widespread effects on other brain systems. Also illustrative of this problem are drugs targeting the neurotransmitter acetylcholine; this was a substrate for PD medications years ago. Neurons releasing acetylcholine as their neurotransmitter are called *cholinergic*. Such cholinergic neurons are present in the striatum and appear to function opposite to the dopaminergic nigrostriatal system. Consequently, drugs that block acetylcholine mildly improve certain aspects of parkinsonism. However, the benefit of anticholinergic drugs is usually overshadowed by side effects, as acetylcholine neurotransmission occurs in memory circuits, as well as in the gastrointestinal tract. Thus anticholinergic drugs are no longer used to treat PD.

Changes Outside the Brain: The Autonomic Nervous System

The symptoms of PD may include problems of bladder, bowels, sexual functioning and low blood pressure. These problems reflect involvement of the autonomic nervous system.

THE AUTONOMIC NERVOUS SYSTEM

We have a series of internal monitoring devices in our body that are constantly assessing and correcting basic internal functions, such as blood pressure and heart rate. These sensors are part of complex reflexes that make adjustments in response to what is being detected. This is done unconsciously, without our awareness. This internal regulatory network is called the *autonomic nervous system*. It regulates our bowels, bladder, sweat glands, sexual functioning, heart rate, and blood pressure. When these sensors detect that we are getting too hot, we sweat. When they sense that our stomach is full, this triggers the opening of a valve allowing food to pass into the small intestine. With standing, gravity tends to pull our blood supply into our leg vessels;

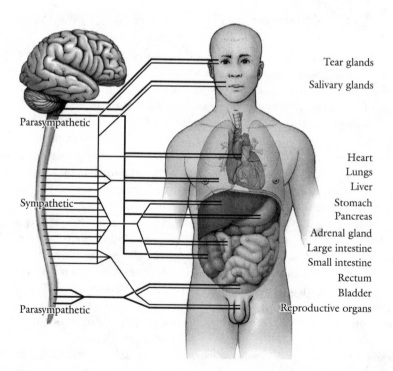

Tear glands

Salivary glands

Parasympathetic

Sympathetic

Parasympathetic

Heart
Lungs
Liver
Stomach
Pancreas
Adrenal gland
Large intestine
Small intestine
Rectum
Bladder
Reproductive organs

3.2 The autonomic nervous system modulates the activity of many internal organs and functions, as listed.

when this is internally sensed, heart and blood vessels reflexively respond to keep the blood pressure constant. Thus, the autonomic nervous system continuously monitors internal systems and makes adjustments to meet our body's needs.

The autonomic nervous system is a large network that includes centers in the brain and circuits distributed throughout our body. Brain centers are located in the hypothalamus (an area just below the thalamus) and the brainstem. Broad-ranging nerve circuits connect these areas with the heart, blood vessels, stomach, intestines, genitalia, and sweat glands. Thus, we have sensors and effectors of the autonomic nervous system throughout our bodies. A general schematic is shown in Figure 3.2. As you can see, this is divided into two primary components, the *sympathetic* and *parasympathetic* autonomic nervous systems.

INVOLVEMENT OF THE AUTONOMIC NERVOUS SYSTEM IN PARKINSON'S DISEASE

Problems of the autonomic nervous system are common in those with PD. They are often mild or minimal early in the disease course. With time, they

Table 3.1.   Autonomic Nervous System Involvement in Parkinson's Disease

Organ	Problem	Symptoms
Blood pressure regulatory systems	Low blood pressure when standing (orthostatic hypotension)	Lightheadedness, faintness when standing; if severe, fainting or near-fainting
Bowels	Slowed transit through the large intestine	Constipation
Stomach	Delayed passage of food from the stomach to the small intestine	Bloating, gas, heartburn (acid reflux)
Bladder	1. Excessive bladder contraction 2. Poor bladder contraction	1. Urinary urgency and frequency (strong urges to void and void often); incontinence 2. Hesitant and delayed voiding; susceptibility to urinary tract infections; incontinence
Sweating	Reduced or inappropriate sweating	Heat intolerance; excessive sweating
Male genitalia	Erectile dysfunction	Impotence

may become more prominent. Furthermore, medications used to treat PD or other conditions often aggravate these problems.

Impairment of the autonomic nervous system is part of the neurodegenerative process of PD. As we have already learned, this neurodegeneration is not confined to the dopaminergic neurons of the substantia nigra. Lewy bodies like those found in the substantia nigra are also found in neurons of the autonomic nervous system. However, the chemistry of the autonomic nervous system is quite different from that of the substantia nigra. Hence, replenishing dopamine, which reverses the movement problems due to substantia nigra degeneration, does not improve autonomic symptoms.

PD may affect the autonomic nervous system very early in the course of the disease, even before the movement problems (e.g., constipation). Typically, however, these autonomic symptoms remain mild until PD is longer-standing. Common symptoms referable to autonomic dysfunction in PD are summarized in Table 3.1. These are described in more detail in subsequent chapters.

PART TWO

◆ ◆ ◆

Parkinson's Disease: Diagnosis and Prognosis

4

♦ ♦ ♦

How Do I Know If I Have Parkinson's Disease?

The diagnosis of Parkinson's disease (PD) is not always simple, sometimes challenging even seasoned physicians. Some people with PD may not initially recognize that something is wrong, given the insidious onset; the symptoms may blend into the routine. Although tremor may suggest the diagnosis, many do not experience tremor as an early PD symptom (about 20% of people with PD never experience tremor). In others without PD, tremor or other signs may be incorrectly attributed to PD. In fact, the majority of people with tremor do not have PD. Some manifestations of PD may be written off to age: "Of course I'm slowing down; I'm getting older." Or some other explanation may seem plausible: "I walk bent over because my back hurts."

Parkinson's disease is a clinical diagnosis made in the doctor's office. The story plus the findings on the examination provide the evidence. There are no blood tests that will tell us that someone has PD. Tests are primarily for the purpose of excluding other disorders and often are not needed. In this chapter, we focus on the clinical evidence that points to the diagnosis.

Parkinsonism versus Parkinson's Disease

The term *parkinsonism* is commonly confused with *Parkinson's disease*. Parkinsonism is a broader term relating to anything that has the appearance of Parkinson's disease (e.g., slowness, rest tremor, or shuffling gait) but is not necessarily true PD. Not everything that looks like PD is that disorder, and these outward signs may occur in other conditions. The most common cause of parkinsonism is PD, but clinicians recognize that other causes of parkinsonism may masquerade as PD.

The History and Examination

The diagnosis of PD is primarily made by the clinician's interview and examination. There are three logical steps in making the PD diagnosis:

1. Parkinsonism must be present (symptoms and signs, as detailed later in this chapter).

2. There should be no unusual features that suggest another condition.

   Comment: Certain unexpected findings, such as frequent falls early in parkinsonism, suggest not PD.

3. The parkinsonism should markedly improve with medications that replenish brain dopamine.

   Comment: The fundamental basis for most PD symptoms is loss of brain dopamine; restoring brain dopamine should be strikingly effective.

Common things being common, if you have parkinsonism, the odds are that you have PD. The last two steps here help confirm PD.

Is it necessary to start medical treatment to prove the diagnosis of PD? The answer clearly is no. The decision whether to start a medication and choice of medication should be based on whether the symptoms are interfering with your life. If the symptoms are mild and do not demand treatment, patience is in order. This will sort itself out in time.

Symptoms versus Signs

In the language of medicine, symptoms are *experienced* by patients and described to the clinician. Signs are *observed* by the clinician. We will address PD symptoms first, which in a broader sense, are the symptoms of parkinsonism.

Symptoms of Parkinson's Disease

People with PD experience a wide variety of symptoms. Some of these are unique to parkinsonism, whereas others are less specific. A list of common symptoms is shown in Table 4.1.

The initial entries in Table 4.1 relate to tremor. *Tremor* is broadly defined as a repetitive, rhythmic movement that precisely repeats itself. It is a back-and-forth movement that goes on and on and on (although it may start and stop). Most commonly, tremor affects the hands, but it may occur in other areas of the body.

In general, tremor has many causes besides PD. The specific tremor characteristics are important in making the diagnosis. Neurologists categorize hand tremor on the basis of whether it is present when the hand is activated or at

Table 4.1. Parkinson's Disease Symptoms*

Specific Parkinsonian Symptoms That Tend to Suggest Parkinson's Disease
- Resting hand tremor (tremor when the hand is relaxed or at one's side when walking)
- Resting thumb or finger tremor (e.g., apparent when your hand is resting in your lap)
- Chin or lip tremor (also a resting tremor, meaning that it is seen when sitting quietly but not when talking or chewing)
- Tremor of a leg when seated (also a resting tremor)
- Toes curling or turning up
- Shuffling gait
- Feet get stuck (gait freezing)
- Less animated (facial appearance not expressive; reduced blinking; loss of expressive movements of the hands)
- Reduced arm swing
- Slowness of movements (it takes longer to do things)
- Softer voice and less distinct speech
- Smaller handwriting

Less Specific Symptoms (They May Have Other Explanations)
- Sense of overall weakness
- Fatigue
- Mild imbalance
- Sense of restlessness, nervousness
- Stiffness of limbs
- Stooped posture
- Difficulty rising from seated position
- Slowed thinking
- Difficulty buttoning buttons or using eating utensils
- Difficulty turning over in bed
- Difficulty brushing teeth
- Drooling or sense of increased saliva

*The early symptoms and signs of PD are often on only one side of the body, or are asymmetric.

rest. If the hand is tremulous when it is lying in your lap, or at your side when walking, this is classified as *at rest*. Tremor at rest is typical of PD but uncommon in other disorders. Tremor when the hand is activated, such as writing or holding a newspaper, is termed an *action tremor*. Action tremors may occur in PD, but also in other conditions. Sometimes a parkinsonian rest tremor affects only the thumb or the fingers; an old term for this is a *pill-rolling tremor*, in which the rhythmic movements of the fingers and thumb give the appearance of a pill being rolled back and forth between these digits.

Table 4.1 also lists a rest tremor of the chin or lip as suspicious for PD. Similarly, a parkinsonian rest tremor in the legs may be apparent when seated, with the knee going up and down when the feet are resting on the floor. Or, the foot may move back and forth if the feet are dangling off the floor.

Another parkinsonian foot symptom is involuntary curling or spasm of the toes. We all experience cramps at times and, rarely, our toes may cramp. However, if curling of the toes is frequent and recurrent, this is suspicious for parkinsonism. This is not to be confused with hammer toes, where the toes chronically develop a fixed bent position. Hammer toes are not a sign of PD. Frequent leg cramps have many causes; parkinsonism is one of them.

Certain walking abnormalities suggest parkinsonism, specifically when taking on the appearance of a "shuffling" gait. Normally when we walk, we step by cocking up our lead foot and planting the heel as we stride forward. We then push off with the ball and toes of that foot as we continue with the step. This alternates from one foot to the other to generate a typical human gait. In contrast, the parkinsonian gait is characterized by loss of the normal heel strike; rather, the foot tends to slide along the floor. Typically coinciding with this is reduced stride length; that is, the steps are shorter. Sometimes, a parkinsonian foot seems stuck to the floor when trying to take a step; this is termed *gait freezing*.

Parkinsonism is also associated with loss of normal facial animation. Humans are very expressive in their facial appearance—we smile, frown, grimace, and convey a variety of subtle communications with our faces. This activity tends to be dampened or lost in PD, termed *facial masking*. Facial masking is rarely appreciated by the person with parkinsonism but rather by the spouse or friends. Obviously, people who are depressed also tend to have bland facial expressions; this should not be confused with the facial masking of parkinsonism.

A component of facial masking is a reduced blink rate. We normally blink around 17 times per minute (slightly more when conversing and less when reading). Parkinsonism is associated with less frequent blinking, perhaps only half the normal rate. This may give the appearance of staring. Reduced blinking or attenuated facial expression is part of a broader loss of unconscious spontaneous movement in PD. This often includes reduced arm swing when walking or loss of gesturing when talking.

Slowness of movement, termed *bradykinesia*, is a highly characteristic feature of parkinsonism. This may be most apparent in one limb, one side, or the body in general. Movements are made as if in done in a swimming pool, slow and laborious. When walking, one leg may lag behind the other; movement overall may seem far too slow for age.

Voice and speech changes may also suggest the diagnosis. Typically, the voice becomes softer and more difficult to hear. Speech may be less precise and may take on a subtle stammering quality; the normal inflections of speech may attenuate, as if speaking in a monotone. Occasional PD patients develop a hoarse voice, although a hoarse voice may have a variety of other causes.

Writing is often a clue to parkinsonism, with the handwriting becoming smaller, known as *micrographia*. It may start out normal but then become progressively smaller by the end of a long word or a sentence.

The last portion of Table 4.1 includes a variety of symptoms that are less specific for PD and also commonly occur in other disorders or with normal aging. For example, fatigue is present in many conditions, and primary care physicians hear this complaint several times a day. Mild imbalance or a stooped posture is common with normal aging. The arthritis of aging (osteoarthritis) may cause stiffness of limbs or difficulty buttoning and doing other activities.

Parkinson's Disease Is Usually Not Symmetric

PD is occasionally confused with other neurological conditions, such as strokes, because of the asymmetry of symptoms and signs. PD often starts in one limb, such as an arm. With progression, the remaining limb on that same side of the body (arm or leg) becomes involved. The diagnosis may be further obscured if there is pain or aching in that limb, as often occurs with PD.

The asymmetry of PD is curious and not what one would intuitively expect in a neurodegenerative disorder. One might expect that such a degenerative process should be more uniform and affect both sides of the body and perhaps all four limbs at the same time. The reason for the asymmetry is unknown.

As PD progresses, the other side of the body eventually will become involved. However, PD typically remains an asymmetric condition; the first side to be affected remains a little worse than the other side over the years.

Signs That Point Toward Parkinson's Disease

Signs are what the physician finds by observing and examining. Although physicians perform a formal examination, the observation of the patient starts as soon as the doctor enters the room. Physicians are trained to be good observers, and parkinsonism may be suggested early in the visit by subtle clues.

Let us assume the perspective of a clinician first meeting and evaluating the patient. No special tools are required. Imagine that you are the doctor and you enter the room where your patient, Mr. Jones, has been waiting. Subtle clinical clues may be quickly apparent:

- Does he have trouble rising from his chair to greet you? Difficulty rising from the seated position is common in PD (despite normal leg strength).

- Do you get a sense of overall slowness (bradykinesia)?

- Is he poker-faced, with little facial animation? Loss of facial expression is a hallmark of parkinsonism.

- Is there a tremor of the hand in his lap? This may be subtle, such as a thumb moving back and forth or a resting chin or lip tremor.

- Is one arm and hand postured stiffly in the lap?

- Is his voice soft? ... Is his speech less articulate than normal? ... Does he speak in a monotone? A decline in voice volume is common in parkinsonism, as are loss of the normal inflections and precision of speech.

- Is he not very animated, such as not gesturing when talking? An important clue is loss of automatic movements, such as gesturing when speaking or arm swing when walking.

These initial observations are summarized in Table 4.2 and matched with the formal medical term for the corresponding sign of parkinsonism.

Once you have had a chance to visit with Mr. Jones (and to make your observations), you then proceed to the more formal parkinsonism examination. It requires no tools, just open eyes. Here is what to ask Mr. Jones to do and how to interpret what you are seeing.

- Have him stand up. Is he slow? Does he require several tries to get up? Does he need to push off or obtain help?

- Have him walk through the office door, down the hall, and come back.

Analyze the different components of gait.

1. Did he hesitate with the first step or when walking through the doorway? Do his feet seem stuck to the floor when he first tries to take a step?

   Comment: Gait freezing is apparent with the first step but typically abates once walking is ongoing; it often recurs when approaching doorways or making a turn.

Table 4.2. Signs of Parkinsonism Apparent from Simple Observation*

Sign	Medical Term
Trouble standing up from the seated position to shake hands	
Moves slowly	Bradykinesia
Poker-faced	Facial masking or hypomimia
Tremor when hand is in lap (also tremor of chin, leg, or foot when in relaxed posture)	Rest tremor
Arm or hand held stiffly in lap or at the side	Rigidity (stiffness) and bradykinesia (slowness and reduced spontaneous mobility)
Voice is softer and speech is less articulate, often devoid of inflections (monotone)	Hypokinetic dysarthria or hypophonic voice (parkinsonian speech and voice)
Lack of gesturing when talking	Loss of automatic movements

*What your doctor observes when first greeting and talking to you.

2. Observe the posture when walking. Is he stooped?

   Comment: As we age we may get a little stooped. However, with parkinsonism, it may be more than expected for age.

3. Is he slow as he walks down the hall?

   Comment: Bradykinesia (slowness) is a cardinal sign of parkinsonism, where movements are slower than expected for age.

4. Observe foot placement as he walks. Is the stride length shortened? Are the feet moving parallel to the floor instead of planting with the heel and pushing off with the ball of the foot? Does the gait appear shuffling? Does one foot lag behind?

   Comment: In those with parkinsonism, the normal heel strike may be lost and the stride length shortened. When severe, the foot never leaves the floor, and this constitutes shuffling.

5. Watch the hands when walking. Is arm swing normal? Is a subtle tremor (rest tremor) present in a hand, thumb, or fingers?

   Comment: PD tends to be an asymmetric disorder, and the reduced arm swing may be only on one side. Observation during walking is one of the best times to look for the hand rest tremor, which may be only on one side.

6. Watch Mr. Jones turn. Instead of pivoting, does he take several steps to turn? Is there gait freezing?

Comment: Instead of making a smooth pivot, those with parkinsonism often will need to stop and replant their feet several times to complete the turn. This may also unmask the tendency for freezing, with the feet briefly stuck in place.

7. Is there unsteadiness?

Comment: Early in PD balance is preserved or only mildly impaired. It may be more of a problem later. Severe imbalance with fall risk early in parkinsonism suggests a parkinsonism look-alike condition.

- Having completed observation of walking, test balance by the "pull test." To do this, stand behind Mr. Jones and tell him to resist being pulled backward. You then pull back on Mr. Jones' shoulders. The pull should be forceful enough to pull the shoulders back slightly, but not so vigorous that it would cause a normal person to fall back. Does he fall backward into your arms? (Be prepared to catch him.)

Comment: People with parkinsonism and imbalance have a tendency to fall backward when pulled; this is termed *retropulsion*. Such imbalance is usually minimal in early PD.

The remainder of the examination is conducted with Mr. Jones seated on the examining table (or in a chair).

- Assess for rigidity, which is stiffness of the limbs (and neck) when moved by the examiner; the patient is encourage to relax. To properly interpret this, these maneuvers should first be performed on normal people to get a sense of normal limb tone. Rigidity can be assessed wherever there is a joint. To test for rigidity, move the joint back and forth, asking Mr. Jones to allow the limb to "go floppy." Start with the wrist, then elbow, then shoulder, and repeat on the other side. Next, rigidity can be similarly assessed at the knee joints. After the limbs have been examined, gently move the neck, again asking Mr. Jones to relax as best he can. Is there resistance to movement of these joints? Do they feel stiff?

Comment: Increased limb tone is one of the hallmark features of parkinsonism. Obviously, Mr. Jones must relax to allow this to be properly assessed. A normal relaxed joint should move like a well-lubricated hinge. Rigidity feels like a rusty hinge with resistance when moved by the examiner. Sometimes the rigidity of PD has a tremulous quality, which is termed *cogwheel rigidity*. Minor degrees of rigidity may be difficult to determine. If there are major joint problems (arthritis), then this cannot be easily analyzed.

- *Alternate motion rate* testing is the last set of tasks (also called *rapid alternating movements*). First, have Mr. Jones rapidly and repetitively tap his index finger and thumb, one hand at a time, for perhaps 10 seconds. The focus here is on both the speed of movements as well as the amplitude (amplitude implies the size of movement excursions).

Comment: In parkinsonism, these repetitive movements slow, and the amplitude diminishes with repetition. The first few movements may have normal excursions but become smaller with continued tapping. They may dampen to the extent that the thumb and finger freeze in place. Since PD is an asymmetric condition, one hand often performs better than the other.

Now have Mr. Jones pat his knee with his hand, alternating between the palm and back of the hand (so-called pronation-supination). Do this one hand at a time.

Comment: Those with parkinsonism may do this slowly and the movements may become impeded (stopping-starting).

Finally, have Mr. Jones tap each foot repetitively and rapidly (like one does when listening to music). Do this one foot at a time. Is he slow? Does the movement break down?

Comment: If Mr. Jones has a leg tremor, the repetitive foot tapping may be driven by the tremor. In that case, have him tap his heel.

The formal parkinsonism examination is summarized in Table 4.3. To that may be added a handwriting sample, to look for micrographia.

We can now consider the totality of our results, including our initial observations, plus what we witnessed on the formal examination. Those with PD will not necessarily display all the signs in the assessment just described. What we are looking for is whether there are enough of these signs to put Mr. Jones into the parkinsonism category. Only one or two of these signs, especially some of the less specific ones, will not necessarily support a diagnosis of parkinsonism. Some of the findings carry more weight than others. For example, a resting tremor of the hand is extremely suspicious; it typically cannot be attributed to other factors. Conversely, a mildly stooped posture may simply be due to age. Reduced arm swing could reflect a shoulder problem. Mild slowness in tapping the foot, if not accompanied by many other signs, may not be very informative. Parkinsonism may be diagnosed only if there are enough of these signs and, especially, those that cannot be written off to other things.

Occasionally, the signs are mild and the physician is simply unable to say for certain whether parkinsonism is truly present. In those cases, time sorts this out. With evolution of the condition over the ensuing 6 to 12 months, those with PD will probably become a little worse, and the diagnosis more apparent.

Table 4.3.   The Formal Parkinsonism Examination

Task	Things to Look for That Suggest Parkinsonism
Standing up from sitting	• Hesitant, slow; requires help; may have to push off with hands (nonspecific sign, since lower limb pain or weakness might also impair standing)
Walking	• Hesitant (gait freezing; feet stuck to the floor) • Stooped posture • Slowness (bradykinesia) • Does not plant the heel and push off from the ball of the foot with each step; feet move parallel to floor (when pronounced, gait is shuffling; feet barely leave the floor) • Stride length shortened • Reduced arm swing • Hand, thumb, or finger tremor when walking (rest tremor) • Turns with several steps rather than with smooth pivot (cannot "turn on a dime") • Imbalance (should not be severe early in PD)
Pull test	• Falls backward with moderately forceful tug on shoulders (usually maintains balance in early PD)
Assess rigidity	• Movement of the joints by the examiner encounters resistance (the person being tested must relax); if superimposed tremor, this gives it a ratchety feel, termed *cogwheel rigidity*
Alternate motion rate testing (tapping of finger, thumb; hands, feet)	• Slow • Amplitude of the excursions is reduced (sometimes apparent only after 5–10 seconds of repetitions); hesitation

Neurologists' Diagnostic Schemes

Neurologists have a short-hand strategy for making the diagnosis of parkinsonism. This requires attention to the four cardinal signs of parkinsonism:

- Resting tremor

- Rigidity

- Bradykinesia

- Characteristic gait disorder or imbalance

Two of these four signs are sufficient to meet the criteria for parkinsonism (but not necessarily for PD). Remember that prominent imbalance with falls should not be seen as an early sign of PD; it suggests another parkinsonian disorder (discussed in Chapter 6).

Specialists also employ a scoring system for PD, called the *Unified Parkinson's Disease Rating Scale* (UPDRS). In the motor examination portion of this scheme (Part III of the UPDRS), each of the observations and tasks we just discussed are given a rating on a 4-point scale. When the motor score is added, this is assumed to correlate with the severity of parkinsonism. While the UPDRS is primarily a research tool for investigators assessing PD treatments, some neurologists use this in the clinic.

Are There Red Flags for Another Parkinsonian Disorder?

The evaluation described earlier in this chapter will tell us if parkinsonism is present. The next step is to determine whether there are other signs to suggest another condition besides PD (see also Chapter 6). For this additional neurological examination, firsthand clinical experience is necessary; hence, we will be brief in considering this.

Once the physician recognizes the findings of parkinsonism, the examination is expanded to determine whether other brain systems are involved. These other brain systems can be broken down into distinct categories:

- Corticospinal tract—Are there signs of spasticity with abnormal reflexes?

- Cerebellar—Are there signs of incoordination (ataxia)?

- Praxis—Are complex movements of the hands (or feet) impaired?

- Eye movements—Is movement of the eyes impaired (especially looking down)?

- Cognition—Is thinking and memory impaired?

In PD, there should not be any substantial abnormalities in these areas. The neurological assessment of these categories is summarized in Table 4.4.

The clinician may also learn facts during the interview that suggest that the parkinsonism may not be PD. Just like the signs discussed in the previous paragraph, the patient may describe symptoms that point to another disorder. Some of these more common red flags that physicians look for in this setting are summarized in Table 4.5.

Certainly, the physician will also review the medication list. A variety of drugs may cause parkinsonism, which resolves when the drug is stopped. This is discussed in detail in Chapter 6.

Table 4.4.   The Extended Neurological Examination*

Brain System	Evidence Found by the Neurologist
Corticospinal tract	• Increased tendon reflexes (assessed with a reflex hammer) • Babinski sign (response of the great toe when the bottom of the foot is scratched). The normal reflexive response is for the toe to go down; if the toe goes up, this represents the Babinski sign. • Characteristic changes in gait and certain unique changes in limb tone
Cerebellar	Signs similar to someone who is inebriated with alcohol: • Imprecision when asked to point back and forth from nose to examiner's finger (incoordination) • Garbled speech (ataxic dysarthria) • Unsteady and wide-base gait; unable to walk heel-to-toe
Praxis	• Inability to perform patterned movements correctly, such as imitating the peace sign, waving goodbye
Eye movements	• Inability to move the eyes, especially downward
Cognition	• Prominent and early thinking and memory problems

*Assessment of other brain systems that are expected to be spared in PD. If prominent signs in these categories are found, the parkinsonism may not be PD.

Testing

Tests will not tell us if someone has PD, but they may help determine if the parkinsonism is due to some other cause. Since degeneration of the substantia nigra does not change the normal contours of brain structures, magnetic resonance imaging (MRI) brain scans are normal in PD. However, they may be abnormal in other parkinsonian conditions. Blood studies may exclude other causes for certain symptoms, such as the fatigue, which could be due to a low thyroid state or anemia.

The integrity of brain dopamine systems can be documented with nuclear medicine scanning. However, it has limited practical utility, as it is abnormal not only in PD but also in other parkinsonian disorders. Recently it was approved for routine clinical use by the U.S. Food and Drug Administration. With this approved technology, striatal dopaminergic projections (terminals) are visualized by vein injection of a radioactively labeled compound that binds to the brain *dopamine transporter*, a biological protein found only in dopaminergic neurons. The first such approved radioactive compound has the brand name DaTscan (ioflupane I-123);

Table 4.5. Features Raising Suspicion That Parkinsonism Is Not Typical Parkinson's Disease

Category	Symptoms	Alternate Possibilities
Age at onset	First symptoms before age 40 years	Although this still could be PD, very young onset indicates the need for more thorough investigation and may justify genetic testing.
Time course	Sudden changes	Sudden onset of symptoms raises question of stroke.
	Rapid deterioration	Suggests not PD unless there is some second causative factor, such as superimposed pneumonia
	Symptoms began after starting a medication	Medication could be responsible.
Gait	Many falls, early in the disease course	Progressive supranuclear palsy, multiple system atrophy, or other cause*
Autonomic nervous system	Low blood pressure leading to faints or near-faints, plus prominent other autonomic symptoms*	Multiple system atrophy* if medications are not the cause for the very low blood pressure

*See Chapter 6 for more details.

the scanning is done using single photon emission tomography (SPECT), which is widely available. The dopamine transporter protein regulates the amount of dopamine in the synapse and is not found in neurons utilizing other neurotransmitters. In PD, the brain dopamine transporter signal is progressively lost as the nigrostriatal system degenerates; this is apparent on the scan. This technique distinguishes PD from normal and from essential tremor (see Chapter 6 for further discussion of essential tremor). It is not useful, however, for distinguishing PD from other parkinsonian disorders such as multiple system atrophy or progressive supranuclear palsy, since dopaminergic neuron loss also occurs in those disorders (these conditions are discussed in Chapter 6).

To summarize, the clinical history and examination are the crucial factors in making the diagnosis of PD. Testing may not be necessary when the symptoms and signs are typical of PD. We discuss testing in more detail in Chapter 7.

Diagnostic Confirmation: The Response to Medications

The symptoms and signs that are the presenting features of PD primarily reflect a deficiency of dopamine within the brain. Hence, administering a medication that restores dopamine (or the dopamine effect) should reverse the symptoms. Thus, the treatment turns out to also be a useful diagnostic test, and is the third step in the diagnostic process outlined at the beginning of this chapter.

But what about those parkinsonian look-alike conditions just mentioned (i.e., multiple system atrophy, progressive supranuclear palsy)? These are also associated with dopamine deficiency; should they not also respond to dopamine replacement therapy? Unfortunately, patients with these disorders have more widespread involvement of other nondopaminergic basal ganglia systems. Fixing only the dopaminergic link in the dysfunctional basal ganglia circuitry is insufficient (analogous to fixing only one link in a chain with two broken links). In contrast, the movement problems of PD are predominantly due to dopamine loss; restoring dopamine allows nearly complete restoration of basal ganglia function, especially early in the disease process.

The two classes of drugs used to restore the dopamine effect are levodopa and dopamine agonists. These are discussed in detail in later chapters. An excellent response to one of these drugs will not only tell us that a brain dopamine deficiency state is present but also that other brain basal ganglia circuits are largely intact.

Levodopa is the natural substance that brain cells directly convert to dopamine. In pill form, it is combined with carbidopa, which protects levodopa from premature metabolism in the circulation. It is prescribed as generic carbidopa/levodopa (brand name, Sinemet).

Dopamine agonist drugs act like synthetic forms of dopamine. Those approved for chronic use do not bind to all the dopamine receptors and hence are not nearly as potent as carbidopa/levodopa. The dopamine agonist pills available in the United States are pramipexole (Mirapex) and ropinirole (Requip); a dopamine agonist is also formulated as a patch—rotigotine (Neupro).

Which drug should you take to test the response, levodopa or a dopamine agonist? Levodopa is more potent and, thus, is a better test. However, an excellent response to a dopamine agonist drug also confirms the diagnosis of PD. Be aware that a single dose is not a sufficient trial; for both carbidopa/levodopa and the dopamine agonists, several weeks of dose escalation are required to adequately test the response. They are conventionally started at low doses and require chronic use to establish benefit. Dosage schemes for these drugs are detailed in Chapters 11–13.

Does an initial response to these drugs guarantee that PD is the diagnosis? Usually, this is the case, but there are exceptions. Some of the conditions that resemble PD respond partially or briefly (see Chapter 6). In PD, the beneficial response is substantial and sustained.

What about My Other Symptoms? (PD Problems Are More Than Movement and Tremor)

A wide variety of additional symptoms may be experienced as direct manifestations of PD; the most common of these symptoms are listed in Table 4.6. You need to recognize these as possibly PD related so that treatment is appropriately tailored.

AUTONOMIC SYMPTOMS

As we discussed in Chapter 3, the autonomic nervous system programs many internal functions, such as bowels, bladder, and blood pressure. Autonomic problems are common in PD, and Lewy body microscopic changes are found in autonomic neurons. Usually, autonomic symptoms are mild in early in PD and sometimes never very problematic.

AUTONOMIC GASTROINTESTINAL PROBLEMS: CONSTIPATION AND BLOATING

The digestive system processes food in successive stages. When food is swallowed, it goes down the esophagus to the stomach, where the digestive process starts. From there, food products pass into the small intestine and nutrients subsequently enter the bloodstream. Ultimately, waste is transmitted down to the colon (large intestine) to form feces. Contractions of the stomach and intestines are crucial to this process (peristalsis), and these contractions are programmed by the autonomic nervous system. When this system malfunctions, the contents back up. A sensation of abdominal bloating occurs if food cannot exit the stomach to the small intestine. Heartburn may develop if the acidic stomach contents back up into the esophagus. On the other end, constipation ensues when the colon does not contract normally to produce bowel movements. Constipation is extremely common in PD, whereas the other gastrointestinal symptoms occur to variable degrees.

DIFFICULTY SWALLOWING, DROOLING

The first step of the digestive process is swallowing, and difficulty swallowing may be a symptom of PD. Typically, this is not severe. Unlike constipation or bloating, difficulty swallowing especially reflects the brain dopamine deficiency; it often improves with dopamine replacement

Table 4.6. Non-Movement Symptoms of Parkinson's Disease

Category	Symptoms
Autonomic Nervous System Gastrointestinal	• Constipation • Bloating • Heartburn (reflux)
Swallowing (arguably, a primary PD motor symptom, rather than autonomic)	• Impaired swallowing • Drooling
Bladder	• Hesitant urination • Sudden uncontrollable urges to void (urgency) • Incontinence • Frequent urination • Recurrent urinary tract infections
Genitalia	• Male impotence
Blood pressure	• Orthostatic hypotension (low blood pressure when standing; faintness, fatigue or faints when standing, walking)
Psychiatric	• Depression • Anxiety • Panic attacks • Inner restlessness (akathisia)
Cognitive	• Slowed thinking (bradyphrenia) • Dementia • Hallucinations, delusions
Sleep	• Insomnia • Daytime sleepiness • Acting out dreams (REM sleep behavior disorder)
Sensory Symptoms	• Sciatica or other limb pain • Pain or discomfort in neck, trunk, or abdomen • Numbness, tingling • Cramps (painful) • Sensation of heat or cold
Other Symptoms	• Fatigue • Shortness of breath

therapy (e.g., carbidopa/levodopa). Major swallowing problems early in the course of PD raise a question of a parkinsonism look-alike condition, such as progressive supranuclear palsy or multiple system atrophy (see Chapter 6).

Drooling is common in untreated PD. It is not caused by excessive saliva production but is due to a reduction in reflexive swallowing. Swallowing saliva is done unconsciously and without thinking, whereas this reflexive function diminishes in PD. This is similar to the reduction of other automatic movements in PD, such as blinking, or arm swing when walking. Drooling, like reduced arm swing and blinking, reflects brain dopamine deficiency and improves with dopamine replacement therapy such as carbidopa/levodopa.

AUTONOMIC BLADDER PROBLEMS: HESITANT URINE FLOW OR LOSS OF CONTROL

The bladder is the reservoir where urine is stored after it has been produced by the kidneys. Neurological reflexes are triggered when the bladder is full, priming it to contract and expel the contents (hopefully, into the toilet). Signals reach the brain indicating the need to get to the bathroom. Normally, we are able to suppress these urges until we are ready. When the autonomic control of the bladder malfunctions in PD, one of several symptoms may occur:

- Difficulty passing urine (hesitant urination)

- Sudden compulsions to void (urgency)

- Incontinence (inability to prevent expulsion of urine)

- The need to urinate often, even when the bladder is only slightly full (frequency); this may require multiple trips to the bathroom at night (nocturia)

- Frequent urinary tract infections (if there is poor urine outflow, the backed-up, stagnant urine is a breeding ground for bacteria)

Sometimes, one cannot be certain if the urinary symptoms are due to PD. It is common for men over the age of 60 to experience prostate problems, resulting in an impeded, slowed urinary stream. Women may experience stress incontinence such that coughing or sneezing provokes urine leakage. This is commonly due to altered anatomy from prior delivery of babies. Urological testing can help determine whether bladder problems are due to PD and can guide appropriate treatment, as discussed in Chapter 27. These urinary problems tend not to be helped by dopamine replacement therapy, apart from minor benefit for urinary urgency.

IMPOTENCE

Male erectile dysfunction (ED) is common in normal aging and is more common in PD; the latter reflects autonomic nervous system involvement. ED may also relate to other factors, such as medications or other medical conditions. Female sexual dysfunction may also occur in PD, although this has been poorly studied. Carbidopa/levodopa and related medications do not directly treat such sexual conditions, although the symptoms may worsen in the complete absence of dopamine replacement treatment. Sexual dysfunction is addressed in Chapter 28.

AUTONOMIC CONTROL OF BLOOD PRESSURE: LOW BLOOD PRESSURE WHEN UPRIGHT

PD may predispose to low blood pressure during standing, termed *ortho-static hypotension* (*orthostatic* implies the upright position; *hypotension* means low blood pressure). The medications used to treat PD often exacerbate this tendency. Orthostatic hypotension tends to cause lightheadedness and, if severe, fainting.

Orthostatic hypotension may go undetected. Blood pressure is conventionally measured in the sitting position. Among those with orthostatic hypotension, the *sitting* blood pressure might be normal, whereas the *standing* pressure might be extremely low. If you think you may be experiencing symptoms of orthostatic hypotension, be sure to read Chapter 21.

Psychiatric Conditions and Parkinson's Disease

DEPRESSION

Depression is common among those with PD. In the mildest form, this may simply be feeling blue most of the time. In more severe forms, people may become terribly disabled by hopelessness and despair.

Diagnosing depression among those with PD is a little more complicated than for the general public. In general, depression causes a variety of symptoms, such as loss of appetite, insomnia (or excessive sleep), loss of initiative, inability to concentrate, irascibility, and even impotence. Among those with PD, however, these symptoms may have other origins. For example, poor appetite or impotence may be due to medications or to problems within the autonomic nervous system. Insomnia and sleep problems are part of PD, as addressed in Chapter 20. Apathy may be a direct consequence of PD, manifesting as reduced initiative and interest. The characteristic loss of facial expression that is common in PD ("masking") may be misinterpreted as evidence of depression.

True depression may have more than one cause among those with PD. Obviously, people with PD may be discouraged by their illness, having reduced abilities and capacities. Hobbies may no longer be possible or enjoyable; golf scores may increase, or competitive tennis may no longer be feasible. However, the PD neurodegenerative process also may involve brain regions responsible for stabilizing affective states (i.e., positive and negative feelings). This certainly includes not only dopamine systems but also those of related neurotransmitters, such serotonin and norepinephrine, as discussed in Chapter 22.

ANXIETY AND PANIC ATTACKS

Anxiety is a common symptom of PD. In its mildest form it may be experienced as simple nervousness or a sense of foreboding that seems out of proportion for the circumstances. At the other extreme are anxiety states or even panic attacks that may be primary symptoms of PD. Anxiety is common in the general population; most people with anxiety do not have PD. However, when anxiety begins with or comes after parkinsonian symptoms, PD may be the cause. Unlike anxiety in the general population, PD-related anxiety usually responds to dopamine replacement therapy (e.g., carbidopa/levodopa).

People with PD often experience a sense of inner restlessness, termed *akathisia*. They describe feeling tense and uncomfortable when sitting still or lying in bed. Sometimes this is difficult to distinguish from anxiety, since the lay term for each of these is often *nervousness*. This may be a factor in the insomnia of PD. Akathisia and insomnia both tend to respond to treatment of the dopamine deficiency of PD—that is, the same medications we use to treat the other symptoms of PD. This is discussed in Chapter 19.

Cognitive Function and Parkinson's Disease

SLOWED THINKING

Like slowness of movements (bradykinesia), thinking may be slowed in PD; this is termed *bradyphrenia*. Among those with bradyphrenia, questions are correctly answered, but with long delays. Bradyphrenia is *not* necessarily an early sign of dementia and does *not* necessarily indicate that major cognitive problems are imminent. Bradyphrenia often improves with the usual medications for PD, such as carbidopa/levodopa.

DEMENTIA

Major thinking and memory problems (dementia) may develop among those with PD. However, many individuals with PD do not experience dementia. When it does occur, it typically is much later in the disease course. It is more likely with advanced age, as in the general population.

When dementia develops in PD, the cause is usually the Lewy body neurodegenerative process, with proliferation of Lewy pathology into cognitive brain regions. It is then termed *Parkinson's disease with dementia*. It is very similar to another condition, dementia with Lewy bodies. Dementia with Lewy bodies is strikingly similar to PD with dementia; the primary difference is that the dementia and parkinsonism develop at around the same time in dementia with Lewy bodies. These and other causes of cognitive dysfunction are discussed in Chapter 23.

HALLUCINATIONS AND DELUSIONS

Seeing things that aren't there (hallucinations) may be caused by PD, but is often provoked by certain of the medications used to treat parkinsonism. In the mildest form, illusory bugs or some nondescript, shadowy image appears in the periphery of vision. However, hallucinations of people, children, or animals may also be experienced. Hallucinations are uncommon in early and even intermediate stages of PD; they tend to be late manifestations. As discussed in Chapter 24, provocative medications should be considered.

Delusions are beliefs that have no validity and often are nonsensical. Like hallucinations, delusional thinking tends to occur late in PD, if it occurs at all. Some delusions are benign, such as being convinced that guests are coming for supper. Others may be disruptive, such as believing that one's spouse is unfaithful. Occasionally, they are bizarre, such as thinking that the FBI has bugged the phones. Delusions, like hallucinations, tend to be caused or exacerbated by certain of the mediations used to treat PD. They respond to the same drugs used to treat hallucinations (see Chapter 24).

Sleep

INSOMNIA

Insomnia is common in the general population, but it is much more common among those with PD. People with PD frequently experience problems both getting to sleep and staying asleep. Most often, this is secondary to a variety of symptoms that are part of PD, which include the following:

- Anxiety

- Akathisia

- Sense of stiffness (rigidity)

- Tremor (present at rest)

- Difficulty turning in bed to get into comfortable position
- Night cramps (see later discussion)

Since these are primary manifestations of PD, they respond to carbidopa/levodopa, as discussed in Chapter 20.

DAYTIME SLEEPINESS

People with PD may experience daytime drowsiness. This is usually caused by some other factor:

- Insomnia with poor nighttime sleep (resulting in secondary drowsiness during the day)
- Medications
- Inability to achieve deep sleep; this may be due to disordered breathing (sleep apnea).

Sometimes, excessive sleepiness is due to PD per se, although treatable causes should first be considered, as discussed in Chapter 20.

ACTING OUT DREAMS (REM SLEEP BEHAVIOR DISORDER)

Normally during dreaming, our body remains in a relaxed state and we don't move; despite experiencing vivid dreams, we lie still in bed. This is because once the dream starts, the connection between the brain's dreaming center and the rest of the brain is switched off. In those with PD, this connection tends to remain open; the dreaming brain remains partially connected to brain movement centers. Thus, people with PD tend to act out their dreams. The medical term for this is *REM sleep behavior disorder*; REM stands for rapid eye movement. REM sleep is a deep stage of sleep during which much dreaming occurs. The body is normally limp and unmoving during this sleep stage, except for our eyes. Thus, the normal person acts out dreams only with their eyes. However, among many with PD, a vivid dream may provoke a variety of vigorous nighttime behaviors known only to the sleep partner. Not only is REM sleep behavior common in PD, it may precede the usual PD symptoms by years or even decades. See Chapter 20 for more details.

Sensory Symptoms

NUMBNESS AND TINGLING

People with PD often experience a variety of uncomfortable or unusual sensations, especially in the limbs first affected by PD. Descriptions include numbness, tingling, pins and needles, or a more nondescript sense that something is not right in that area of the body. A feeling of heat or cold may also be experienced. These sensations sometimes respond to dopamine replacement medications.

PAIN AND CRAMPS

Pain is common among those with PD but is often overlooked as a component of this disorder. Parkinsonian pain often manifests as a cramp-like sensation and usually responds to levodopa or related medications. Limb pain characteristic of sciatica may be a symptom of PD, as may pain experienced in the neck, trunk, or abdomen.

Obviously, pain is common, and we should not jump to the conclusion that any and all pain is due to PD. Our body uses pain to tell us that something isn't right and other causes may need to be investigated. However, if the pain completely resolves with levodopa treatment, it is likely due to PD. Chapter 19 discusses this issue further.

Other Symptoms

FATIGUE, WEAKNESS, LETHARGY

Poor energy and loss of the usual stamina are typical of PD. People with PD find that they are less able to burn the candle at both ends. They may function satisfactorily at moderate activity levels but cannot switch into high gear or work long hours as they could previously. Similarly, people with PD may complain of feeling weak, but without any true muscle weakness apparent on examination. The medications for PD may be helpful for these symptoms but often are only partially effective.

Apathy implies loss of initiative and interest. Activities that previously captured interest no longer seem exciting or worth the effort. This occurs to variable degrees among those with PD and is exacerbated in the absence of dopamine replacement medications.

SHORTNESS OF BREATH

Shortness of breath is not uncommon later in life and usually suggests heart or lung problems. However, shortness of breath may also be due to PD (see Chapter 19). One shouldn't jump to the conclusion that PD is responsible; your physician must first consider other more common causes. Shortness of breath due to PD typically responds to carbidopa/levodopa treatment.

OTHER NON-MOVEMENT SYMPTOMS
IN PARKINSON'S DISEASE

A variety of non-movement symptoms occur in PD. Some of the more common symptoms have already been discussed in this chapter, but this is not an all-inclusive list. As a general rule of thumb, if a particular symptom disappears, time-locked to carbidopa/levodopa doses (or related medications), it may well represent a symptom of PD.

5

◆ ◆ ◆

Prognosis

Being told that you have Parkinson's disease (PD) can be psychologically devastating. Often the first thing that comes to mind is an image of some relative or acquaintance with terrible, end-stage problems. We tend to remember worst-case scenarios. Mentioning "Parkinson's disease" may evoke a mental image of Uncle Frank with PD, who was in a wheelchair and died in a nursing home. However, a colleague in the workplace, still leading a full life after 10 years of PD, may be forgotten. Furthermore, Uncle Frank may not have had PD; perhaps he had one of those other disorders that only looks like PD (described in Chapter 6), or possibly his course was complicated by a stroke. Also, Uncle Frank may have developed PD before effective medications became available.

Stories in the lay press may raise unnecessary concerns. Newspaper articles on PD frequently begin with statements such as, "The medicines for Parkinson's disease only work for a few years." Is this true? Will I have no effective treatment in a few years? In fact, the press sometimes takes major liberties with the facts, at least when it comes to writing about PD. This may be necessary to make the story interesting. However, this can be disconcerting if you have PD.

What are the facts? How can we predict how you will do over the long term with PD? Although precise predictions are not possible, the collective experience with PD over the last several decades provides a framework for looking into the future.

Life Expectancy

Will I die from PD? Will it shorten my life? These are often questions people ask their doctor when first given their diagnosis. Clearly, there are neurodegenerative disorders in which lives are cut short. For example, people with Lou Gehrig's disease (ALS, amyotrophic lateral sclerosis) typically succumb to their disorder within a few years. Thankfully, PD does not fall into this category, even though it is also a neurodegenerative disorder.

You may have read that people with PD do not live as long as the rest of us. Whereas that is true, the average reduction in life span associated with PD is relatively small. Bear in mind that how long we are expected to live depends on our current age. A normal person of 50 may be expected to live about 30 years; a person of 30 should live about 50 years. Consequently, any figures cited for PD longevity must be relative to the age of the person.

We examined longevity among residents of Olmsted County, Minnesota, where the Mayo Clinic is located. Over a 20-year span, from the mid-1970s to the mid-1990s, approximately 200 Olmsted County residents were diagnosed with PD. These people with PD lived an average of 10 years after diagnosis. If you saw this figure in insolation, it might be a bit disconcerting if you are currently 60 years old with PD. However, consider that the average age of this group was 71 years. In comparison, a group of Olmsted Country residents without PD but of similar age lived only slightly longer—on average, a total of 13 years. Thus, these Olmsted County residents with PD lived 3 years short of their actuarial predictions; this translates into a near-normal average life span.

Levodopa and Longevity

In the early 1960s, before we had any effective medications for PD, mortality statistics revealed a much different story. Studies from that era documented that people with PD did not live nearly as long as the rest of us (although the figures were not as dismal as for ALS). The introduction of levodopa therapy in around 1969–1970 changed all that. It revolutionized treatment, pulled people out of wheelchairs, and increased longevity. Over a half-dozen independent studies examined mortality rates among those with PD in the first several years after levodopa was introduced compared to the years just prior. These studies all reported mortality rates were substantially improved immediately following the introduction of levodopa therapy. This is not all that surprising, given its often dramatic effect in reversing parkinsonian: people previously confined to a sedentary existence became mobilized.

There was a simple beauty to this story. Administration of a natural substance, levodopa, replenished a deficient brain neurotransmitter (dopamine) and substantially extended life spans.

Progression of Parkinson's Disease: The Levodopa Response

When the initial symptoms of PD first become apparent, there is about a 50% loss of dopaminergic neurons within the substantia nigra. At that time, the surviving dopaminergic terminals within the striatum are able to adequately replenish dopamine with the supplementary levodopa. Thus, administered levodopa is taken up into these surviving striatal terminals, transformed into dopamine, stored, and released in a physiological fashion.

Unfortunately, more of these neurons die over the ensuing years and eventually fewer than 10% remain. With prominent loss of these neurons, there no longer is a uniform distribution of dopaminergic terminals within the striatum. At some point, the few remaining nigrostriatal terminals can no longer compensate. Administered levodopa is erratically handled by these surviving neurons, resulting in unstable medication responses; striatal dopamine concentrations are no longer physiological and well modulated.

At that time, other neighboring brain cells come into play. Certain non-dopaminergic neurons within the striatum have the capability of taking up levodopa and converting it into dopamine. It is these other cells that then take on most of this task. However, they are not ideally designed or positioned for this purpose. They are distant from the dopamine recep-tors; that is, they are not located precisely at dopaminergic synapses. They do not have the capability of the chronic, slow dopamine release onto the receptor, nor do they have the capacity for removing the excess that nor-mally should allow consistent dopamine stimulation. Thus, they are not in a position to control the amount of dopamine stimulating the recep-tor. The receptor may consequently see both dopamine insufficiencies and excesses.

So what does this mean for the person with PD? During the early years, the compensation from the remaining substantia nigra neurons allows a stable response to levodopa. These surviving neurons take up the admin-istered levodopa, synthesize dopamine, release it at the site of the receptor, and control the concentrations. The levels are neither too high nor too low. Because there are no sudden fluctuations in the dopamine concentrations at the receptor, there are no ups or downs in parkinsonism control. At this stage of PD, the timing of the levodopa doses is not critical. One can take the doses earlier or later in the day without noticing any difference. This is because there is adequate nigrostriatal dopamine storage capacity and a well-regulated release rate at the receptor. Clinicians term this stable, persis-tent levodopa benefit the *long-duration response*.

Years later, the situation changes; with few surviving dopaminergic nerve terminals to modulate dopamine levels, the clinical responses become erratic. Rather than precisely timed and programmed dopamine release, huge dopamine fluxes occur at the synapse. This is when the parkinsonism control starts to become unstable in two respects:

1. Because the amount of dopamine at the receptor can no longer be tightly regulated, it may be intermittently excessive. At times, too much dopamine stimulates the receptor and the slow movements of parkinsonism transform into exaggerated, involuntary movements called *dyskinesias*. Thus, the person with PD who otherwise moves slowly now moves too much from excessive dopamine stimulation.

2. Dopamine is no longer efficiently stored in terminals and continuously released at the receptor sites; this results in episodic loss of dopamine influence. The backup brain cells, which normally are not part of this system, make and release dopamine only when levodopa is administered. They are incapable of longer-term storage or slow, regulated release. For the person with PD, the benefits become tightly time-locked to each dose of levodopa. The continuous, long-lasting responses become overshadowed by briefer bursts of benefit, lasting a few hours or less. This is the "short-duration" levodopa response, manifest as alternating loss of parkinsonism control, termed *motor fluctuations* or "on" and "off."

This later-developing lability of the levodopa response varies from person to person. Some with PD never experience very troublesome complications of this type. There are others in whom it is extremely difficult to maintain a consistently beneficial response. Young-onset PD patients (onset before age 40 years) are especially prone to levodopa fluctuations and dyskinesias; conversely, those with PD starting after age 70 are usually not very troubled by this.

The likelihood of developing these levodopa complications is quite variable. In general, about 4 people in 10 (40%) will experience at least modest levodopa-related dyskinesias after 5 years of treatment. The 5-year risk of motor fluctuations is about the same (40%).

Saving the Best Levodopa Responses for Later?

Some have suggested that the stable responses can be saved for later by deferring levodopa treatment. However, there is no evidence to support this assertion. The substrate for such later-developing unstable responses is the progressive loss of nigrostriatal neurons. If we had a strategy for preventing further degeneration of the nigrostriatal system we could prevent these levodopa complications. However, the fundamental problem relates to the ongoing PD neurodegenerative process and not to the duration of levodopa treatment.

These fluctuating levodopa responses and dyskinesias are the basis for published statements in the lay press, such as, "The medications for Parkinson's disease only work for a few years." In fact, the medications continue to work; however, it is the consistency of the response that is the problem. Such levodopa response instability usually can be effectively treated. This requires levodopa dosage adjustments and sometimes supplementary medications, which we will address in later chapters.

Increasing Parkinsonism after Many Years

A reduced response to levodopa does tend to occur much later in the course of the disease. Whereas the initial levodopa response may result in an almost normal function and appearance, this may be less complete after a number of years. This is not to say that the response is lost in PD. The dopamine system is still responsive. However, the Lewy neurodegenerative process often extends to nondopaminergic neurons in the basal ganglia. Since the neurotransmitter in these circuits is not dopamine, levodopa has no influence. Imbalance is one such problem, perhaps requiring a cane or other gait aids after many years. Balance systems in the brain appear not to use dopamine as a neurotransmitter. Whereas levodopa can normalize walking, it cannot reverse the tendency to fall if this develops. For some with PD, the levodopa response does not substantially decline over years of PD, especially among those with young-onset Parkinson's disease. Those who develop PD later in life may not do as well, consequent to the additive effect of brain aging.

Other Modes of Progression

PD may progress in other ways besides movement problems, although this can be quite variable. In the last chapter, we discussed non-movement symptoms that may develop in PD. Most tend to occur later in the course of PD.

Dementia may slowly develop after a number of years; the prevalence in PD clinics ranges from 10 to 40%. Some people will also experience disordered perceptions or hallucinations. We do have medications to treat hallucinations; unfortunately, however, medications for major memory and thinking problems are only modestly beneficial.

Problems of the autonomic nervous system become more likely in long-standing PD (bowels, bladder, low blood pressure). Usually, these are minimal during the early years but become more apparent over the subsequent course of PD. These are variably treatable; later chapters (e.g., Chapters 21, 25–27) address therapy.

Early- versus Later-Onset Parkinson's Disease: Effect on Progression

Those who develop PD very early in life tend to progress differently than those with later-onset PD. *Young-onset PD* is defined as PD starting before age 40 years; this often has a different course than that of later-developing PD. Levodopa instability (dyskinesias and short-duration levodopa responses) tend to become apparent within the first few years among those with such young-onset PD. Usually, the levodopa benefit tends to be very robust, with near resolution of parkinsonism. If dyskinesias can be controlled, these patients often pass for normal. Commonly, those with young-onset PD remain within the mainstreams of their lives for many years, continuing to work, cut the grass, and play golf. However, they tend to be at the mercy of their medications, often requiring complex medication regimens, which may still leave gaps in coverage. As we will discuss in Chapter 33, deep brain stimulation (DBS) has proven especially helpful for these problems when medication responses cannot be stabilized.

At the other extreme, those who develop PD after age 75 years often do not experience substantial problems with dyskinesias or motor fluctuations. However, their response to levodopa may be incomplete; in other words, despite maximal levodopa therapy, they may still experience some parkinsonian symptoms, especially imbalance. This group is also more likely to experience cognitive problems. One contributor relates to aging effects in the brain, which affect nondopaminergic neurons; this is additive with the Lewy neurodegenerative process.

The experiences of most people with PD falls somewhere in between these two extremes of age. However, given that PD is such a variable disease, there are many exceptional cases.

How Best to Prognosticate

We have discussed general PD progression and basic principles. What about you, however, the person with PD? How will you do over the next 10 years, 20 years?

Medical prognostication is educated guesswork, and this is also true for PD. Predictions based on the averages of others with PD are a starting point. However, we have already emphasized that PD is an extremely variable disorder. The course in any given person tends to remain fairly consistent for at least the next several years. One can predict how someone will do, based on the parkinsonism progression up to that time. For example, if a person is still doing well after the first 5 years of PD, playing tennis and working full time, the next 5 years should go well. Long-term prognostication well beyond 5 years is less certain, in part because of the superimposed problems of aging and other medical conditions.

Much Is Spared in Parkinson's Disease

We have addressed the standard problems that occur in PD. But is that all? What about other brain regions or the major organs, such as heart, liver, and kidneys? Are they affected by PD?

In most cases, the regions of the brain that degenerate in PD are confined to certain areas. This includes the substantia nigra and several related basal ganglia regions, whereas much of the remainder of the brain is minimally affected in most people. The exception is among those who develop dementia, in whom thinking and memory regions in the cortex are affected. Dementia risk increases primarily with a combination of long duration of PD (e.g., well beyond 10 years) and increased age (e.g., over age 70 and especially over age 80); however, a few unfortunate people experience cognitive difficulties early in PD and before age 70. More information about this is provided in Chapter 23.

People with PD also need to know that the internal organs, such as liver, heart, lungs, and kidneys, are not involved. Although the autonomic system is affected in PD, the internal organs are spared. Shortness of breath can occur in PD, but this does not reflect a primary lung or heart problem (see Chapter 19). If urinary difficulties develop, this is not a kidney problem but is due to reduced autonomic system control of the bladder (discussed in Chapter 27). People with PD are not substantially more likely to experience heart attacks or strokes.

Cancer rates among those with PD have been debated, with some studies suggesting a lower rate and others a higher rate. Recent studies have indicated that people with PD are more likely to have had or later develop melanoma. Evidence indicates that this is linked to PD per se, and not to the medications used to treat PD. No major trends in other cancers have surfaced.

Medications and Long-Term Toxicities

For the most part, the medications we use to treat PD have no long-term toxicities. Levodopa had been the subject of debate, but the cumulative evidence over four decades has failed to reveal any long-term toxicity with this drug (see Chapter 9). None of the drugs currently used to treat PD carry any substantial potential for liver or kidney damage or compromise blood counts. The only exception is tolcapone, which has potential liver toxicity and requires monitoring of blood tests. This drug is rarely prescribed because of that problem.

Will I Develop All These Problems I Am Reading about?

A myriad of symptoms are described in this book. Do not assume that these are your destiny. Many of these symptoms develop in only a minority of people with PD. You need to be aware of these diverse potential problems so that if they do occur, they can be recognized and appropriately treated. However, you may be spared many or most of them.

Will My Children Get Parkinson's Disease?

Passing PD to offspring is a concern for many with PD. For the vast majority of individuals with PD, the risk is very small. Let us look at the statistics. In Olmsted County, Minnesota (where Mayo Clinic–Rochester is located), the general individual lifetime risk of PD is 2% for all males and 1.3% for females. If you have a parent or other immediate relative with PD, your risk triples, which sounds worrisome upon first hearing this; however, 3 times a small number is still a small number. Thus, if you have PD, the lifetime PD risk for your sons is 3 times 2% = 6%. Similarly, your daughter's risk is 3.9% (3 times 1.3). If multiple other family members are affected with PD, the risks will increase, but there are no tables to precisely predict these risks. If many are affected, this might justify further investigation and should be discussed with your physician.

As we will discuss in Chapter 8, we do not know what causes PD. There may be both environmental and genetic influences. In the vast majority of people with PD, the genetic contribution seems unlikely to come from one gene. Many genetic investigations have explored this possibility and come up with scant evidence for single-gene causes (except in rare families or certain ethnic groups). Likely, there is a strong genetic component, but probably manifested by small contributions from many genes.

PART THREE

◆ ◆ ◆

Distinguishing Parkinson's Disease from Other Disorders

6

♦ ♦ ♦

Conditions Mistaken
for Parkinson's Disease

Not all parkinsonism is Parkinson's disease (PD). In this chapter we review disorders that are commonly confused with PD, including the following:

- Prescription drugs that induce parkinsonism

- Essential tremor and other tremor syndromes

- Parkinsonism-plus syndromes that resemble PD, but have additional features

- Parkinsonian gait disorders (lower-body parkinsonism)

- Dementias with parkinsonism

- Manganese or copper toxicity, including Wilson's disease

In most cases, these conditions can be easily distinguished from PD, provided the clues are recognized.

Check Your Medications: Drugs That Cause Parkinsonism

A variety of medications may induce a *reversible* syndrome of parkinsonism that appears identical to PD; these are listed in Table 6.1. Note that all of these medications require a prescription; no over-the-counter medications cause parkinsonism.

Nearly all of the prescription drugs that cause parkinsonism block the binding of dopamine to brain dopamine receptors.

DRUGS THAT BLOCK DOPAMINE

These dopamine-blocking drugs are called dopamine *antagonists*; that is, they antagonize the dopamine signal. Contrast this to the dopamine *agonist* drugs that activate the dopamine receptors after binding to them (much like dopamine). Dopamine *agonists* are used to treat parkinsonism, and dopamine *antagonists* tend to cause parkinsonism.

Drugs that block dopamine receptors are commonly prescribed for treatment of several conditions:

- Major psychiatric disorders, such as psychosis or schizophrenia

- Nausea or problems with bowel motility

- Migraine with nausea

- Tourette's syndrome (a disorder of twitches and tics)

When one of these dopamine-blocking drugs is discontinued, the parkinsonism usually does not resolve immediately and may take several weeks. There have been rare cases where it took up to 6 months to resolve.

Occasionally, the parkinsonism never goes away after stopping the dopamine antagonist medication. In this case, the drug was probably not the primary cause of parkinsonism but rather unmasked PD that was destined to develop. There is no compelling evidence to indicate that *permanent* parkinsonism is caused by medications that block dopamine receptors.

It may be unwise to discontinue one of these medications in certain cases, such as when used to treat schizophrenia. Among the medications for psychosis and schizophrenia, two do not induce parkinsonism: quetiapine (Seroquel) and clozapine (Clozaril).

Note that drugs used to treat depression do not block dopamine receptors, except for amoxapine (Asendin) and the combination drug perphenazine/amitriptyline (Triavil). These two drugs are now rarely prescribed.

Table 6.1. Common Prescription Medications That May Induce Parkinsonism

Indications for the Drug	Drug	Brain Mechanism Causing Parkinsonism; Comments
Major psychiatric disorders, psychosis, schizophrenia; also used for Tourette's syndrome	Aripiprazole (Abilify) Chlorpromazine (Thorazine) Fluphenazine (Prolixin) Haloperidol (Haldol) Loxapine (Loxitane) Lurasidone (Latuda) Mesoridazine (Serentil) Molindone (Moban) Olanzapine (Zyprexa) Paliperidone (Invega) Perphenazine (Trilafon) Triavil (perphenazine with amitriptyline) Risperidone (Risperdal) Thioridazine (Mellaril) Thiothixene (Navane) Trifluoperazine (Stelazine) Ziprasidone (Geodon)	Block dopamine receptors
Depression	Amoxapine (Asendin)	Block dopamine receptors
Nausea and related gastrointestinal problems; also used for migraine	Metoclopramide (Reglan) Prochlorperazine (Compazine) Promethazine (Phenergan) Thiethylperazine (Torecan)	Block dopamine receptors
Seizures, migraine, psychiatric disorders	Valproic acid (Depakote)	Unknown mechanism; commonly causes tremor; rarely mild parkinsonism
Heart rhythm disturbances	Amiodarone (Cordarone)	Unknown mechanism; rarely causes tremor, imbalance, cognitive impairment, or parkinsonism
Tourette's syndrome	Pimozide (Orap)	Blocks dopamine receptors

WHAT TO DO IF TAKING A DOPAMINE-BLOCKING DRUG

If you are taking one of the dopamine antagonist drugs listed in Table 6.1 and suspect that it is the cause of parkinsonism, your physician may consider discontinuation. A few rules of thumb apply to this situation, as follows.

- Only discontinue a drug if it seems safe to do this.

- Chronically used drugs should be tapered off rather than abruptly stopped.

- Once off the drug, allow sufficient time to determine if the parkinsonism will resolve; often this requires about 1 month of abstinence.

- Avoid drug treatment of parkinsonism (e.g., carbidopa/levodopa) immediately after discontinuing the offending drug; it will probably not be effective until dopamine blockade has dissipated.

NON-DOPAMINE-BLOCKING DRUGS THAT (RARELY) CAUSE PARKINSONISM

The two drugs listed in Table 6.1 that do not block dopamine receptors are valproic acid and amiodarone. These two drugs rarely are the cause of parkinsonism, although valproic acid frequently causes action tremor. Neither drug blocks the effect of carbidopa/levodopa and related drugs. If they have an important medical indication, they often should be continued. Valproic acid (Depakote) is used to treat seizure disorders (epilepsy), migraine, and mood instability (including bipolar disorder). Amiodarone (Cordarone) is used to treat serious heart rhythm disorders.

SSRI DRUGS

Years ago, rare cases of parkinsonism were linked to the prescription of selective serotonin reuptake inhibitor (SSRI) medications. This class of drugs includes Prozac (fluoxetine), Zoloft (sertraline), Paxil (paroxetine), and numerous others. These may have represented chance associations. I have frequently prescribed these antidepressant medications over many years and cannot recall anyone experiencing new or worsened parkinsonism as a side effect. I believe they are safe to use in PD. Depression is discussed in detail in Chapter 22.

Essential Tremor and Other Tremor Syndromes

The lay public often carries the mistaken impression that tremor is synonymous with PD. However, tremor has a variety of origins, and PD is not even the leading cause. The most common tremor disorder is *essential tremor*, which is often confused with PD.

ESSENTIAL TREMOR

Tremor is "essentially" the only symptom of essential tremor (ET). In contrast to PD, ET is *not* associated with slowness, walking problems, or any other prominent neurological symptoms. ET is more common than PD, about 3–5 times more frequent. It may start in childhood but more often begins in adulthood, and at any age. The majority of people with ET have another family member with tremor and a genetic cause is suspected.

The tremor of ET fundamentally differs from that of PD. Like PD tremor, ET most commonly affects the hands, but in a different form. ET hand tremor appears when the hand is active, such as holding a cup to drink, writing, or eating with a utensil. Except in rare cases, the tremor of ET is absent with the hand at rest in the lap or at the side when walking; that is, there is no resting tremor, in contrast to PD. ET is usually present when the hand is moving, such as when reaching, pointing, or bringing a spoon to the mouth. In contrast, the hand tremor of PD markedly attenuates when the hand is moving. PD hand tremor predominantly or exclusively affects only one upper extremity in the beginning, which contrasts to ET, where most often both hands are affected.

One clue to ET is the presence of a head or voice tremor. Head and voice tremors are not seen in PD but are fairly common among those with ET. Although a chin or lower lip tremor may develop in PD, the entire head does not shake. These distinctions are summarized in Table 6.2.

Table 6.2.   Essential Tremor Compared to Parkinson's Disease with Tremor*

Tremor	Essential Tremor	Parkinson's Disease
Head	Yes	No
Voice	Yes	No
Hand tremor at rest	Uncommon	Yes
Hand tremor with movement	Yes	Attenuates or disappears with movement
Hand tremor: one or both hands?	Usually both	One side predominant
Jaw tremor or lower lip tremor	Uncommon	More common (minority)

*Some with Parkinson's disease have no tremor.

Occasional people with PD also have the typical tremor of ET. In some cases, this may be a coincidence. Both ET and PD are common disorders and, by chance, may occur in the same person. There also are rare individuals where Parkinson's disease begins as ET and within a few years evolves into more typical PD. However, the vast majority of people with ET do not develop PD, and ET is not considered to be an early sign of this disorder.

A few people with ET develop a rest tremor, but this typically is minor or occurs after many years. The very rare exceptions are those in whom a rest tremor is present early in the course of ET; this is termed *resting-postural tremor* or *mixed-tremor syndrome*. Similar to ET, there are no parkinsonian features (other than the resting tremor). This rest tremor does not respond to the medications used to treat PD.

ET responds to different drugs than those used to treat PD. The primary medications for essential hand tremor are drugs that block one type of adrenalin responses, termed *beta-blockers*; this includes propranolol and nadolol. These should not be used in people with asthma, low blood pressure, or low pulse rates. The barbiturate mysoline (Primidone) is also prescribed for ET, although sedation and imbalance may limit the tolerability. Head and voice tremor usually do not benefit from these drugs; however, they often respond to injections of botulinum toxin into involved muscles. Medical treatment of tremor is discussed in greater detail in Chapter 14.

Marked essential tremor that fails medication therapy can be controlled with deep brain stimulation (DBS). This is major brain surgery and is reserved for those with the most problematic tremor; see Chapter 33 for related discussion.

BENIGN TREMULOUS PARKINSONISM

This syndrome is uncommon and is usually recognized only after several years of neurological follow-up. Initially, patients have a prominent resting and postural hand tremor plus mild signs of parkinsonism. After several years, it becomes apparent that tremor remains the most prominent feature, whereas the parkinsonism is not very progressive. Even after a decade, walking tends to remain normal or near-normal except for reduced arm swing. Usually, the response to carbidopa/levodopa is partial at best, and it is difficult to treat this syndrome with medications. If the tremor is severe, DBS can be gratifying (see Chapter 33).

OTHER TREMOR SYNDROMES

Strokes, tumors, traumatic injuries, inflammation, or other insults to certain specific brain regions may also cause tremor. Rarely are these confused with PD, because the symptoms develop more abruptly and often with features pointing to the cause. An MRI brain scan may reveal the insult in brain areas known to cause tremor, whereas in PD, the brain scan is normal for age.

Tremor may also be caused by a variety of metabolic or toxic problems, such as thyroid hormone excess or major systemic illnesses (e.g., kidney or liver failure). These induce a tremor that resembles ET, with a prominent hand tremor during posture and movement; this contrasts with tremor in PD. Certain drugs also provoke this type of tremor, such as valproic acid (see previous discussion), lithium, or medications that enhance adrenalin responses, for example, certain asthma medications or stimulants.

Parkinson's-Plus Syndromes

Parkinson's-plus relates to a group of neurodegenerative disorders with prominent parkinsonism, plus other features not seen in PD. These often respond partially or not at all to carbidopa/levodopa and have a less favorable prognosis. Brain regions beyond the substantia nigra degenerate in these conditions, which gives them their unique clinical features. These PD imitators include the following:

- Multiple system atrophy

- Progressive supranuclear palsy

- Corticobasal syndrome

How can you distinguish these from PD? Testing may help, but the physician's history and examination are keys to making the correct diagnosis. These conditions are much less common than PD, and most people with parkinsonism do indeed have PD.

MULTIPLE SYSTEM ATROPHY (MSA)

Multiple system atrophy (MSA) was previously called Shy-Drager syndrome, for the physicians who initially described this disorder. It usually results in more widespread and varied degeneration of brain motor control systems than that in PD. Besides parkinsonism, people with MSA typically have associated features, which may include the following:

- Incoordination (ataxia) from cerebellar degeneration

- Signs of spasticity and increased deep tendon reflexes from damage to the corticospinal tract

- Prominent and early involvement of the autonomic nervous system with symptoms including orthostatic hypotension (with fainting or near-fainting), bladder dysfunction, and loss of male erections

- Stridor (abnormal breathing sounds) during sleep

These associated features may not be very evident in the beginning of the disease course, and that is when MSA can easily be mistaken for PD. The parkinsonism of MSA may not respond to levodopa therapy, or it may only respond partially; this is often a clue, provided the carbidopa/levodopa trial was adequate.

The components of MSA occur together in varied combination, and the diagnosis requires a savvy clinician. Common clinical components are summarized next.

Cerebellar Ataxia

Some individuals with MSA have signs of cerebellar degeneration, resulting in ataxia (refer to Figure 2.3 in Chapter 2 for a picture of the cerebellum). Ataxia is not seen in PD; if it is identified, this argues against the diagnosis of PD.

Ataxia implies incoordination. This typically manifests as clumsy hand movements and a wide-based, unsteady gait resembling someone who is drunk. The speech also resembles someone who has consumed too much alcohol, given the difficulties coordinating lips, tongue, and palate.

Physicians evaluate hand coordination by observing finger-to-nose movements, in which patients alternately touch their nose and the examiner's outstretched finger. Ataxia is apparent when these movements are made imprecisely. People with PD may be slow in doing this exercise, but they precisely hit the targets. Similarly, people with PD may walk slowly or shuffle their feet, but this pattern is distinct from the wide-based, clumsy gait of ataxia. In MSA, imbalance may be severe, resulting in falls. Frequent falls are not expected in early PD unless the patient is very elderly.

Corticospinal Tract Signs

The corticospinal tract is another brain motor control circuit frequently affected in MSA, but spared in PD. If there are prominent corticospinal tract signs on examination, parkinsonism may not be PD. One clue is excessively reactive (brisk) reflexes when the physician uses the reflex hammer. For example, striking the knee with this rubber hammer normally elicits a slight kick of the leg; those with corticospinal tract problems explosively kick high into the air. Also, scratching the bottom of the foot normally elicits reflexive curling of the toes downward; those with corticospinal tract problems reflexively extend their great toe upward (Babinski sign).

Autonomic Dysfunction in MSA

The autonomic nervous system tends to be severely affected by MSA and this may be an early clue. In men, complete loss of erectile function may predate other symptoms by a few years. Bladder problems, such as urinary urgency and incontinence, also tend to occur early in the MSA course. The most obvious clue is often orthostatic hypotension, where the blood pressure plummets when upright. This may result in fainting or near-fainting. Of course, the physician must check the medication list to exclude drugs that cause low blood pressure (see Chapter 21). These same autonomic problems may develop in PD but are mild early in the course and only become troublesome much later, with rare exceptions.

Stridor

MSA may result in *stridor*, a type of abnormal vocal cord movement. This occurs primarily or exclusively at night, while asleep. This is not present in PD. Stridor is heard as a screeching, high-pitched sound while inspiring (breathing in). It is due to the vocal cords tightly coming together while inhaling (normally they should separate to allow air to pass). Stridor suggests potential for serious breathing disruption during sleep. Confirmation is necessary from breathing studies done during a formal sleep study (polysomnography; see Chapter 7).

Two types of MSA

MSA is subdivided into two categories, based on the primary manifestations, cerebellar ataxia (incoordination) or parkinsonism. The cerebellar form should not be mistaken for PD since incoordination (ataxia) fundamentally differs from parkinsonism. This cerebellar type of MSA is termed *MSA-c*, with the *c* standing for "cerebellum" or "cerebellar." When MSA presents with prominent parkinsonism, it is termed *MSA-p* (*p* for "parkinsonism"). It is this form that is often misdiagnosed as PD, especially early in the disease course. Frequently, ataxia and parkinsonism occur together in MSA, although one problem usually predominates.

Parkinsonism Variant of MSA

The older term for MSA-p is *striatonigral degeneration*, implying that the degeneration affects not only the substantia nigra but also the next link in the circuit, the striatum. In the initial stages, MSA-p may be identical to PD, although an incomplete response to levodopa therapy may suggest the diagnosis. Because MSA neurodegeneration extends to the striatum, levodopa (and related drugs) often provides only a partial response. This may be a clue to MSA, provided that the carbidopa/levodopa trial is adequate (see Chapter 12).

Testing for MSA

MRI brain scans may be subtly abnormal in MSA and provide distinctive clues to the diagnosis. Some medical centers offer special tests of autonomic function, which are useful in identifying the more severe autonomic involvement of MSA. Sleep centers may document the nighttime stridor of MSA. No one test makes the diagnosis but rather the aggregate of findings.

Treatment of MSA

The individual problems of MSA are variably treatable. For example, many of the autonomic symptoms have treatments available, some being quite effective (see Chapters 21, 26, 27). Unfortunately, if the parkinsonism of MSA has a poor response to adequate doses of carbidopa/levodopa, other medications are unlikely to provide substantial motor benefit. We have no good medications for cerebellar ataxia, falls, or spasticity (spasticity implies corticospinal tract problems). Stridor may result in serious breathing difficulties at night and should be addressed by sleep specialists.

PROGRESSIVE SUPRANUCLEAR PALSY (PSP)

The prominent parkinsonism of progressive supranuclear palsy (PSP) often resembles PD in the beginning. Time typically provides the clues as additional symptoms and signs surface.

PSP was initially described by three physicians, Drs. Steele, Richardson, and Olszewski, who were impressed by the abnormal eye movements of these patients. That was the basis for the name; the "palsy" refers to paralysis of eye movements. "Supranuclear" relates to specific features of the impaired eye movements, which indicated that the problem was higher in the brain than the last link in the eye movement system. This last link is the brainstem nucleus of neurons that activate eye muscles. The character of the eye movement problem suggested that the damaged site was above this nucleus, or, supranuclear.

Eye movements may be relatively normal early in the course of PSP, which may delay the diagnosis. Once this problem develops, people with PSP cannot easily move their eyes. When severe, the eyes are fixed straight ahead, and changing the direction of gaze is done by moving the head. When less pronounced, the eyes move very slowly. The primary hallmark of PSP is an inability to look down.

The recognition of PSP is by the neurological history, examination, and sometimes subtle changes on MRI brain imaging. Some of the clinical clues are summarized in Table 6.3.

The most important and early clue to PSP is falling. People with PD may complain of imbalance but rarely, if ever, fall down (unless they are very elderly or perhaps after 15–20 years of having PD). Those with PSP may

Table 6.3.   Distinguishing Progressive Supranuclear Palsy from Parkinson's Disease*

Symptom	Progressive Supranuclear Palsy	Parkinson's Disease
Eye movements	Often severely impaired; inability to look down is a hallmark feature. May be normal in early PSP	Able to move eyes in all directions, except occasionally looking upward is affected
Falls	Frequent early in the disease course	Rare until many years elapse or in very elderly
Resting tremor	Often absent; if present, usually not very prominent	Occurs in majority
Eye blinking	Severely reduced; often prominent wide-eyed staring expression	Reduced, but not as much as PSP
Neck and trunk movement	Often very slow neck, head, and trunk movements; person tends to plop into chairs; severe difficulty rising from sitting	Rigidity and slowness of movement more prominent in the limbs than in trunk and neck
Levodopa response	No, or partial response that does not persist	Consistently very responsive

*Parkinsonism is present in both.

topple over while walking, unable to maintain their balance if their body's center of gravity is perturbed. People with PSP usually report falling at least several times monthly or use a walker or wheelchair to avoid falls. MSA may also be associated with early falls.

The limited eye movements of PSP may confirm the diagnosis, but sometimes not until after several years have elapsed. The inability to look down may especially compromise reading or eating, although eye movements in all directions are often affected. People with PSP may mistakenly think that they need new glasses and often go first to their eye doctor. Double vision may be a very early symptom.

The facial appearance may also help to distinguish PSP from PD. People with PD usually have reduced facial animation (masking) and blink less than normal. These signs are usually much more striking in PSP, with a wide-eyed staring expression, rarely blinking.

People with PSP also tend to have very stiff-appearing trunk movements. To sit, they typically plop into their chair. Conversely, they rise from the seated position with great difficulty. When engaged in conversation and looking from one person to another, they do this very stiffly and slowly; as they turn to speak, their whole upper body turns like a statue, instead of just moving the eyes or neck. Rigidity of the neck is often pronounced in PSP, exceeding that in PD. Most people with PSP do not have a prominent rest tremor.

The response to levodopa therapy is also an important clue. It is effective in perhaps 20% of people with PSP, and even when it does work, the benefit wanes after a year or two. Again, this assumes that the carbidopa/levodopa trial was adequate, as will be discussed in Chapter 12.

CORTICOBASAL SYNDROME (CORTICOBASAL DEGENERATION; CORTICOBASAL GANGLIONIC DEGENERATION)

Corticobasal degeneration was originally named for the brain areas that degenerate in this condition, which includes the cortex and basal ganglia. To refresh your memory, the cortex is the outer layers of the brain where human thought, language, perception, and complex actions are organized at their highest level (see Figure 2.3 in Chapter 2). In the corticobasal syndrome, not all of the cortex is involved; the degeneration is primarily in limited areas of the front half, especially those involved in programming complex limb movements. This cortical damage results in apraxia, which implies inability to perform patterned movements, most apparent in the hands; movements such grasping a fork, saluting, or waving goodbye are done extremely awkwardly. The problem lies in brain programming of sequential muscle activation to generate complex movements. The performance of simple hand gestures, such as making the peace sign, may take many seconds and even then, done clumsily and incorrectly. People report that they cannot make their hand do what they want it to do. The parkinsonism of this syndrome is due to degeneration of certain portions of the basal ganglia. Thus, limb movements are stiff (rigid) and slow (bradykinetic).

For unknown reasons, corticobasal syndrome is extremely asymmetric, disproportionately involving one side of the body. Usually in the beginning, only one limb is affected. With progression, both sides of the body are involved, but always much more prominently in the initially affected limb. Although PD is asymmetric, it is much less so than the corticobasal syndrome. The final clue is the lack of response to levodopa therapy; no medications are very helpful for this disorder. The features distinguishing corticobasal degeneration from PD are summarized in Table 6.4.

The initial published report of corticobasal ganglionic degeneration in 1968 included description of the neuropathological findings on postmortem (autopsy) examination. It was later recognized that the microscopic pattern often varied from the original report, despite the same clinical picture. Hence, the term *corticobasal syndrome* is now the preferred term for the

Table 6.4.   Corticobasal Syndrome versus Parkinson's Disease

Clue	Corticobasal Syndrome	Parkinson's Disease
Asymmetry	Pronounced; starts in one limb, which persistently is most affected	PD is asymmetric and often starts in one limb, but not to the degree seen in corticobasal degeneration
Rigidity (stiffness)	Marked limb muscle tension; eventually the limb may become immobile	Rigidity is less than the severe rigidity of corticobasal syndrome
Apraxia*	The hallmark of this disorder	Not seen in PD
Myoclonus resembling tremor	Common; repetitive myoclonic jerks of the outstretched hand are not truly rhythmic; i.e., not true tremor**	Rest tremor (rhythmic)
Levodopa response	No substantial response ever seen	Prominent levodopa benefit

* This is most apparent in the hands, and is characterized by an inability to easily perform simple tasks, such as waving, saluting, and imitating the peace-sign, despite good strength.

** This can be difficult to visually determine, but is confirmed with special electromyography (EMG) techniques.

clinical diagnosis; that is, it does not imply a specific microscopic pattern, which cannot be known in life.

Parkinsonian Gait Disorders (Lower-Body Parkinsonism)

Physicians occasionally encounter people with a shuffling gait, just like that in PD, but without other parkinsonian signs. These patients have no tremor; their faces are not masked and they do not have a soft voice as in PD. Typically, they have no symptoms above the waist. Sometimes freezing of gait (feet stuck to the floor) is a component of this problem. This has been called *lower-half parkinsonism*, although other (confusing) names have been applied, such as frontal lobe gait or gait apraxia.

Among those with this lower-half parkinsonian syndrome, additional signs may further distinguish this syndrome from typical PD. The gait is often wide-based with the feet spread apart (in PD, the base is normal). Arm swing during walking is usually preserved, in contrast to the reduced arm swing of PD. This lower-half parkinsonism typically represents one of three conditions:

1. Normal pressure hydrocephalus;

2. Multiple small strokes affecting basal ganglia connections with the frontal lobes of the brain (hence the term *frontal gait*); or

3. An indeterminate neurodegenerative condition that affects the basal ganglia–frontal lobe brain circuits, which often cannot be further characterized.

Let's consider each of these.

NORMAL PRESSURE HYDROCEPHALUS (NPH)

Normal pressure hydrocephalus (NPH) is a condition that potentially has a neurosurgical treatment. The problem is impeded flow of spinal fluid. We make most of our spinal fluid within *ventricles* within our brain, depicted in Figure 6.1. Humans make approximately a third of a milliliter of spinal fluid per minute. Spinal fluid generated within the ventricles flows toward the back of the brain, passing through the third and fourth ventricles. There are openings for passage near the bottom of the brainstem, where spinal fluid then flows into the space that surrounds the brain and spinal cord. Thus, the brain and spinal cord float in spinal fluid. Ultimately, the dynamic flow of spinal fluid is completed by passage into the large cranial veins, via a system behaving like one-way valves.

In people with NPH, the flow of spinal fluid is partially obstructed, but not enough to raise the pressure inside the skull; hence the term *normal pressure*. The obstruction to the flow of spinal fluid is presumed external to the ventricular system, at the interface between the spinal fluid and bloodstream where the spinal fluid passes into the veins.

The term *hydrocephalus* essentially translates into "water on the brain." This term is used whenever there is obstruction to the flow of spinal fluid. NPH fundamentally differs from certain other forms of hydrocephalus, such as that occasionally occurring in infants due to developmental defects, or when the ventricles are obstructed by tumors; these are urgent neurosurgical problems. Although NPH is neurosurgically treated, it is not an urgent problem.

Basically, NPH is a plumbing problem. The treatment focuses on providing an alternate route to vent the impeded spinal fluid. Neurosurgeons do this by inserting a hollow tube, or *shunt*, through the brain into one of the lateral ventricles; the other end of the shunt is placed elsewhere in the body where the spinal fluid can drain. This shunt contains a valve that allows appropriate amounts of fluid to exit when the pressure builds up.

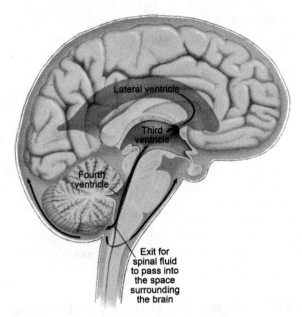

6.1 The brain and spinal cord float in a large sack of spinal fluid. Most of the cerebrospinal fluid is generated within the ventricular system. These cisterns include the large lateral ventricles and the smaller third and fourth ventricles. The slow flow within these brain channels leads to the lower end of the brainstem, where the spinal fluid exits to fill the sack enveloping the brain and spinal cord. Ultimately, the spinal fluid surrounding the brain is slowly channeled into the large veins on the surface of the brain, via a mechanism functioning like a one-way valve. Thus, there is normally continuous spinal fluid flow.

The suspicion that someone might have NPH comes from the neurological history and examination. There are three clinical features that suggest this diagnosis:

- A lower-half parkinsonian gait;

- Urinary incontinence (unable to control urination with substantial leakage); and

- Cognitive impairment (typically not severe).

This clinical picture will usually prompt the physician to order a brain scan, with attention to the brain ventricles. The obstruction to flow of the spinal fluid causes it to back up, leading to enlarged ventricles. Thus, the hallmark feature of NPH is large brain ventricles.

This diagnostic strategy sounds simple; however, the picture is often confused by the fact that normal aging results in enlarged brain ventricles due to brain shrinkage. With aging, we slowly lose brain cells, which becomes increasingly apparent by ages 70–80 years. Since the skull does not proportionately shrink, the spaces in and around the brain enlarge. This includes the "spaces" inside the brain, that is, the ventricles. The physician must decide whether the enlarged ventricles are disproportionately expanded or whether they are enlarged in proportion to the age-related brain shrinkage.

There are a variety of strategies for determining who truly has NPH and will likely respond to shunting. This commonly includes a lumbar puncture in which a large volume of spinal fluid is removed on a trial basis. If walking (or other symptoms) markedly improves after this procedure, treatable NPH is thought more likely. Unfortunately, even with the best tests available, physicians cannot always predict who will respond to shunting. Sometimes the shunt fails to improve symptoms despite fulfilling all the diagnostic and predictive criteria.

Shunting sounds simple but it is not risk-free. Even with the most experienced neurosurgeons, bleeding within the brain can occur, resulting in stroke-like symptoms. Fortunately, this is quite infrequent, whereas slightly more common are problems with the shunt, which can get plugged or become infected.

TINY STROKES CAUSING LOWER-HALF PARKINSONISM

Multiple small strokes that go unrecognized may result in a parkinsonian gait (lower-half parkinsonism). Frequently this is associated with intellectual impairment and other neurological signs. The clues are on the MRI scan of the brain. Small, discreet strokes and related MRI changes are thus seen in the basal ganglia and connected structures.

Often this syndrome occurs in people with uncontrolled high blood pressure (hypertension). Persistent and uncontrolled hypertension damages blood vessels, including smaller arteries. Another name for this is *atherosclerosis* (hardening of the arteries). Diabetes mellitus may also predispose to this problem. If the small arteries in the front half of the brain become plugged, damage to basal ganglia–related brain circuits may result in lower-half parkinsonism as well as intellectual impairment. Other factors besides hypertension or diabetes may also promote atherosclerotic small-artery occlusion, and sometimes this occurs in the absence of such risk factors. When this clinical syndrome is identified, focus should be on control of atherosclerotic risk factors, such as elevated blood pressure or cholesterol and diabetes.

Although this gait problem does not represent PD, carbidopa/levodopa is sometimes administered, as outlined in Chapter 12. There is no downside to trying this, and it can be discontinued if there is no benefit.

OTHER NEURODEGENERATIVE DISORDERS RESULTING IN LOWER-HALF PARKINSONISM

There are occasional people with lower-half parkinsonism in whom clues point to no specific cause. They do not have the other features of NPH and the MRI brain scans reveal no small strokes. There are three possible conditions this might represent:

1. Atypical PD;

2. An indeterminate neurodegenerative disorder that might become apparent with passage of time, such as a variant of PSP; or

3. A nonspecific syndrome of brain aging, as discussed in the next section.

These conditions may warrant a trial of carbidopa/levodopa therapy, as outlined in Chapter 12. There is nothing to lose, and it can be discontinued if not beneficial.

The Gait of Aging

Our bodies age, and so does our brain. It may be discomforting to learn that our brain shrinks with passing decades of life, which is very apparent on MRI brain scans. Substantial differences in brain size can be seen between MRI scans of typical people in their 30s and those in their 80s.

In otherwise normal people, subtle decline of brain function becomes apparent by mid-life. Elite athletes can no longer compete at a high level by the time they reach 40 years of age. Major league baseball hitters can no longer catch up to a fastball. Mathematicians solving the most challenging mathematical problems typically do this in early adulthood. The senior years are often marked by "senior moments."

This brain aging especially affects walking and balance. Although some octogenarians are still playing tennis, others are using canes for balance. Progressively into the 80s and 90s, brain aging causes increasing problems with walking. Joint problems are a factor for some, but the gait of advanced seniors often starts to take on some of the features of parkinsonism, with shuffling.

Although a shuffling gait would be a good reason to consider a trial of carbidopa/levodopa, the gait of aging rarely responds. Nonetheless, it is reasonable to try this (Chapter 12). Unfortunately, we have no medications for imbalance, which is a common problem in people at advanced ages.

Dementia with Parkinsonism

Dementia is defined as a loss of intellectual abilities sufficient to interfere with activities of daily living, typically irreversible. This includes problems with memory, judgment, or abstract reasoning. Dementia is the central feature of certain neurodegenerative disorders, such as Alzheimer's disease.

Dementia is an early feature of the Lewy neurodegenerative condition termed *dementia with Lewy bodies.* This disorder includes the typical features of Parkinson's disease but with dementia as an initial problem.

DEMENTIA WITH LEWY BODIES; LEWY BODY DEMENTIA

Dementia with Lewy bodies (DLB) is the second most common cause of dementia, second only to Alzheimer's disease. This disorder resembles advanced PD with dementia.

Recall that after many years of otherwise typical Parkinson's disease, dementia may develop, especially among the aged. This reflects the progression of the Lewy neurodegenerative process, spreading to cognitive regions of the brain. When this occurs, it is termed *Parkinson's disease with dementia.* DLB differs in that the dementia is among the earliest symptoms. The changes in the brain (i.e., Lewy body neurodegeneration) are essentially identical to those in PD with dementia. Clinical researchers have arbitrarily defined these two syndromes on the basis of when the dementia developed. If cognitive impairment starts before or within 1 year of parkinsonism, this qualifies as DLB. If the dementia starts more than 1 year after Parkinson's disease, this is termed PD with dementia. This overlap of PD and DLB begs the question as to whether these conditions have common origins or are variations of a single disorder.

The hallmark features of DLB may include the following:

- Dementia as an initial feature

- Parkinsonism (often responsive to levodopa therapy, like PD)

- Hallucinations

- Autonomic symptoms (e.g., urinary urgency, constipation)

- REM sleep behavior disorder (acting out dreams)

Also, a common observation by family members is fluctuating mental clarity.

Treatment of DLB parallels the treatment of PD and, more specifically, PD with dementia. The same treatment strategies discussed in this book for PD are also appropriate for Lewy body dementia. However, a notable caveat cannot be overemphasized: carbidopa/levodopa alone is advisable to treat the parkinsonism of Lewy body dementia (guidelines in Chapter 12); the other PD drugs tend to provoke hallucinations.

The later developing dementia of PD that overlaps with DLB is discussed in Chapter 23. Diagnosis and treatment of these dementing disorders is addressed in more detail in another book: *Dementia with Lewy Bodies and Parkinson's Disease Dementia* (J.E. Ahlskog; Oxford University Press, 2014).

ALZHEIMER'S DISEASE

Alzheimer's disease is the most common cause of dementia, with memory loss as the most prominent feature. Alzheimer's disease is not typically associated with prominent motor problems such as gait disorders. However, since Alzheimer's disease occurs later in life, age-related gait and balance problems may coincidentally develop. Thus, slowness, stooped posture, or imbalance may surface and occasionally raise a question of DLB.

Manganese or Copper Toxicity Causing Parkinsonism

Toxic causes of PD are very rare. Here we address two elements that under unique circumstances accumulate within the brain to induce parkinsonism.

MANGANESE TOXICITY

Massive environmental exposure to the metal manganese can induce parkinsonism. Usually, the parkinsonism differs from typical PD and tends not to respond as well to carbidopa/levodopa.

Welding generates manganese fumes, which are not problematic if there has been good ventilation of the workplace. Long-term welding in poorly ventilated environments may lead to the buildup of brain manganese; this tends to accumulate within the basal ganglia (especially globus pallidus), causing parkinsonism. Welding is an extremely rare cause of parkinsonism in the United States, where the Occupational Safety and Health Administration (OSHA) standards minimize the likelihood of substantial manganese exposure in the workplace.

An important clue to manganese-induced parkinsonism is seen on MRI brain scans. Specifically, the globus pallidus becomes bright with certain MRI techniques (so-called T1 imaging); only rarely is this pattern seen in other disorders and never in typical PD.

MANGANESE TOXICITY DUE TO LIVER FAILURE

Brain manganese accumulation may occur in the setting of liver failure. Note that manganese in trace amounts is present in most of our meals. Our body requires tiny amounts of manganese for certain biochemical processes, and the excess is normally excreted through the liver's bile system. However, the bile system often malfunctions in those with liver failure; hence manganese accumulates in the body, especially in the brain, where it has a predilection for the basal ganglia. MR brain imaging will document increased globus pallidus signal on routine T1 sequences, corresponding to the manganese.

Treatment of manganese-related parkinsonism of liver failure is not simple. Purging the manganese from the body through chelation therapy appears to be ineffective. Manganese is present in so many of our foods that meaningful dietary therapy is not practical. Liver transplantation appears to be an effective treatment, as it improves the capacity for the body to eliminate manganese through the restored bile system. Carbidopa/levodopa therapy may be tried to treat the parkinsonism of liver failure, with uncertain benefits.

WILSON'S DISEASE

Wilson's disease is a disorder of copper metabolism, almost always developing in younger people. It is extremely rare; I have never diagnosed a new case, despite ordering thousands of screening tests for this condition. However, it is important to recognize because it can cause irreversible brain and liver damage if left untreated. In Wilson's disease, copper from the diet is not adequately excreted via the liver-biliary system. When this occurs, more copper enters the body than leaves it. Eventually, the buildup of copper reaches toxic levels, primarily in the brain and liver.

The neurological syndrome may include tremor, parkinsonism, as well as psychiatric or cognitive problems. Liver failure may also herald the diagnosis. Most people with Wilson's disease develop the neurological symptoms by early adulthood, although rare cases have been documented in late middle age. The MRI brain scan is typically quite abnormal. A usual screening workup includes blood tests (serum copper and ceruloplasmin) and a 24-hour urine collection for copper, as well as a special eye examination using a device called a slit-lamp. This ophthalmological examination involves looking for copper deposits around the iris, termed *Kayser-Fleischer rings*.

7

♦ ♦ ♦

Testing

The clinician makes the diagnosis of Parkinson's disease (PD) primarily from the history and the neurological examination. Laboratory tests and scans have only a limited role in routine cases. However, when there are unusual or unexpected findings, these studies may be appropriate. Also, testing is done in the evaluation and treatment of conditions linked to PD, such as urinary problems or memory impairment. The discussion here will proceed along these lines, first addressing tests that may be used to establish the diagnosis; the evaluation of problems related to PD will be discussed last.

Tests to Determine Parkinson's Disease versus Another Disorder

The appearance of parkinsonism does not necessarily assure us that someone has PD. However, this is usually the case if there are no atypical or unusual features. In typical cases, limited or no testing is often appropriate. What constitutes a typical case of PD? If the condition meets the following criteria, the workup could be kept simple:

- Parkinsonism onset over 50 years of age

- Symptoms and examination findings are only those of parkinsonism, that is, no ataxia, corticospinal tract signs, or apraxia (discussed in Chapter 4)

- Balance adequate to avoid falling (except very late in the course or in those of age greater than 80 years)
- No major thinking or memory problems
- No sudden change in symptoms (as occurs with strokes)
- No major problems with low blood pressure or orthostatic hypotension (unless explained by medications)
- No other active major medical issues

If these criteria are met, no neurological testing is usually necessary. However, the medication list should have been reviewed to make certain that there are no causative medications, as listed in Chapter 6.

PD is often associated with certain less specific symptoms such as extreme fatigue or weight loss. When such symptoms are present, a general medical examination by a primary care clinician is appropriate, including routine blood studies. Routine blood studies include a complete blood count, thyroid, and a chemistry panel. PD may start before age 50 years, but in this age group, additional tests are often done and may include an MRI brain scan and perhaps a screening test for Wilson's disease (e.g., serum ceruloplasmin).

FURTHER TESTING, BASED ON ATYPICAL FEATURES

Additional testing is based on specific medical and neurological findings keeping company with parkinsonism. Some of the more common features that lead to testing are listed in Table 7.1. This is not an exhaustive list and other clues may push the testing in different directions.

Most parkinsonism represents PD. However, a careful history and exam may suggest other causes and the need to proceed with testing, as summarized next.

Table 7.1. Symptoms and Signs Occurring with Parkinsonism That Justify Further Testing

Symptoms and Signs	Possible Condition (see Chapter 6)	Tests: MRI Brain Scan* Plus
Sudden onset of symptoms	Stroke	• Brain imaging, plus further tests if a stroke or bleed is identified

(continued)

Table 7.1. Continued

Symptoms and Signs	Possible Condition (see Chapter 6)	Tests: MRI Brain Scan* Plus
Cognitive impairment	Dementia linked to PD versus a separate cause (see Chapter 23)	• Routine blood studies, including complete blood count, chemistry profile, vitamin B12, thyroid • CT, rather than MRI head scan, may be sufficient • The history may suggest other tests (e.g., if recent-onset confusion, fever, consider lumbar puncture)
Prominent autonomic problems, such as: • Orthostatic hypotension not due to medications • Urinary incontinence • Severe and early male erectile dysfunction	Multiple system atrophy	Studies of autonomic nervous system Urinalysis and urological evaluation
Typical triad of symptoms: • Shuffling gait but with parkinsonism sparing upper body • Urinary incontinence • Cognitive impairment	Normal pressure hydrocephalus	Lumbar puncture to drain spinal fluid with assessment of the response before and after
Other neurological signs: • Frequent falls • Ataxia • Corticospinal tract signs • Apraxia	1. Parkinsonism-plus (progressive supranuclear palsy, multiple system atrophy, corticobasal degeneration) 2. Other rare brain disorders	Workup depends on initial impression of the physician

*A brain scan is usually indicated when parkinsonism departs from the expected. An MRI scan is preferred, as it provides substantially higher resolution and often reveals subtle clues to parkinsonism-plus disorders.

Cerebrovascular Causes (Strokes, Brain Hemorrhages)

Sudden onset of major neurological symptoms may suggest a stroke, albeit a rare cause of parkinsonism. When a stroke or brain hemorrhage causes parkinsonism, this typically damages other brain regions, resulting in additional neurological symptoms and signs; the neurological examination is therefore important. When a stroke is suspected, an MRI brain scan is typically done. A CT head scan is less sensitive but may be sufficient in some cases if an MRI scan cannot be done. Parenthetically, people with typical PD often report that their tremor abruptly became apparent; as an isolated symptom, this does not necessarily indicate a stroke-like process.

Aging and hardening of the arteries (atherosclerosis) is occasionally associated with multiple small stokes, visible on the MRI brain scan and often affecting the basal ganglia. Because these strokes are tiny, they may not be heralded by sudden symptoms but rather accumulate to insidiously become symptomatic. Such multiple small strokes are especially common among smokers or those with uncontrolled hypertension, diabetes mellitus, or high cholesterol. Since these small strokes are not confined to only parkinsonian brain regions, other neurological symptoms and signs may signal a clue to this process. When identified, it may be unclear whether such small stroke-like changes on an MRI scan are the cause of parkinsonism. In that case, the response to levodopa therapy will often sort this out; parkinsonism due to strokes typically responds poorly to levodopa treatment.

Intellectual Impairment with Parkinsonism

If cognitive impairment is present, further testing is always appropriate; one should not jump to the conclusion that it is simply a component of the neurodegenerative process. Seniors are especially susceptible to impaired thinking from certain routine medical conditions. For example, an underactive thyroid, marked anemia, or a urinary tract infection may cause someone with marginal cognitive impairment to decompensate and become confused. Furthermore, occult brain lesions, such as a blood clot (subdural hematoma), or benign tumor (such as a meningioma) may impair thinking and cause motor symptoms. Appropriate tests when thinking is impaired include the following:

- A head scan (MRI or CT)
- Complete blood count
- Sedimentation rate (a clue to an infectious or inflammatory process)
- Chemistry profile (sodium, potassium, calcium, glucose, liver and kidney function tests)

- Thyroid (e.g., sensitive thyroid-stimulating hormone [TSH])

- Vitamin B12 (a low B12 level can result in a variety of neurological problems and be due to selective malabsorption of this vitamin)

- Urinalysis

Other tests may also be appropriate based on the history; for example, if the patient is coughing and running a fever, a chest X-ray should be checked. If there has been fairly rapid development of confusion, a lumbar puncture for spinal fluid analysis should be considered.

Parkinsonism-Plus Disorders

Atypical parkinsonism with unexpected features (e.g., frequent falls, faints, ataxia) requires further assessment. These parkinsonism-plus conditions of multiple system atrophy (MSA), progressive supranuclear palsy (PSP), and corticobasal syndrome were discussed Chapter 6. An MRI brain scan often provides subtle clues to these diagnoses.

Prominent symptoms of autonomic nervous system dysfunction raise a suspicion of MSA and autonomic testing may be considered. These autonomic studies include tests of sweating as well as reflexive changes in blood pressure and heart rate in response to certain stimuli. If MSA seems likely, then evaluation at a sleep center is appropriate to determine whether stridor is present during sleep (stridor is characterized by screeching sounds during inhalation; in the setting of MSA this has serious implications).

Normal Pressure Hydrocephalus (NPH)

NPH is a consideration in the setting of a wide-based, shuffling gait, cognitive impairment, and urinary incontinence; parkinsonian signs are absent above the waist (see Chapter 6). A brain scan, preferably an MRI scan, is the appropriate screening test. To help confirm the diagnosis of NPH, physicians often perform a lumbar puncture (spinal tap). If removal of a volume of spinal fluid markedly improves walking and other symptoms, this provides further evidence of NPH. The definitive treatment of NPH is the neurosurgical insertion of a shunt tube into the brain ventricular system (see Figure 6.1 in Chapter 6).

NUCLEAR MEDICINE SCANS: PET, SPECT

Special scans image the dopamine-containing neurons in the brain, as discussed in Chapter 4. Various techniques of this type have been used for years as research tools. In general, they employ the vein injection of a specific substance that passes from the bloodstream into the brain and is uniquely taken up by the dopaminergic neurons. A radioactive tag attached to the injected substance gives off tiny amounts of radioactivity; this generates a brain picture of dopaminergic neurons on the scanning screen. The radioactive signals are read and processed using one of two techniques: positron emission tomography (PET) or single photon emission computed tomography (SPECT). With these techniques, deficiencies of dopaminergic neurons are detected. However, they cannot distinguish between PD and one of the parkinsonism-plus disorders (where dopaminergic neurons also degenerate).

Only one such technique, dopamine transporter imaging using SPECT, has been approved for routine clinical care. The *dopamine transporter* is a molecule that modulates dopamine concentrations in the synapse. It is unique to dopaminergic neurons and is especially localized in the dopaminergic terminals in the striatum (see Figure 2.5 in Chapter 2). The sole approved indication for a dopamine transporter scan is to distinguish PD from essential tremor (per the U.S. Food and Drug Administration [FDA]). FDA approval is important as these studies are very expensive. Such imaging is not routinely used to diagnose PD.

GENETIC TESTING

Genetic assessments are a very important research tool and have led to many very important insights into the mechanisms playing a role in PD, as will be addressed in the next chapter. However, among people with routine PD, a causative gene can be identified in only 1–2%. The percentages increase in certain ethnic groups, most notably Ashkenazi Jewish people and others with Middle Eastern heritage, as well as in very young-onset PD.

Having two family members with PD does not substantially increase the likelihood of detecting a genetic basis. However, when many within a single family have PD, a causative gene may be found. Such families have been the basis for important discoveries and are of major research interest.

Should genetic testing be considered as part of routine care in the absence of other affected family members with PD? The primary negative factors include the following:

- Substantial expense (e.g., a comprehensive Parkinson genetic panel currently costs approximately $10,000)

- Current inability to translate genetic findings into treatment

- Implications for other family members who may not wish to know genetic risks

Genetic testing is not currently routinely advised in PD clinics. If done, it should be with the help of genetic counsellors to put genetic findings into the proper context. Obviously, if multiple living family members are affected with PD, researchers are very interested.

Testing to Diagnose and Treat Conditions Linked to Parkinson's Disease

A variety of symptoms may be associated with PD. We will not address testing of each and every complication but confine this discussion to some of the more common problems.

URINARY SYMPTOMS

Impaired bladder control is common among those with PD and is discussed in detail in Chapter 27. For simpler problems, the clinician will start with a routine examination of the urine via urinalysis. For more troublesome problems an urologist should be consulted. The urologist can look inside the bladder (cystoscopy) and test the neurological reflexes of the bladder (urodynamics). Measurement of residual urine after routine voiding can help guide the therapy.

Those with bladder dysfunction are predisposed to bladder infections. Burning during urination may signal such an infection, which can be evaluated with a urinalysis and a urine culture for bacteria. Using the culture, laboratory personnel can identify which antibiotic(s) will potentially kill the bacteria.

CONSTIPATION

Most individuals with PD are constipated sooner or later (see Chapter 26). If this pattern is stable and long-standing, no testing may be necessary. However, if there has been a recent substantial change in bowel habits, the colon should be examined to rule out cancer or other internal problems. The colon is the last part of the intestine, which ends in the rectum, emptying through the anus. In general, if there has been a history of colon polyps (growths) or prior cancer, or if there is a family history of colon cancer, the colon needs to be examined periodically. The most sensitive way of examining the colon, colonoscopy, is with a tube that is passed through the colon, allowing the physician to see the internal features.

LOW BLOOD PRESSURE

Low blood pressure in the standing position (orthostatic hypotension) is common among those with PD (see Chapter 21). It is typically due to problems within the autonomic nervous system that are exacerbated by certain medications. It is appropriate to check a complete blood count to make certain that anemia is not contributing. If there are other active medical problems, a complete battery of blood chemistry tests may be considered. As discussed earlier, there are special studies that can assess function of the autonomic nervous system, which are primarily appropriate when MSA is being considered.

SWALLOWING PROBLEMS

Minor swallowing problems are common among those with PD (see Chapter 25) and do not require testing. Only if the problems become disabling or are atypical is further study necessary. Fortunately, this is very rarely the case in PD, and serious swallowing disorders raise concerns about PSP or MSA.

Testing may include swallowing a substance that can be seen via X-ray, demonstrating passage from the throat to the stomach. Also, a tube (endoscope) can be used to look beyond the throat into the esophagus, the passageway between the throat and stomach.

DAYTIME SLEEPINESS

Drowsiness during the waking day is common in PD. Frequently, this is due to poor sleep at night and may respond to levodopa and related treatment. Alternatively, certain prescription drugs may also induce daytime drowsiness. These problems are discussed in Chapter 20. Not uncommonly, daytime drowsiness is due to sleep apnea (intermittent breathing interruptions during sleep). Sleep apnea is unrecognized by the sleeper, whereas the sleep partner may hear loud snoring.

A screening test for sleep apnea can be done at home using an oximeter. This device includes a sensor attached to one fingertip; it is connected to a digital recorder, which registers the ongoing blood oxygen saturation overnight during sleep. Frequent reductions in blood oxygen saturation suggest sleep apnea, which is then appropriately followed up with overnight assessment at a sleep center. However, if sleep apnea seems likely it would be appropriate to proceed directly to *polysomnography*, where the patient is monitored overnight in a sleep laboratory. Physiological monitoring of various body processes with videotaping may then confirm sleep disordered breathing and lead to treatment.

SHORTNESS OF BREATH

Shortness of breath may occasionally be a consequence of PD, as will be discussed in Chapter 19. This does not reflect a primary problem with the lungs or heart. Rather, this is the consequence of dampened breathing movements (diaphragm, rib cage muscles) from parkinsonism. It is not a dangerous problem for those with PD, but it can be very uncomfortable. Fortunately, it responds to levodopa therapy.

When such breathing symptoms are experienced, one should not simply jump to the conclusion that PD is the cause. Rather, the clinician will want to make certain that there are no primary heart or lung problems. A variety of breathing and heart tests can be employed; the choice of test depends on the person's symptoms and the clinician's level of suspicion.

OSTEOPOROSIS

Weakening of the bones is not a problem directly linked to PD. However, this is especially common among those with PD relating to several factors, including age and reduced physical activity. Also, those with PD often have insufficient blood levels of vitamin D, which is crucial for calcium absorption and bone health (see Chapter 30). Because PD may affect balance, strong bones are important in case of falls.

Bone strength is assessed with a special nuclear medicine bone density scan (DEXA scan). A minimally radioactive substance that binds to bones is injected into a vein. When this substance enters bones, a scanner can measure how much is bound, documenting whether the bone is dense or porous. This test allows an estimate of fracture risk and is important for guiding therapy. Testing may also include blood measurement of vitamin D, plus calcium and related substances.

PART FOUR

◆ ◆ ◆

The Cause and Progression of Parkinson's Disease

8

◆ ◆ ◆

Clues to the Cause(s):
Genes, Environment

Parkinson's disease (PD) is a neurodegenerative disorder. Neurodegenerative conditions encompass a variety of disorders, such as Alzheimer's disease and amyotrophic lateral sclerosis (ALS, or Lou Gehrig's disease). To date, we have not identified the cause(s) for these conditions, despite major research efforts in many laboratories and clinics around the world.

For decades, theories have been proposed for the cause of PD, but with modest support from hard facts. Blame has been placed on everything from viruses and bacteria to the food we eat. Each hypothesis has had enough supporting evidence to stimulate research, but most of these have been dead ends. What we need are creditable clues to point us in the right direction. These clues are slowly accumulating, although some may be red herrings. The answer is likely buried in what we already know, but putting this puzzle together has been both challenging and frustrating.

Over the last quarter century, 11 large clinical trials have tested drugs that were hoped to slow the progression of PD (discussed in more detail in Chapter 9). Most of these trials were funded by the U.S. federal government and were carried out with "cautious optimism." Despite these good intentions, nothing has come of this. We still have no drugs proven to slow the progression of PD. We have learned many things from these trials, especially routes to therapeutic dead ends that should be avoided in the future.

Nonetheless, we still have no disease-slowing drug to offer those with PD. Why have we collectively failed despite so many smart clinician-scientists doing research backed by generous funding? Obviously, selection of the tested drugs has been the problem. Criticism is easy in retrospect, but how do we make better selections in the future? The answer lies in the funding of research directed at the *cause* of PD. You cannot fix a car unless you understand how the engine works, and the same principle applies to PD. If we had a clear understanding of the causative mechanisms, scientists could come up with treatments.

To put this into further perspective, let us wind back the clock 25–35 years. At that time, clinicians and scientists had a very limited view of PD, trying to make sense of what they knew about this disorder. Levodopa therapy had recently been discovered, which was revolutionizing the treatment of PD. This discovery was borne of the recognition that degeneration of the dopaminergic substantia nigra caused most PD symptoms. We know now that PD encompasses much more than dopamine, but at that time this was not so obvious. With the focus on dopamine and the substantia nigra, it was easy to assume that the neurodegenerative mechanism must be linked to dopamine. Perhaps dopamine is a substantia nigra toxin! This leap of faith led to the proposal that "oxidative stress" generated by dopamine metabolism killed substantia nigra neurons. Note that oxidative reactions are ubiquitous components of all human cellular biochemistry, with many biological checks and balances. Regardless, this theory was widely accepted at the time, and considerable research was directed at that hypothesis. This included several early clinical drug trials hoping to slow PD progression by reducing this oxidative process; these studies all generated negative results.

This narrow view prevailed until landmark studies were published by Heikko Braak and colleagues about a decade ago. A crucial starting point for identifying the cause(s) of PD requires an understanding of the evolving pattern of the neurodegenerative process in the brain; this is what Braak and colleagues importantly put into context.

Braak's Important Contributions

Braak, a neuroanatomist in Frankfurt, Germany, conducted his research using microscopic examination of postmortem brains of people with PD. However, he did not simply restrict his study to those who died midway in PD. Using special stains to identify Lewy bodies, the biological marker of PD, he examined brains from a broad spectrum of affected people. He already knew that about 15% of seniors without clinical signs of PD have postmortem Lewy bodies. He proposed that these Lewy body–affected patients without signs of PD represent the earliest stage of PD. This early stage is now called *incidental Lewy body disease.*

The Lewy body–affected brain regions in those with incidental Lewy body disease fit with symptoms often preceding PD: loss of the sense of smell, constipation, and dream enactment behavior. Restated, otherwise normal people with one or more of these three symptoms are at a significantly greater risk of later developing PD. At the other end of the spectrum, people with very advanced PD and dementia were noted by Braak and colleagues to have Lewy body changes invading cognitive brain regions.

Based on these findings, Braak provided a staging scheme for PD, spanning decades. The earliest stage is localized to limited regions of the nervous system:

- Lower brain stem

- Autonomic nervous system

- Olfactory brain regions (smell sense)

In this scheme, the dopaminergic substantia nigra is affected midway in the course. Late stages reflect the spread of Lewy changes well beyond nondopaminergic areas and especially the cortex (the cortex is illustrated in Figure 2.3, Chapter 2). This proliferation of Lewy pathology correlates with the late development of dementia and levodopa-refractory movement symptoms.

In this scheme, PD is a slowly evolving process, starting years or decades before the first motor symptoms of PD. This broad view takes us away from the focus on dopamine and the substantia nigra. The relevance of the dopaminergic nigrostriatal system for symptomatic treatment cannot be overstated; however, dopamine may have been one of the red herrings that arguably sidetracked the search for the cause of PD.

Braak's contributions would not have been possible without other crucial discoveries years prior, especially the potentially important role of *alpha-synuclein* in PD. Recall from Chapter 3 that this normal brain protein is concentrated in great abundance in Lewy bodies. Thus, special alpha-synuclein tissue stains allowed Professor Braak to easily visualize Lewy bodies under the microscope. Beyond that, alpha-synuclein now appears to have major relevance to the cause and, perhaps, ultimate treatment of PD.

Genetic Contributions to Parkinson's Disease

ALPHA-SYNUCLEIN

The alpha-synuclein story starts in Contursi, a small village in southern Italy. Early in the last century, a number of its sons and daughters immigrated to the East Coast of the United States. Some 50 to 75 years later, offspring began appearing with parkinsonism in neurological clinics, including the neurology clinic of the Robert Wood Johnson Medical School in New Jersey. At that center, Professors Lawrence Golbe and Roger Duvosin astutely recognized the common heredity, with parkinsonism passed from one generation to the next. Through careful medical detective work they traced the condition back to two original Italian Contursi families. Notably, the parkinsonism was nearly identical to typical PD, including being highly responsive to levodopa therapy; moreover, it was associated with Lewy bodies on postmortem brain examination. The family trees revealed PD affecting multiple generations, one after the other, typical of dominant inheritance. Hence, one abnormal gene was thought to be causative.

The responsible gene was ultimately identified, coding for the protein alpha-synuclein. Investigators failed to find this abnormal alpha-synuclein gene outside those families in people with typical PD. However, special tissue stains that selectively mark microscopic alpha-synuclein revealed high concentrations of this substance within Lewy bodies in typical PD patients. Restated, normal alpha-synuclein was accumulating in brain cells of those with PD, represented by microscopic Lewy bodies. Although the Contursi genetic mutation turned out not to cause usual PD, it suggested that alpha-synuclein per se may play a causative role. This is not quite that simple, since nearly 300 other substances are also contained within Lewy bodies, although alpha-synuclein appears to be among the most abundant. The story does not stop there, however.

Inherited Parkinsonism from Too Much Alpha-Synuclein

The potential relevance of alpha-synuclein to the cause of PD became especially apparent when one or two *extra* alpha-synuclein genes were linked to inherited PD. The first such family had been followed at the Mayo Clinic for years, with multiple PD-affected members, spanning multiple generations (i.e., dominant inheritance). The cause did not turn out to be an abnormal alpha-synuclein gene; rather, two *extra* (but normal) alpha-synuclein genes were found, thanks to researchers at Mayo Clinic–Jacksonville. Subsequently, a half dozen similar families have been recognized, some with one and others with two extra normal alpha-synuclein genes. All have been levodopa-responsive, and when postmortem examinations have been done, Lewy bodies were documented.

Of special relevance, those with *two* extra alpha-synuclein genes experienced earlier PD onset and a more aggressive course than those with only one extra gene. These extra genes translated into substantially more alpha-synuclein production, with the two-gene variant generating more than those with one extra gene. Extra genes have not been found in usual people with PD. These studies demonstrate, however, that too much alpha-synuclein is sufficient to cause PD.

Alpha-Synuclein at the Molecular Level

Alpha-synuclein is widely found in the brain. It is present in the terminals of all neurons. While the normal role for this brain molecule is debated, it does appear to play a role in synaptic transmission. Normal alpha-synuclein is soluble (i.e., it dissolves in brain fluids) and is quite mobile at the cellular level. However, the mutated alpha-synuclein from the Contursi families is prone to aggregate and become insoluble. Although the alpha-synuclein of those with PD is not mutated, it also is in the aggregated form in the Lewy bodies of affected neurons. Thus, aggregation or clumping of alpha-synuclein appears to be fundamental to the Lewy neurodegenerative process.

Microscopic alpha-synuclein aggregates include not only Lewy bodies but also much smaller accumulations, termed *Lewy neurites* and *Lewy dots*, as mentioned in Chapter 3. These Lewy products represent the aggregated, insoluble accumulations of alpha-synuclein as well as other substances. Normal brain cells are able to dispose of unwanted protein products through natural mechanisms; however, it appears that excessive concentrations of insoluble, aggregated alpha-synuclein may overwhelm the neuronal disposal mechanisms. Once alpha-synuclein accumulates, it may disrupt cell function, perhaps leading to neuronal death.

Where Will the Alpha-Synuclein Story Take Us?

We now have an important clue to the cause of PD. Alpha-synuclein deposition parallels the Lewy neurodegenerative process and may be an integral component of the causative mechanism. However, the story is unlikely to be simple. We have no confirmation that alpha-synuclein is unequivocally causative in typical PD. Even if causative, is it the sole factor or one among many? Does it only initiate the neurodegenerative process or does it continue to drive the progression? As an extension of that question, will lowering brain alpha-synuclein slow the progression of PD? Complicating such therapeutic challenges is the fact that the brain has countless biological compensatory mechanisms that tend to offset external and internal perturbations. Moreover, the body's complex metabolic processes are difficult for researchers to *selectively* target, often resulting in unintended adverse therapeutic consequences. Despite these caveats, we are hopefully moving toward treating the cause of PD.

OTHER GENES CAUSING LEVODOPA-RESPONSIVE PARKINSONISM: *parkin*, *PINK1*, AND *DJ-1*

In the first edition of this book, this chapter (i.e., Chapter 8) included discussion of three gene mutations that were then thought to provide clues to typical PD: *parkin*, *PINK1*, and *DJ-1*. Our collective thinking has changed since then. While these three (recessive) gene disorders do result in levodopa-responsive parkinsonism, they are substantially different from usual PD; the syndromes caused by these genes are uniquely characterized by the following:

- Parkinsonism onset is nearly always before age 40 years.

- There is no microscopic Lewy body pathology (with occasional exceptions).

- They have a different long-term course from that of usual PD

The disease course differs in that people with these mutations tend to have a nearly fully preserved levodopa response for decades, but complicated by early levodopa fluctuations and dyskinesias. They usually do *not* develop dementia or autonomic problems. This young-onset disorder is largely restricted to degeneration of the dopaminergic nigrostriatal system without progression to other brain regions. In sum, the condition caused by mutations in one of these three genes appears to be fundamentally different from PD.

The functions of *parkin*, *PINK1*, and *DJ-1* appear to be important for maintaining the integrity and function of mitochondria. In fact, mitochondrial dysfunction has been proposed as the primary substrate for the development of parkinsonism associated with these gene mutations. Could this have any relevance to typical PD?

Mitochondrial abnormalities have been consistently documented in common PD. Mitochondrial dysfunction does not appear to represent the sole or primary cause of common PD; however, it may be a contributing factor. At this juncture, mitochondria deserve further comment, starting with discussion of their normal role in cellular function.

MITOCHONDRIAL ABNORMALITIES

Mitochondria are small structures contained within all human cells. They are critical to the life of the cell and, in essence, are each cell's power source; they are what makes all humans and animals aerobic organisms. Their primary role is to generate the high-energy molecule ATP (adenosine triphosphate), used to fuel many crucial cellular reactions. Mitochondria complete the metabolism of products of our digestion in this process (carbohydrates, fats, protein). Like fire in a furnace, oxygen is critically necessary for mitochondrial function. Several mitochondrial complexes (I through IV) are linked in a biochemical series to generate ATP from ingested metabolic products and oxygen.

Mitochondrial complex I is dysfunctional in people with typical PD, not only in the brain but also within muscles and blood cells. While this fact has been known for over 25 years, it has not translated into any further insights into the cause of PD. Although mitochondrial dysfunction appears to play a primary role in the more limited parkinsonian disorders of *parkin, PINK1,* and *DJ-1,* the role in typical PD is unknown. It may be a susceptibility factor, or even just a noncausative association, rather than the primary cause. The problems of mitochondria, in general, have proven very difficult to study.

In the first edition of this book, a small clinical trial was cited that found high-dose coenzyme Q10 administration to be efficacious in PD. Coenzyme Q10 is a cofactor that facilitates mitochondrial complex I activity; hence it was proposed as treatment for typical PD. Two subsequent large, federally funded studies have now failed to replicate those initial favorable results, including with the same high doses and also twice those amounts. It now appears that coenzyme Q10 has no proven role in PD treatment.

LRRK2 MUTATIONS CAUSING PARKINSON'S DISEASE IN SPECIFIC POPULATIONS

An enzyme with multiple functions, leucine-rich repeat kinase 2 (LRRK2), was identified as the cause of dominantly inherited PD in certain families from North Africa and the Middle East. This *LRRK2* mutation was reported to be responsible for approximately 40% of PD cases in North African Arab populations, 10–20% in Ashkenazi Jewish patients, and 3–8% in Spanish and Portuguese patients. Outside of those localities and ethnic groups the frequency is much lower—about 1–2% of all people with PD. It is the most frequent genetic cause of PD overall but obviously rare, except in these populations.

The *LRRK2* gene has been intensively studied, with the expectation that understanding its function would provide clues to the cause of PD. This is still a work in progress because of the diverse biological roles of LRRK2 in neurons. It appears to be relevant to more than just PD, since *LRRK2* mutations have also been associated with different neurodegenerative syndromes (i.e., not PD), with microscopic patterns other than Lewy bodies. It also appears that not all those who carry this gene mutation will develop PD or any neurodegenerative disorder.

THE GAUCHER'S GENE: AN UNEXPECTED LINK WITH PARKINSON'S DISEASE

Gaucher's disease is a recessive disorder causing blood, liver, and bone abnormalities, typically early in life. The abnormal (deficient) glucocerebrosidase protein is an enzyme located in lysosomes, which are small compartments within cells that degrade waste products. Since Gaucher's disease is genetically recessive, each of the two genes coding for the affected glucocerebrosidase protein must be abnormal. Individuals carrying only one abnormal glucocerebrosidase gene do not develop Gaucher's disease.

Carriers of only one glucocerebrosidase mutation do not have any manifestations of Gaucher's syndrome. However, having one such glucocerebrosidase gene mutation increases the risk of PD by at least five-fold. This is interpreted as a risk factor for PD rather than a true Mendelian genetic cause, since this same single gene mutation is also found in normal people without PD, albeit much less frequently. This is the most common genetic risk factor for PD.

Glucocerebrosidase mutations are not uniformly distributed across all ethnic groups. About 6–8% of Ashkenazi Jewish people carry one such abnormal gene, whereas in most other populations the carrier frequency is around 1%. Unlike *LRRK2*, this genetic mutation is uncommon in North Africa, which suggests that these two genes have different evolutionary histories.

As mentioned, glucocerebrosidase is found in lysosomes. The normal function of lysosomes is to break down certain unwanted or excessive cellular products, and this includes alpha-synuclein. Reduced lysosomal degradation of alpha-synuclein products might play a role in the formation of Lewy aggregates in neurons. These findings are generating a new research focus, possibly targeting alpha-synuclein degradation.

GENOME-WIDE ASSOCIATION STUDIES SUGGEST SMALL CONTRIBUTIONS TO PARKINSON'S DISEASE FROM MANY GENES

Genome-wide association studies (GWAS) are now commonly used to study the genetic contributions to many diseases. GWAS involves typing all the genes on all chromosomes and comparing two large groups of people: (a) patients with a given disease (e.g., PD) and (b) normal control subjects. Precise genotyping of all DNA genetic sequences on such a large scale is not currently feasible; rather, GWAS entails assessing genetic markers across the entirety of cellular DNA. The intent is to determine if any specific gene (gene marker) is significantly more frequent in the disease group than in the control group. Conducting meaningful individual comparisons of hundreds of thousands (or millions) of genetic markers between those with the disease (e.g., PD) and control subjects is an enormous statistical undertaking. Complex statistical methodology is necessary to generate meaningful results; this is because the more comparisons, the greater the likelihood that any given gene will be more frequent in one group by chance. Genes assumed relevant to the disease process are those shown to be significantly more frequent after statistically correcting for the many comparisons.

A number of GWAS analyses of patients with PD compared to control subjects have been performed, and each new study seems to implicate a few new genes. This is a work in progress, and there may be many more genetic contributions to PD remaining to be discovered. At present, nearly

30 genetic susceptibility regions have been identified in GWAS assessments of PD; variants in the genetic code of these loci increase the risk of developing PD. The identified genes include alpha-synuclein and *LRRK2*. Further complicating these analyses is the observation that GWAS in differing ethnic groups do not necessarily identify precisely the same genes.

OVERVIEW OF GENETIC CONTRIBUTIONS TO PARKINSON'S DISEASE

Single-gene mutations (or gene duplications) are the cause of no more than 2% of all PD, except in certain ethnic groups. GWAS suggest that there is a major genetic component to PD, but it is mediated via small contributions by many genes. To put this into perspective, recall that any given genetic factor that doubles or even triples the PD risk still generates a small number. With a general lifetime PD risk of 2% for males, doubling that yields only a 4% risk. Conceivably, many, many genes may be at play.

The genetic contribution to PD may be even more complex than simply many small contributions from numerous causative genes. First, there likely are "good" genes that work to offset the risk. Second, the location of these PD-risk genes within specific biological pathways may be very relevant. Thus, two PD-risk genes in the same biological pathway may lead to pathway failure, whereas PD-risk genes in different biological pathways may be compensated for, and tolerated. Note that the numerous risk genes in GWAS appear to be in several different biological systems, suggesting complex disease interactions between different biochemical pathways. Finally, there may be culpable genes interacting with environmental exposures, further complicating this issue.

ARE GENETIC STUDIES LEADING US TO ANSWERS?

We do not know the full aggregate genetic contribution to PD. Does it account for most of the cause of PD, or does it play a minor role? With each genetic discovery it seems that the picture becomes more complex and sometimes more confusing. Is research money better spent elsewhere?

Taking a broader view, each discovered gene is one piece to a very complex jigsaw puzzle. These identified genes code for specific biological proteins, each implicating a biological mechanism and telling us something about the disease process. The discovery of the alpha-synuclein mutation in the Contursi families revealed a disease-related protein that had never been considered previously. Discovery of the glucocerebrosidase (Gaucher) genetic PD-risk factor was unexpected and implicated another mechanism: protein degradation by lysosomes. Each of the genes surfacing in GWAS is telling us something about Lewy body disorders. Each newly recognized gene provides scientists with a potentially causative biological clue to study and understand. You do not need every piece in a jigsaw puzzle to recognize the picture. You just need enough pieces in place to perceive the pattern.

Environmental Contributions to Parkinson's Disease

PD is more likely to develop with each passing decade of life. It is rare before age 40 years, leading to speculation that perhaps cumulative environmental exposures may be causative. The interest in environmental factors accelerated some years ago when studies of twins failed to document significant differences in PD concordance when identical twins were compared to nonidentical twins. Specifically, if PD is genetic, one identical twin with PD should also have a twin-mate with PD, in contrast to nonidentical twins, who share only half their genes. However, the frequency of PD twin pairs was similar among identical and nonidentical twins.

IS PARKINSON'S DISEASE MORE LIKELY IN CERTAIN TOWNS OR LOCALITIES?

Epidemiologists are the researchers who study disease patterns to identify causes and risk factors. One important starting point for epidemiologists is the recognition of "clusters" of affected individuals in a workplace or living close together sharing common exposures. However, despite an intensive search for such clusters of PD, none have surfaced, apart from rare families with genetic causes.

PRACTICES AND HABITS ASSOCIATED WITH PARKINSON'S DISEASE

Hundreds of studies have examined lifestyles and exposures among people with PD compared to those without PD of the same age and gender. Certain associations have been documented, but the aggregate risk-ratios have been modest, never more than two- to three-fold (recall that 3 times a small number is still a small number; e.g., the lifetime PD risk for men is 2%; 3 times 2 = 6%). Note an important caveat when interpreting these studies: an association does not necessarily imply cause and effect. The common associations that have been consistently found may be summarized as follows.

Factors That Increase PD Risk

- Pesticide exposure has been associated with PD risk on the order of two- to three-fold. This may also account for associations of

PD with rural living as well as farming, although with even smaller risks. No particular pesticide has been identified as the primary culprit. The herbicide Agent Orange, widely used for defoliation during the Vietnam War, has been accepted as a contributor to PD by the Veteran's Administration; however, this has not yet been documented in controlled epidemiological studies.

- Prior brain trauma requiring medical evaluation has been associated with the later development of PD in most but not all studies. It is unclear if simple concussions, such as those experienced in sports, predispose to PD; if they do, it is unlikely to be a major risk factor.

- Adiposity (overweight) was associated with an increased risk of PD in two large surveys, although with a relatively small risk. Note that once PD has occurred, it is common for patients to complain of unexplained weight loss.

Men are more likely to develop PD, raising concerns about workplace risks. However, PD clusters have not been identified in factories or specific workplaces and occupational exposures do not appear to confer prominent risks. As mentioned, farming appears to be associated with a modestly increased PD risk. Welding has also been reported as linked to PD, but not in well-controlled studies. Although long-term welding with poor ventilation can cause parkinsonism with MRI brain changes, this is not PD; rather, this reflects brain manganese accumulation (see Chapter 6). Limited studies have suggested that major exposure to organic solvents may be linked to PD in rare cases (e.g., trichloroethylene, carbon tetrachloride).

Commonly, people worry about exposures in the environment that might be disease-causing. In the case of PD, hundreds of epidemiological studies have closely explored this issue and, gratifyingly, major risks have not surfaced.

Factors That Reduce PD Risk

- Smoking earlier in life has been found to reduce later risks of PD by about half in nearly all epidemiological studies where this has been assessed (which now number over 50). This has been consistently found even when controlling for the fact that smokers tend to die before nonsmokers. At first glance, this finding suggests that there may be something in cigarette smoke that protects against PD. However, one study found that current smokers with PD were more likely to have cognitive impairment, whereas another reported that smoking failed to slow PD progression. Perhaps the same inherent brain chemistry that confers a lower risk of PD also makes smoking pleasurable. In other words, those destined to develop PD may have early-life aversion to smoking or experience less enjoyment from smoking. Consistent with that proposition is a recent retrospective study documenting that people who would later develop PD had more easily stopped smoking in mid-life compared to those not destined to develop PD. Smoking, in general, is bad for the human body, and no physician advocates smoking as a treatment for PD.

- Coffee drinking is also associated with a lower likelihood of PD in most but not all studies. Similar to smoking, this could be explained by common brain chemistry that both confers a lower PD risk and makes coffee consumption pleasurable. Like nicotine, caffeine has direct effects in the basal ganglia. Note that dopamine is a prominent neurotransmitter in brain reward systems and that the dopamine deficiency of PD might start years before the first signs of PD. There is no evidence that coffee slows the progression of PD once it starts, although this has not been adequately studied.

- Midlife exercise has been reported as reducing the later risk of PD in several investigations, including an aggregate analysis of these studies. There is also compelling indirect evidence from a variety of sources to support the benefit of vigorous exercise once PD begins. The possibility that aerobic exercise may slow PD progression will be addressed in more detail in Chapters 9 and 31.

MORE ABOUT TWIN STUDIES

The twin studies documenting infrequent concurrence of PD in identical twins suggested that genetics was a minor factor in PD. Thus the research focus shifted to external influences. However, the failure to find highly prevalent environmental causes ostensibly leaves us at a dead end. If neither genetic nor environmental factors play a prominent role in the development of PD, what is left? It is time to rethink these issues, and perhaps the PD twin studies need to be revisited.

We now know that mild and limited Lewy body disease may be present without the clinical symptoms or signs of PD; this condition is sometimes termed *incidental Lewy body disease*. It is found in around 15% of neurologically normal people over age 60, which is many times more common than recognized PD. In the Braak scheme, this represents the earliest stage of PD. Extending this finding to twin studies, when only one identical twin has PD, might the other have this early-stage Lewy body condition, incidental Lewy body disease? Obviously, the earlier twin studies could not take this into account.

Interactions of Genes and Environment

Genes and environmental exposures are not necessarily mutually exclusive. There is now increasing recognition of a potential role of genetic factors that protect against or enhance the influence of environmental factors. For example, some people may have better inherent defenses against toxins or viruses. PD researchers are increasingly focusing on such interactions.

Complicating the genes-versus-environment discussion is the fact that family members typically live in the same household for portions of their lives. Hence, when PD occurs in more than one family member, a genetic basis is not necessarily the cause; these individuals have also shared common environmental exposures.

Reason for Optimism

This chapter paints quite a complex picture of conceivable mechanisms by which PD may occur. Understanding these causative mechanisms is crucial to finding a cure for PD, or at least a means of halting progression. Science often progresses in sudden leaps, triggered by a novel discovery that allows previously incoherent findings to make sense. There is no shortcut to this process, and smart people also need providence to make those discoveries. They are coming, but who can predict when and what they will be?

9

◆ ◆ ◆

Are There Drugs or Strategies to Slow Parkinson's Disease Progression?

We have effective medications for treating the symptoms of Parkinson's disease (PD), and this will be the focus of subsequent chapters. Nonetheless, PD slowly progresses over many years and *non*-dopamine neurons become increasing affected. This renders levodopa and related drugs less helpful overall. Parkinsonism symptoms that do not have a dopamine substrate tend to be poorly controlled, such as imbalance. Cognition and autonomic symptoms are not dopamine-based and become more problematic. This progression reflects the spread of Lewy neurodegenerative processes outside of the dopamine domain. We need drugs to at least slow, if not halt, this progression.

The process by which the PD neurodegeneration might theoretically be slowed is often characterized by the terms *neuroprotection* or *disease-modifying*. To develop drugs for this purpose, we need reliable means of measuring true PD progression in clinical trials. This sounds simple, until you consider our experience to date.

Measurement of PD Progression in Clinical Trials

Clinical trials for assessing drug influences on PD progression have proven to be expensive and complicated, with results often difficult to interpret. Typically, enrolled PD patients are randomly assigned to receive the study drug or a similar-appearing placebo ("sugar pill"). Whether a patient has been assigned the study drug or placebo is not disclosed to either the patient or the clinician until after the study has ended; this is termed a *double-blind study* (patients and clinicians are both "blinded").

Clinical trials assessing PD neuroprotection are challenged by multiple factors:

- PD progression is very slow, over many years, requiring long-term trials.

- With long-term trials subjects gradually drop out, for a variety of reasons. Major biases can be introduced when the dropout rate is substantial (e.g., disproportionate dropouts in one group may leave only those with the mildest condition in that group).

- The rate of progression varies widely among people with PD, requiring large numbers of enrolled subjects to average out this variability; complex statistical analyses are required to analyze the outcomes.

- PD progression takes many different forms, for example, predominantly affecting balance in some people and cognition in others, or causing autonomic problems.

- Levodopa and related mediations effectively treat PD symptoms and signs, confounding many outcome measures. One could forbid patients from taking these mediations, but that would be unrealistic in long-term studies, if not unethical. Researchers have attempted to work around this problem by having patients hold levodopa for 12–24 hours before examination; however, this drug has a "long-duration" effect spanning approximately a week, as we will discuss in subsequent chapters.

These problems also challenge those trying to interpret published reports of such clinical trials. Summaries in the lay press overlook many of these key issues.

An obvious solution to this problem would be the discovery of a "surrogate marker" of PD progression, such as brain imaging or a blood test. To date, we have no biological markers that reliably reflect PD progression. Brain dopamine transporter imaging (discussed in Chapters 4 and 7) was used to assess progression in several earlier trials. This brain imaging technique documents striatal dopamine terminals, which decline over years of PD. Unfortunately, these imaging outcomes were confounded by the effect of levodopa and dopamine agonist drug treatment.

Drug Trials to Slow PD Progression

We have no medications that we can direct at the cause of PD, since we do not know the cause. This has not stopped clinical researchers from proposing and testing a variety of drugs hoped to have neuroprotective properties, based on educated guesses. In the last quarter century, 11 large, randomized, controlled clinical trials have assessed 11 different drugs on PD progression (Table 9.1). The names of the trials are mostly acronyms and are listed in Table 9.1, in case you encounter these in other reading. None of these trials have documented convincing evidence of slowed PD progression.

Table 9.1. Large* Randomized, Controlled** Clinical Trials of Drugs Directed at PD Progression

Clinical Trial Name	Drugs Assessed
1. DATATOP	Selegiline (MAO-B inhibitor); vitamin E
2. CALM-PD	Pramipexole (dopamine agonist)
3. REAL-PET	Ropinirole (dopamine agonist)
4. PRECEPT	CEP-1347 (inhibits programmed cell death: apoptosis)
5. TCH346	TCH346 (inhibits programmed cell death: apoptosis)
6. ADAGIO	Rasagiline (MAO-B inhibitor)
7. QE3	Coenzyme Q10 (mitochondrial cofactor)
8. MitoQ	Coenzyme Q10 analogue (lipid-soluble to increase brain concentrations)
9. FS-1	Creatine; minocycline (antibiotic)
10. FS-TOO	Coenzyme Q10; GPI-1485 (immunophilin, thought to have neurotrophic properties)
11. LS-1	Creatine

* All these trials had more than 100 patients.

** "Controlled" implies use of a placebo group; patients were randomly assigned to either the medication group or a placebo group.

The most recent such trial assessed the body-building supplement creatine, which had generated promising results in a preliminary study. Unfortunately, the subsequent large 5-year creatine trial in PD was terminated in late 2013 due to futile outcomes.

It appears that the next drug to be assessed as a neuroprotective agent in a large clinical trial is *isradipine*. This antihypertensive medication is from the calcium channel blocker class. Theoretically, specific calcium channel–blocking drugs may reduce biological stress on dopaminergic neurons. Isradipine and related drugs have neuroprotective properties in animals whose nigrostriatal neurons have been poisoned with toxins; however, numerous other drugs with efficacy in such PD animal models later failed in PD clinical trials. Several retrospective studies have assessed the later risk of developing PD among people who had been taking calcium channel–blocking drugs; most, but not all, showed reduced PD risk. One other study retrospectively assessed disease progression among PD patients taking brain-penetrant calcium channel–blocking drugs but failed to prove benefit.

The drugs listed in Table 9.1 have been abandoned as neuroprotective agents. However, some clinicians would take exception to that statement, holding out hope for rasagiline, which deserves further comment.

RASAGILINE (AZILECT)

In the first edition of this book (published a decade ago), selegiline was discussed as a drug proposed for neuroprotection. The selegiline story deserves retelling to put the rasagiline story into a more complete context.

The large DATATOP trial (Table 9.1), conducted over 20 years ago, produced initial results suggesting that selegiline delayed progression of the symptoms and signs of PD. These initial results were so compelling that nearly all physicians at that time routinely prescribed selegiline for their PD patients.

In that DATATOP study, early PD patients treated with selegiline were able to delay starting levodopa by many months, which suggested that progression had been slowed. Parkinsonism scores were still better many weeks after selegiline was stopped. Selegiline was assumed to have no effect on PD symptoms, so it was concluded that this drug was "disease-modifying." It was subsequently recognized that selegiline does indeed improve PD symptoms, albeit mildly. Moreover, the effect in the brain is extremely long-lasting, exceeding the duration of selegiline withdrawal in the DATATOP trial. Thus, the symptomatic effect of selegiline appeared to account for the findings in that study. Soon neurologists reversed their conclusions about the benefits of this drug and generally stopped prescribing it, except for the mild symptomatic benefit.

Rasagiline has now supplanted selegiline as a proposed neuroprotective agent. These two drugs are very similar. Both block one of the enzymes that break down brain dopamine, monoamine oxidase type B (MAO-B). The primary difference between these two drugs is that selegiline generates weak forms of amphetamine, unlike rasagiline.

MAO is an enzyme that is present in the brain and elsewhere in the body. By degrading dopamine and related substances, MAO normally prevents the dopamine levels from becoming excessive. MAO is present in two forms, MAO-A and MAO-B. In the prescribed doses, selegiline and rasagiline each selectively block only the B-form, resulting in a mild elevation of brain dopamine. As with selegiline, rasagiline inhibits MAO-B irreversibly and requires new brain synthesis of MAO-B to restore function; this effect has a half-life of about 40 days. Parenthetically, other drugs are available that block both MAO-A and -B but potentially have very serious side effects and require special diets; they are not used to treat PD.

The large ADAGIO trial (Table 9.1), conducted several years ago, assessed rasagiline as a possible disease-modifying agent. The study design differed from the DATATOP trial, which had been seriously confounded. In the ADAGIO trial, comparative parkinsonism scores were assessed after 18 months. Some patients received rasagiline for all 18 months; others had rasagiline delayed by 9 months or stopped after 9 months. This was a very complex study and required sophisticated statistical analyses of the different groups. Paradoxically, the analyses suggested that the lower-dose rasagiline group (1 mg) could have had a disease-modifying effect, but not the 2 mg group. Intuitively, this makes little sense since, pharmacologically, they both should have had a similar effect on MAO-B and both had similar benefits in clinical trials of symptomatic treatment. Moreover, critics voiced numerous concerns about the complexities of the study, which could easily have resulted in spurious outcomes. Ultimately, the U.S. Food and Drug Administration (FDA) reviewed the data and concluded that there was insufficient evidence of a disease-modifying benefit with rasagiline.

Should you take rasagiline (Azilect) as a neuroprotective agent? My view is that the data in support of a neuroprotective effect are not compelling, and the clinical trial results are more readily explained by the symptomatic effect. Rasagiline is expensive. Furthermore, the FDA has issued warnings about possible drug interactions with a variety of commonly prescribed medications, including most antidepressants, narcotics, and certain other prescription pain relievers. If the symptomatic benefit is desired, selegiline should be just as effective and is less expensive.

A FORGOTTEN STORY: LEVODOPA AND LONGEVITY

Levodopa was the first major breakthrough in the treatment of PD. Before the introduction of levodopa in 1969, PD patients had substantially shortened lives. We had no effective symptomatic drugs, and those available (e.g., anticholinergic agents) had many troublesome side effects that often overshadowed the benefits. This situation changed dramatically with levodopa and especially after carbidopa was added a few years later; carbidopa made levodopa tolerable (nausea and often vomiting were common side effects before carbidopa was introduced).

Longevity increased substantially with the advent of levodopa use. This was confirmed in seven independent, published studies that compared life spans just before and after the introduction of levodopa (carbidopa/levodopa). Why should levodopa therapy prolong life? There is no reason to think that levodopa targeted mechanisms causing PD. Almost certainly, improved longevity with the introduction of levodopa was due to improved mobility and function. Prior to levodopa, those with PD were increasingly relegated to very sedentary lifestyles. Without an effective symptomatic treatment, they often became house-bound with very limited activities. Levodopa liberated a generation of people with PD. With treatment, they were often able to resume more normal lives, participate in activities, and re-engage in exercise.

Perhaps there is a lesson to be learned from the levodopa longevity data: staying active tends to facilitate longer lives. Our bodies need to be exercised. Becoming a couch potato is easy in our current culture but likely is not good for humans in the long run.

Aerobic Exercise May Be Neuroprotective

None of the myriad of drugs tested as PD-neuroprotective agents have generated proof of a disease-slowing effect (Table 9.1). That is too bad; we all like quick fixes—just take a pill and continue with the usual routine. Life should always be this easy! Although there is no such pill, there is more here to contemplate.

From the levodopa longevity discussion just summarized, one might surmise that physical activity may tend to prolong the life of those with PD. Before the advent of levodopa, those with PD tended to be sedentary and had shortened lives. Levodopa use often restored the ability to walk and become active; correspondingly, longevity substantially increased. Perhaps we are on to something here. Will physical activity, especially vigorous activity (i.e., exercise), tend to prolong our lives? Might regular vigorous exercise slow the progression of PD? No randomized clinical trial has assessed this question; however, there is voluminous scientific evidence that strongly argues for aerobic exercise as a neuroprotective strategy. We will conclude this chapter with that discussion.

What Is Aerobic Exercise?

Aerobic exercise is vigorous exercise that ultimately tends to lead to physical fitness. It is exercise that tends to make people hot, sweaty, and tired. Physiologists assess this by having subjects run on a treadmill or ride an exercise bicycle. The efficiency of the subject's use of oxygen during peak exercise is the physiological measure; hence the term *aerobic* exercise to characterize this.

Aerobic exercise occurs in many activities and not just formal gym routines. Briskly walking, shoveling snow, and raking leaves all translate into aerobic exercise. Note, however, that not all exercise qualifies as aerobic. Stretching or balance routines may be beneficial, but these are not forms of aerobic exercise. Washing dishes and fixing dinner are important activities but are not aerobic exercise. Swimming laps at a steady pace is a form of aerobic exercise even though you may not generate visible perspiration; stretching in the pool is not aerobic exercise. Aerobic exercise can be done sitting and not just on an exercise bicycle; gyms usually have a variety of machines at which repetitive lifting, pushing, or pulling can be done while sitting. Thus bad hips or knees should not disqualify one from doing aerobic exercise. Weight-lifting using lower weights with more repetitions and less rest tends to build fitness and represents aerobic exercise. Now that we have defined aerobic exercise, what is the evidence for its neuroprotective benefit?

Is There a Neuroprotective Effect from Aerobic Exercise?

The following discussion summarizes findings from over 100 published scientific studies relating to direct beneficial effects of exercise on the brain, with implications for those with PD. There are no randomized clinical exercise trials assessing long-term progression in PD patients; these would be extremely challenging to reliably conduct. However, compelling evidence has converged from a variety of sources, which we will summarize, one by one. (For those interested in exploring this issue further, see the article Ahlskog JE. Does vigorous exercise have a neuroprotective effect in Parkinson's disease? *Neurology* 2011; 77:288–294.)

DOES EXERCISE EARLIER IN LIFE LOWER THE RISK OF LATER DEVELOPING PARKINSON'S DISEASE?

In five independent studies, people who engaged in regular exercise in mid-life were consistently found to have a reduced risk of later developing

PD. Note that some of those who exercised did later develop PD, but at a significantly lower frequency.

If the PD risk is reduced by exercise, is this an effect on the causative process? A cautious view recognizes that this finding could also result from reduced inclination to exercise as an early manifestation of PD. Restated, people destined to develop PD may have subtle manifestations years before, and this might include a reduced interest in exercising.

WILL EXERCISE REDUCE THE RISK OF DEVELOPING DEMENTIA AFTER PD ONSET?

Dementia is perhaps the most feared aspect of PD. It does not develop in all individuals with PD and when it does, it often is after many years and much later in life. Unfortunately, no studies have addressed exercise in early PD and later dementia risk. Thus we must rely on the evidence for exercise and fitness influencing cognition in the general population. There is a sizable volume of data that sheds light on that subject.

EXERCISE AND COGNITION IN THE GENERAL POPULATION

Several very large studies have investigated cardiovascular fitness (the product of aerobic exercise) and later cognitive measures. Among young Swedish military inductees there was a significant correlation between fitness and cognitive scores at the time of induction; fitness scores also correlated with later educational outcomes. In a study of young adults from the United States, treadmill fitness scores correlated with several cognitive outcomes 25 years later. Among seniors, a half-dozen studies have documented physical fitness as being associated with better scores on cognitive testing.

Functional MRI (fMRI) brain scans have revealed more robust brain connections among people who are fit compared to unfit individuals. Moreover, two studies showed improved cortical activation and connectivity after 6–12 months of an exercise program.

EXERCISE AND FITNESS REDUCE LATER RISKS OF DEMENTIA IN THE GENERAL POPULATION

Recent aggregate analyses of all published studies relating midlife exercise and later dementia indicated a significantly reduced dementia risk. More than 10 studies involving thousands of subjects documented that midlife exercise reduced the likelihood of later becoming demented.

Less severe cognitive dysfunction has been categorized as *mild cognitive impairment*, implying that the memory and thinking problems do not prevent routine activities. Risk of mild cognitive impairment was also reduced

ANIMAL STUDIES SUGGEST EXERCISE FACILITATES NEUROPLASTICITY VIA VARIED MECHANISMS

Rats or mice that are exercised manifest an array of brain changes suggestive of enhanced neuroplasticity. *Neuroplasticity* implies the generation of new neural connections within the brain. Memories require such neuroplastic brain processes, as does learning how to operate a computer or play a board game. Scientists have studied this extensively and identified factors and mechanisms that play a role in neuroplasticity. Certainly, these are crucial for intellectual activities and attenuating brain aging. They presumably should play a role in countering neurodegenerative processes. Thus investigations in rats or mice have documented increased brain expression or enhancement of the following:

1. *Brain growth factors* (these facilitate neuroplasticity; similar to fertilizer on your lawn)
   - Brain-derived neurotrophic factor (BDNF): 16 studies
   - Glial cell line–derived neurotrophic factor (GDNF): 3 studies
   - Insulin-like growth factor-I: 1 study

2. *Hippocampal neurogenesis* (the hippocampus is one of the few brain regions where new neurons are produced, i.e., neurogenesis): 9 studies

3. *The electrophysiological correlate of learning, long-term potentiation*: 3 studies

4. *Synaptic proteins or synaptic plasticity genes* (synapses represent the connections between one neuron and another to form brain circuits): 4 studies

5. *Factors and enzymes that promote neuroplasticity*: 5 studies

6. *Dendrite development* (dendrites are on the receiving end of synapses; enhanced synaptic connections are typically associated with increased dendrite length and complexity): 3 studies

This plethora of investigations documenting enhanced neuroplasticity in exercised animals is difficult to ignore. These studies complement those in humans and suggest that the correlation of human fitness (aerobic exercise) with enhanced cognition has plausible substrates.

Levodopa to Facilitate Exercise for Slowing PD Progression

The evidence suggesting that aerobic exercise may counter brain aging and slow PD progression is indirect but converges from a variety of sources. This provides a compelling rationale for not arbitrarily withholding levodopa when parkinsonism threatens to scale back activity. A goal for treating clinicians should be to keep those with PD active and exercising. This should be one of the primary criteria when considering when to start medical treatment (i.e., carbidopa/levodopa). It is difficult to stay active and maintain an exercise routine in the face of the slowness, stiffness, and sometimes pain, which reflect dopamine deficits.

How Much Exercise?

Studies have not adequately addressed the optimum amount of exercise to fully capitalize on this strategy. This will vary among people, and other medical conditions may influence it as well. The American Heart Association advice seems a reasonable prescription for exercise; they suggest "moderate-intensity aerobic physical activity for a minimum of 30 minutes on five days each week or vigorous-intensity aerobic activity for a minimum of 20 minutes on three days each week." They also add that resistance exercises should be considered "for a minimum of two days each week." Resistance exercise improves strength and involves pushing or pulling against a weight (resistance). This is typically done with free weights or machines with adjustable resistances.

CAVEAT: CARDIAC DISEASE

Heart conditions may need to be addressed with your doctor before starting an exercise routine. In general, cardiologists encourage exercise, provided that active heart disease has been treated and stabilized. If exercise provokes upper body pain, especially chest or arm pain, this suggests the possibility of coronary artery disease. In other words, the increased demands on the heart during exercise exceed the capacity of the coronary arteries to supply blood to heart muscle. This must be addressed first and foremost. Also, if congestive heart failure is present, the cardiologist will likely suggest modifications to an exercise program to fit the individual capabilities.

Exercise Has Other Health Benefits

We have focused on exercise influences on the brain; however, that represents only a fraction of the health benefits. Consider the other well-documented effects of aerobic exercise on disorders that accelerate aging, morbidity, and mortality:

1. Cardio- and cerebrovascular health, with benefits directed at various potential conditions:

   • Diabetes mellitus

- Hypertension
- Hyperlipidemia (e.g., cholesterol elevation)
- Obesity

2. Osteoporosis

3. Sarcopenia (muscle shrinkage with aging)

4. Depression

Especially worth noting are two recent large retrospective studies documenting significantly increased longevity among people who exercised.

But I Have Good Excuses

As a full-time clinician, I have heard all the excuses. The most honest and probably most frequent reason for not exercising is "I hate to exercise." Here is a confession: I also do not like to exercise. That was not true when I was young; I love sports, and pick-up basketball and playing catch with my son were excellent outlets. As I grew older, there were fewer and fewer fun options. Also, normal aging saps energy and makes our bodies achy. I have firsthand experience with each of these excuses but nonetheless engage in regular exercise. This is important for health and longevity.

You can adapt to a lot of limitations and still engage in a regular exercise routine. Bad knees or ankles as well as imbalance do not preclude exercising while sitting or exercising the upper body; consider the following:

- Stationary bicycles and rowing machines are widely available and are used in the sitting position.
- Gyms have a variety of machines that involve exercise done while sitting, including various exercises for the upper body. Use these or free weights with the resistance adjusted so that you can do 15–20 repetitions without having to stop to rest. Circuit training involves doing such exercises one after the other without rest or with minimal rest. You can gradually adjust the machine's resistance (or the size of the weights) as you become more fit. You can rest less and complete the routine more and more quickly as you become fit.
- Sit-ups should be tolerated despite many painful joints, as long as your back is not one of them. Push-ups or modified push-ups do not place much stress on lower limb joints.
- Swimming laps provides an excellent workout and is not hard on joints.

Another excuse is also among the most frequently voiced: "I don't have enough time." Bad excuse! This is your life; make time for yourself.

Saving Levodopa for Later?

"My parkinsonism prevents me from exercising. I want to save the best levodopa responses for later."

The Internet and other sources often advise those with PD to "save levodopa until you really need it." While it is true that levodopa works best during the first years of PD, can this response really be saved for later? To address this issue, we need to put it in context.

PD is a progressive disorder that marches along, regardless of whether it is treated or not. With early signs of PD, the dopamine nigrostriatal system has only partially been lost; the residual dopaminergic neurons are able to compensate with the aid of administered levodopa. Over several years, the progressive loss of these dopaminergic neurons increasingly limits their ability to maintain a stable motor response. Shortened levodopa responses lead to motor fluctuations; dyskinesias may develop, reflecting an excessive levodopa effect. This instability presumably parallels the loss of dopamine neurons. These unstable responses can be treated; however, medication adjustments only partially control the symptoms when the instability is prominent. This is especially problematic in younger PD patients.

The admonition to save levodopa assumes that you can always get the "best" responses years later if you defer carbidopa/levodopa treatment. The concept of saving levodopa for later ignores the occurrence of progressive events within the brain as PD progresses. The numbers of dopaminergic neurons continue to diminish, and the Lewy neurodegenerative process spreads to nondopaminergic systems. This occurs regardless of whether levodopa (or related drugs) is administered.

It may seem that the longer you have been treated, the less robust are the levodopa responses; however, this actually reflects how long you have had PD. The crucial distinction between the *duration of PD* and *levodopa treatment duration* was apparent in analyses of levodopa responses when this drug became available, circa 1969. Back then, newly treated patients had often experienced years of untreated PD because levodopa was not available. In one global analysis of these early levodopa treatment trials, half of the levodopa-treated PD patients developed levodopa dyskinesias within only 6 months. This contrasts with the 40% risk after *5 years* of treatment in the modern era. In a Mayo study from 1969 enrolling PD patients with longer durations of PD, 26 of 27 people experienced dyskinesias within the first year of treatment; motor fluctuations were present in nearly three-fourths by 2 years of levodopa therapy. Again, this contrasts with the 40% incidence after *5 years* of levodopa treatment in modern times. Thus, long durations of PD without levodopa translated into unstable levodopa responses soon after levodopa was ultimately instituted.

The natural progression of PD over time predisposes to these levodopa complications.

In summary, there is no good evidence that people can save their best levodopa responses for later, and this strategy may well be fruitless. Rather, it may simply be accepting a poor short-term outcome for no gain.

◆ ◆ ◆

PART FIVE

The Movement Problems of Parkinson's Disease: Medication Rationale and Choices

10

♦ ♦ ♦

Medications for Movement Problems (Gait, Tremor, Slowness): Background and Rationale

Although we do not have drugs that affect the underlying cause or progression of Parkinson's disease (PD), we have very good drugs for controlling many of the symptoms. The progression of PD is extremely slow, and hence the symptomatic treatment is often gratifying for many years. Although the treatment of the symptoms is not always smooth or perfect, optimal adjustment of medications can typically keep people in the mainstreams of their lives and turn back the clock on this disorder.

One important reason for writing this book is to help guide patients in their choices of medications. A variety of drugs are available for treatment of PD with a vast spectrum of benefits and side effects. Some have substantial revenue streams that may give them more attention than they deserve. Table 10.1 summarizes these drug categories and the specific medications. How does one choose which one(s) to take?

The appropriate choices of symptomatic medication(s) should be based on hard facts. In this chapter we will review these drugs and how they interact with brain chemistry. To provide a rational basis for drug treatment, we need to understand basic scientific principles. Subsequent treatment chapters provide details about doses and dosing schemes.

Table 10.1.   Medications for the Symptomatic Treatment of Parkinson's Disease

Class of Medication	Mechanism of Action	Available Medications
Dopamine precursor	Replenishes brain dopamine	Levodopa (carbidopa/ levodopa; Sinemet; in Europe, benserazide/ levodopa; Madopar)
Dopamine agonist	Synthetic form of dopamine	Pramipexole (Mirapex) Ropinirole (Requip) Rotigotine (patch: Neupro) Apomorphine (Apokyn: injection for rescue therapy)
Catechol-O-methyltransferase (COMT) inhibitor	Blocks an enzyme that breaks down circulating levodopa	Entacapone (Comtan) Carbidopa/levodopa and Entacapone: Stalevo (single pill)
Monoamine oxidase B (MAO-B) inhibitor	Blocks an enzyme that breaks down brain dopamine	Selegiline (Eldepryl, deprenyl) Rasagiline (Azilect)
Antiglutamate (glutamate antagonist)	Blocks a specific type of receptor for the brain neurotransmitter glutamate (NMDA)	Amantadine
Anticholinergic (no longer used for PD treatment)	Blocks a specific class of the brain neurotransmitter acetylcholine	Trihexyphenidyl (Artane) Benztropine (Cogentin)

Dopamine

The key region of the brain that degenerates in those with PD is the substantia nigra, as we have learned in Chapters 2 and 3. This substantia nigra connects with the striatum, forming the nigrostriatal system; the nigral projections to the striatum are shown in Figure 10.1.

In the 1960s, the neurotransmitter released by normal nigrostriatal brain cells was identified and confirmed as dopamine. Thus, when the substantia

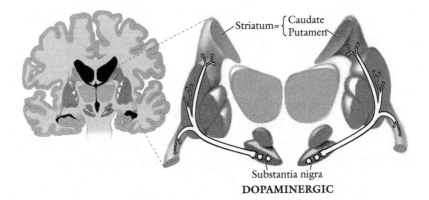

10.1 Substantia nigra neurons send a long, wire-like projection to the striatum. Nigrostriatal terminals in the striatum release dopamine as the neurotransmitter. The striatum includes two components, the caudate and putamen, shown in the figure as two separate nuclei.

nigra degenerates in PD, dopamine levels within the striatum plummet. These insights set the stage for modern-day medical therapy of PD.

The neurotransmitter dopamine is normally released within the striatum from this nigrostriatal connection on a relatively constant basis. In other words, the signaling activity of this system does not start and stop. Rather, the dopamine release seems to provide a persistent and relatively stable modulatory effect.

What is the consequence of losing dopamine within the striatum? There are a variety of experimental means for reducing brain dopamine concentrations in animal models. The experimental animal depleted of striatal dopamine moves slowly and stiffly with a stooped posture and reduced animation. This is very similar to those with PD. When the animal's brain dopamine is replenished, normal movement is restored. Such animal models illustrate the basis for medical treatment of PD, with the main focus on brain dopamine.

Impediment to Raising Brain Dopamine: The Blood-Brain Barrier

It has been known for decades that dopamine taken by mouth or administered by peripheral injection does not get into the brain. There is a natural barrier that prevents the myriad of substances that circulate in our bloodstream from entering the protected brain environment. This is called the *blood-brain barrier*. If it were not for this blood-brain barrier, all the circulating products of our digested meals would flood the brain, perhaps making us all psychotic. The blood-brain barrier allows only selected substances and only limited amounts to cross from the bloodstream to the brain. Certain substances pass readily and others require special transport across this blood-brain barrier; others are absolutely blocked by this barrier. Because of dopamine's chemical structure, it cannot cross the blood-brain barrier.

Actually, dopamine does cross the blood-brain barrier in one small region, the so-called chemoreceptive trigger zone. This is the nausea-vomiting center of the brain. This brainstem region senses when certain undesirable substances are circulating within the bloodstream. Nausea and vomiting are induced if sufficient dopamine passes into this chemoreceptive trigger zone. Hence, if dopamine is administered in pill form or intravenously, it cannot reach the striatum but will pass into the brainstem nausea center, making people sick.

The Role of Enzymes

In the normal state, dopamine is constantly being synthesized within appropriate brain regions. Like most natural substances in our bodies, there is a sequence in which it is continuously being made, used, and then broken down. Hence, there is a continuous cycling of dopamine. The amount produced matches the amount degraded, keeping brain dopamine levels constant. There are metabolic machines for each step in these processes, called *enzymes*. Each enzyme typically performs only one limited task, modifying a specific body chemical. It may add to or delete some portion of that chemical, or it may combine body substances. A sequence of enzymes is responsible for making almost all substances necessary for life, in a series of enzymatic steps. Enzyme systems are analogous to an automobile assembly line, where each worker on the line performs one function, ultimately resulting in the manufactured car.

The Amino Acid L-dopa (Levodopa)

Dopamine is made in our bodies from the immediate precursor dopa, which is more specifically known as *levodopa*, or *L-dopa*. L-dopa is a natural substance that our body manufactures, but this also comes from our diet. To make dopamine, levodopa is transformed by the enzyme dopa decarboxylase. This enzyme changes one small component of levodopa, resulting in dopamine. This enzyme is present not only in the brain but outside of it as well. Unlike dopamine, levodopa is transported across the blood-brain barrier.

Levodopa is from a class of natural body chemicals called *amino acids*, which serve a variety of roles in our body. Perhaps the most fundamental role of amino acids has nothing to do with dopamine or other brain neurotransmitters. Amino acids are the building blocks of the body's proteins. Proteins are responsible for much of the unique structure of our body. Everything from muscle to brain to skin is made up of unique proteins that bond together with other substances to form body organs. Thus, the three basic components of our body's structure include proteins, plus carbohydrates and lipids.

A protein is simply a chain of amino acids strung together. There are 20 specific amino acids in our bodies, each with a unique chemical shape and property. The exact sequence of these amino acids determines the type of protein.

Our diets are rich in proteins. Dietary protein is present in high concentrations in such foods as meat, fish, poultry, and dairy products. When we eat proteins, our digestive system breaks them down into the constituent amino acids. Those amino acids are then released into the bloodstream from our intestinal system. They then go to various places in our body and are used for a variety of purposes, including making new proteins.

Amino acids are also a source of metabolic energy, similar to sugar. Cells are able to transform them into metabolic fuel, yielding energy for that cell.

In the context of PD, we are less interested in how amino acids are made into proteins or burned as fuel by cells. Rather, amino acids serve a third purpose, as a precursor to certain neurotransmitters. The nigrostriatal neurotransmitter dopamine is made from the amino acid levodopa (L-dopa). Substantia nigra neurons are able to take up L-dopa and transform it into dopamine.

WHY THE "L" IN L-DOPA?

Molecules have a three-dimensional configuration. However, any three-dimensional structure may have a mirror image that is identical but oriented just opposite. Similar to gloves, which are both right- and left-handed, natural substances often have two forms, which are right- and left-oriented. Like many chemicals in nature there are two forms of dopa, one the mirror image of the other. The type of dopa that is active in our bodies is the left-oriented form. The term *levo*, which means "left," is the prefix attached to dopa to indicate it is left-oriented; hence the term levodopa, or L-dopa for short.

The other type of amino acid, *dextro* for "right-handed," does not have an important role in our bodies. These dextro-amino acids are relatively inert in terms of body chemistry. Body amino acids are the "L" or left-handed forms. It would be correct to simply refer to "dopa," but L-dopa and levodopa are more specific terms.

LEVODOPA PASSES ACROSS THE BLOOD-BRAIN BARRIER

Amino acids are needed within the brain for all the purposes just noted, including manufacture of proteins, cellular fuel, and as precursors for neurotransmitters. However, their chemical structure prevents them from easily crossing the blood-brain barrier. How, then, does the brain capture adequate amounts of necessary amino acids? It is by way of a chemical transport system. This is analogous to a train that transports coal over a bridge and across a river. Unique transport systems are located at the blood-brain barrier; these recognize critical substances in the bloodstream needed by the brain. Specific circulating molecules selectively bind to the transport mechanism and are carried across the barrier. Each type of transporter binds one specific type of molecule; other substances are not picked up.

Levodopa is transported by one such transport system located at the blood-brain barrier. This specific transport mechanism picks up not only levodopa but also other amino acids of a similar type; these amino acids share a similar chemical structure (the so-called large neutral amino acid class). Although no other substances bind to this specific transporter, a variety of other transporters carry other necessary substances into the brain.

Levodopa as a Treatment for Parkinson's Disease

Half a century ago, with the discovery of dopamine depletion in PD, scientists debated strategies to restore brain dopamine. Attention focused on levodopa, since this was known to be one step removed from dopamine and is transported across the blood-brain barrier. Early trials generated mixed results. The doses were either too low to provide benefit or caused nausea. The nausea was due to levodopa being converted into dopamine in the bloodstream: circulating dopamine easily penetrated the brainstem nausea center where the blood-brain barrier is absent, the chemoreceptive trigger zone.

Fortunately, most individuals with PD were able to tolerate therapeutic doses of levodopa, using a strategy of low initial doses and slow dose escalation. Large clinical trials performed in the late 1960s ultimately confirmed striking success in treating the symptoms of PD with levodopa therapy. These outcomes often bordered on the miraculous. Some people with PD who had not walked for years were again mobile. Disabling tremor suddenly came under control. Some were able to leave nursing homes and return to their families. This discovery of levodopa therapy for PD was revolutionary and heralded a new era of symptomatic treatment.

More to the Story: Carbidopa

Nausea and vomiting was a limiting factor for some PD patients during the early years of levodopa therapy in the early 1970s. Although this nausea is not associated with damage to the stomach (it does not cause ulcers or injure the stomach lining), it often prevented adequate dosage. As we discussed earlier, nausea is caused by premature conversion of levodopa to dopamine outside the brain. Once dopamine is generated within the circulation, it is unable to cross the blood-brain barrier, but it does pass into the brainstem nausea center (the chemoreceptive trigger zone).

Cleaver scientists quickly recognized how to block this premature conversion of levodopa to dopamine outside the brain. The solution was the creation of a substance that would block the conversion of levodopa to dopamine in the circulation but not in the brain. The enzyme, dopa decarboxylase, is present on both sides of the blood-brain barrier, that is, both within the brain and also in the bloodstream. For levodopa therapy to treat PD symptoms, the brain dopa decarboxylase must not be inhibited; however, to prevent nausea, dopa decarboxylase outside the brain must be blocked. This was accomplished by creating a dopa decarboxylase–blocking drug that would not cross the blood-brain barrier. Two such agents were identified, carbidopa and benserazide. Neither crosses the blood-brain barrier, but each inhibits dopa decarboxylase. Thus circulating levodopa was protected from premature conversion before it crossed the blood-brain barrier.

The combination of carbidopa and levodopa has been the mainstay of PD treatment within the United States. The brand name given this combination drug was Sinemet, derived from the Latin *sine emesis*, meaning "without emesis" (emesis = vomiting). In certain European countries and elsewhere, benserazide, rather than carbidopa, is combined with levodopa for the same effect; one common brand name is Madopar. Sinemet and Madopar are essentially identical medications. Carbidopa has no advantages over benserazide and vice versa. Neither carbidopa nor benserazide appears to have any effect apart from blocking the enzyme dopa decarboxylase (outside the brain). Neither has toxicity, even when administered in relatively high doses.

Since this book is targeted to a North American audience, it focuses on carbidopa/levodopa rather than benserazide/levodopa. However, these two combination drugs are essentially interchangeable when the amount of levodopa is the same.

Levodopa in the absence of carbidopa (or benserazide) is no longer used for PD treatment. Whenever we talk about levodopa therapy, treatment with carbidopa/levodopa is implied (or in Europe, benserazide/levodopa).

Despite carbidopa (or benserazide), nausea is still experienced by occasional people with PD taking levodopa. Often this resolves with continued use, provided that one starts with a low dose and only slowly raises it. For more difficult problems with nausea, a number of strategies are available, and these are discussed in detail in Chapter 12.

Levodopa and Diet

Small amounts of levodopa are contained in our dietary proteins. Could increasing our protein intake treat PD? Unfortunately, this does not work. With the breakdown of dietary protein, a variety of amino acids are generated and released into the circulation. The blood-brain barrier transporter that carries levodopa has only a limited capacity. In other words, it is easily filled up; the cars on the train have only a finite number of seats. Other amino acids compete with levodopa for binding sites on the transport mechanism, with only a limited number of such sites. Restated, levodopa is easily prevented from crossing into the brain by competing amino acids. In fact, dietary protein products (amino acids) may completely block the effect of levodopa treatment by this mechanism.

Could PD be treated by any certain foods that are very high in levodopa and lower in other amino acids? There are very few items in our diet with a favorable ratio of levodopa to other competing amino acids. Fava beans, a staple in some southern European and Middle-Eastern diets, do contain proportionately high concentrations of levodopa and are at least mildly beneficial as PD treatment. However, this is an unpalatable and impractical way to treat PD for most people and not very effective when precise doses are necessary.

Levodopa Therapy and Advancing Parkinson's Disease

As experience with levodopa treatment continued into the 1970s it was recognized that there were shortcomings. In long-standing PD, the levodopa benefit was often found to be incomplete. Furthermore, maintenance of stable brain levodopa and dopamine levels became more problematic. With fluctuations in these levels came fluctuations in symptom control. People could be relatively normal one minute and severely parkinsonian several minutes later, as the brain dopamine levels declined. If too much levodopa was administered in an attempt to control these fluctuations, involuntary movements might occur, termed *dyskinesias.*

With the recognition of the problems came strategies for dealing with them. It was appreciated that levodopa dosing and timing were crucial. New drugs were also created for stabilizing the responses, although generally these proved to be less helpful than hoped. Now, 40 years later, levodopa remains the most effective drug we have for PD treatment and the foundation of therapy. However, knowing how to use carbidopa/levodopa, and understanding the role of the adjunctive medications, is crucial to optimal treatment. That is the primary focus of this book.

If the Dopaminergic Neurons Are Lost, Why Does Levodopa Work?

Normally, dopamine is synthesized within nigrostriatal neurons and released within the striatum to signal other neurons in the circuit. Since these nigrostriatal neurons degenerate in PD, why is levodopa effective? After all, the cells where levodopa is converted to dopamine progressively degenerate. Fortunately, there is more than one way this can occur, and the primary mechanism is probably a function of how long one has had PD.

- *The first few years of PD:* In those with early PD, 50–80% of the substantia nigra cells are lost. Conversely, 20–50% of the nigrostriatal neurons have survived during this early stage. These surviving cells are able to increase their production and output of dopamine when bolstered by levodopa therapy. They are able to compensate for what was lost. This is perhaps why those with early PD typically have very smooth and long-lasting responses to levodopa therapy.

- *Late in PD:* The neurodegenerative process is slowly relentless and after a number of years, the loss of dopaminergic terminals may exceed 95% in some areas of the striatum. Despite this, levodopa therapy is still effective, although the smoothness of the response is lost, with fluctuations in the symptoms. The clinical response tends to vary with blood levels of levodopa. At this stage, levodopa conversion primarily occurs within other cells in the striatum, which normally are not involved in dopamine generation. This includes cells that release other neurotransmitters, such as serotonin. Certain of these other brain cells have enzymes capable of converting levodopa to dopamine. The supporting cells of the brain, called *glia,* probably also are involved in the generation of dopamine from levodopa in later-stage PD. Normally, glial cells are not directly involved in the signaling (neurotransmitter) process.

Since nondopaminergic neurons and glia are not part of the usual brain dopamine network, the dopamine they produce from levodopa therapy is released less smoothly and consistently; the synaptic concentrations are not stabilized. This likely plays a role in the unevenness of the levodopa response after many years.

Drugs That Act Like Dopamine: Dopamine Agonists

Scientists have developed drugs that cross the blood-brain barrier and act like dopamine. These are called *dopamine agonists.*

The term *agonist* is applied to drugs that behave like the naturally occurring neurotransmitter; they stimulate the specific receptor because they are chemically similar to the true neurotransmitter. In the case of dopamine agonists, portions of the molecule have chemical configurations that resemble dopamine and hence are able to bind to dopamine receptors. They are analogous to skeleton keys. The real key opens the lock, but skeleton keys have enough of the correct shape to do the same. In this analogy, the lock is the dopamine receptor and the "real key" is dopamine; the dopamine agonist is the skeleton key.

In the United States, four dopamine agonist drugs are available for treatment of PD. This includes the oral medications pramipexole (Mirapex) and ropinirole (Requip), plus a skin-patch formulation, rotigotine (Neupro). A potent, but short-acting dopamine agonist administered by subcutaneous injection is also available, apomorphine (Apokyn).

To understand the properties and roles for these dopamine agonists, we must digress and discuss dopamine receptors. There are five different types of brain dopamine receptors, classified as D1 through D5. Obviously, dopamine binds to all five, and the dopamine agonist, apomorphine, has similar affinities for these receptors. However, pramipexole, ropinirole, and rotigotine have quite specific affinities for the D3 receptor, with much less affinity for the other forms of dopamine receptors. This more limited binding likely accounts for the fact that these three agonists are not nearly as efficacious for PD treatment as levodopa (or apomorphine).

Pramipexole, ropinirole, and rotigotine are used for chronic daily therapy of PD. Although not as potent as levodopa, they have relatively long-lasting effects, especially in the extended-release formulations (pramipexole and ropinirole) or the skin patch (rotigotine). Hence, one role for these drugs has been as a supplement to levodopa, to smooth some of the ups and downs experienced later with levodopa treatment.

Apomorphine is administered by subcutaneous injection (i.e., under the skin), specifically used as "rescue therapy" for people with PD who are trapped in a levodopa-off state (discussed in Chapter 18). The benefit is similar to a full dose of carbidopa/levodopa and occurs within 10 minutes; however, the benefit only lasts 60–90 minutes. Parenthetically, apomorphine administration by mouth results in kidney toxicity, but it is safe when administered by injection.

Dopamine Agonists as Initial Therapy for Parkinson's Disease

Some clinicians advocate starting treatment of PD with a dopamine agonist. You might wonder why a less potent class of drugs would be proposed, when carbidopa/levodopa is readily available and much less expensive. The primary rationale relates to the longer-lasting effect of these agonists and the unproven proposal that early agonist treatment may reduce the later incidence of levodopa fluctuations and dyskinesias. Recall that carbidopa/

levodopa treatment during the first several years produces a stable and long-lasting effect without fluctuations or dyskinesias (with very rare exceptions). After years, when the dopaminergic nigrostriatal system has further degenerated, levodopa benefits tend to become time-locked to each dose; dyskinesias may surface.

The longer-lasting presence of pramipexole, ropinirole, and rotigotine in the circulation rarely translates into such clinical instability. Use of one of these three agonists without carbidopa/levodopa will indeed generate stable responses that continue beyond a few years. However, the lesser anti-parkinsonian benefit is problematic. They do not treat PD symptoms nearly as effectively as carbidopa/levodopa, and after no more than a few years, carbidopa/levodopa is necessary in the vast majority of PD patients. If carbidopa/levodopa is deferred and introduced years later, the response instability may be quickly apparent. Thus, it is not clear that early dopamine agonist use confers any later benefit.

PD onset before age 40 years is termed *young-onset* and is associated with levodopa motor fluctuations and dyskinesias typically surfacing during the first few years. In this group of people, dopamine agonists are often the first choice, with the hope that this will provide adequate control of parkinsonism for several years. On the other hand, this is a group of people likely to be active in the workforce, raising families, and still engaging in sporting activities. Since the available dopamine agonist drugs are much less efficacious than carbidopa/levodopa, they may be a poor choice for some.

Dopamine Agonists Added to Carbidopa/Levodopa to Reduce Instability

Once fluctuations in the levodopa response develop, the later addition of pramipexole, ropinirole, or rotigotine to carbidopa/levodopa therapy may help stabilize control. The longer-lasting dopamine stimulation with these agonists, superimposed on the more potent levodopa effect, may be helpful in some with PD. This is addressed in detail in Chapter 18.

Unique Dopamine Agonist Side Effects

Pramipexole, ropinirole, and rotigotine may produce adverse effects that can easily go unrecognized as related to these drugs. These effects deserve special attention. The side effects discussed in this section relate especially to pramipexole and ropinirole. Rotigotine (administered as a patch) has received less such notoriety, although that may relate to relatively lower conventional doses, plus the fact that it has only been on the market for a few years. The pharmacological properties of all three drugs appear to be similar, with specific affinity for the dopamine D3 receptor. In no particular order, discussion of the unique problems that occasionally develop with this class of medications follows.

SLEEPINESS

Soon after pramipexole and ropinirole were introduced in the 1990s, papers were published documenting "sleep attacks" and consequent car accidents relating to these drugs. In my own experience, a small minority of patients develop drowsiness. With the regular formulations of pramipexole and ropinirole, this was relatively easy to recognize since sleepiness tended to be time-locked to each dose (conventionally taken 3 times daily). With the extended-release formulation (taken once daily with persistent blood levels), the relationship to the drug is less apparent. Often the sleepiness is so prominent that the agonist must be tapered off. Dose reduction to eliminate the sleepiness may require doses so low that any beneficial effect on parkinsonism is lost.

HALLUCINATIONS AND DELUSIONS

Seeing illusory images (hallucinations) or displaying disordered thinking such as paranoia (delusions) may develop in later-stage PD, in relation to the Lewy body process. However, the dopamine agonist drugs may provoke this in even early PD. This is very infrequent with carbidopa/levodopa when used alone; a substantially greater risk is with the dopamine agonists. In clinical trials, pramipexole and ropinirole were approximately 3 times more likely to provoke hallucinations than carbidopa/levodopa. Fortunately, these are infrequent issues until late in the course of PD. Chapter 24 addresses such problems in more detail.

SWELLING (EDEMA)

Leg or foot edema is occasionally provoked by pramipexole or ropinirole. This is not a very important problem unless very prominent. About twice a year, I encounter a PD patient taking one of these drugs with massive leg edema that has failed aggressive conventional therapy. The crucial point is to recognize the cause. The agonist must be tapered off to allow treatment of the edema.

PATHOLOGICAL BEHAVIORS

Recall that the three dopamine agonists used for chronic PD therapy (pramipexole, ropinirole, rotigotine) have a unique affinity for a specific set of dopamine receptors: the D3 receptors. These D3 receptors are predominantly found in the limbic system of the brain, which plays a fundamental role in the experience of reward. Hence, it should not be surprising that chronic treatment with one of these drugs tends to provoke certain compulsive behaviors, such as gambling or sexual ideation, as well as excessive eating, spending, or shopping. It appears that any behavior that is inherently rewarding may become a focus and obsession for affected people taking one of these dopamine agonists. In our clinic, we tabulated a 25% frequency of such pathological behaviors among PD patients taking therapeutic doses of pramipexole or ropinirole. "Pathological" implies that the behavior was sufficiently out of control to impair the life of affected individuals. In our experience, elimination of this problem requires tapering off the agonist. For people starting one of these drugs, family members or the spouse should be made aware of this potential, as those affected often have poor insight.

The dopamine agonists also share side effects with carbidopa/levodopa, which are usually not problematic. They may cause nausea (but not stomach ulcers) or lower the blood pressure in susceptible people (i.e., orthostatic hypotension).

What about the Dopamine Agonists Pergolide and Bromocriptine?

In the first edition of this book, considerable attention was given to the dopamine agonists pergolide (Permax) and bromocriptine (Parlodel). These drugs were in common use until several years ago. They are from a class of medications called *ergots*. A PD drug used in Europe, cabergoline, is also an ergot medication. Subsequent to the publication of the first edition of this book, numerous reports documented that such ergot drugs frequently provoked very serious inflammatory scarring of heart valves as well as other organs, such as the lungs. They are no longer used for PD.

Other Drugs: Blocking Enzymes That Break Down Levodopa and Dopamine

Dopamine and levodopa, like most other body chemicals, are constantly being synthesized and then broken down. Specific enzymes mediate these cyclic processes. If one could block the enzymes that degrade circulating levodopa or brain dopamine, higher levels would result. These higher levels should theoretically translate into reduced symptoms of PD. Two specific enzymes degrade levodopa or dopamine into inactive substances: catechol-O-methyltransferase (COMT) and monoamine oxidase (MAO).

Blocking these enzymes has been an additional strategy for treating PD.

CATECHOL-O-METHYLTRANSFERASE (COMT) INHIBITORS

Two COMT inhibitors are available as treatment for PD, entacapone (Comtan) and tolcapone (Tasmar). Unfortunately, tolcapone was discovered to have potential for life-threatening liver toxicity. Although it is still available, it is rarely used and requires very frequent blood tests of liver function. We will not address tolcapone further in this book and address only entacapone.

Entacapone does not cross the blood-brain-barrier, and its benefits derive from blocking COMT in the bloodstream. This results in a more sustained circulating levodopa level and is primarily used in people with only a short levodopa response (e.g., 2–4 hours). Entacapone prolongs the levodopa response by 30–60 minutes; this is not a huge benefit but is helpful in selected people.

The entacapone effect on levodopa lasts about 4 hours; usually it is taken with every dose of carbidopa/levodopa. If the levodopa dosing interval is very short, for example, 2 hours, it may be taken with every other carbidopa/levodopa dose. Entacapone pills come in only one size, 200 mg. Larger doses are tolerated but confer no additional benefit. Half-doses (i.e., 100 mg) serve no purpose. Note that entacapone in the absence of carbidopa/levodopa has no anti-parkinsonian effect.

Entacapone not only prolongs the levodopa response duration, it also enhances the magnitude of the response. This sometimes translates into dyskinesias. These involuntary movements represent an excessive levodopa effect and can be eliminated by reduction of the levodopa dose. People already troubled by dyskinesias would be wise to avoid entacapone.

A combination of carbidopa/levodopa and entacapone is available under the brand name Stalevo. The primary utility of this formulation is ease of use, since it combines two pills into one. However, it does not easily allow for levodopa adjustments. Often it is preferable to administer carbidopa/levodopa and entacapone separately.

MONOAMINE OXIDASE (MAO)-B INHIBITORS

We have already alluded to the two MAO-B inhibitors, selegiline and rasagiline, in Chapter 9. We will now address the pharmacology of these drugs and monoamine oxidase in more detail.

The two forms of MAO are MAO-A and MAO-B, each of which degrades dopamine. Drugs that block both forms of MAO are occasionally prescribed by psychiatrists to treat severe depression, but these have a serious side-effect spectrum. Blocking MAO-A may result in elevated concentrations of adrenalin-like substances in the bloodstream, potentially provoking severely elevated blood pressures. Special diets are necessary when these drugs are used to reduce such hypertensive risks. These nonselective MAO inhibitors that block both MAO-A and MAO-B are not appropriate for PD treatment and will not be discussed further here.

Brain MAO-B converts dopamine into an inactive substance; blocking this enzyme raises brain dopamine levels. MAO-B does not degrade adrenalin-like substances to any substantial extent. Hence selectively blocking this enzyme does not carry a hypertensive risk or require a special diet. One caveat, however, is that the MAO-B blocking drugs are safe only in conventional doses; if much higher doses are administered, they also block MAO-A, with the discussed risks.

Selegiline (Eldepryl) is an MAO-B inhibitor that previously went by the name *deprenyl* (the name used in the DATATOP clinical trial, discussed in Chapter 9). Selegiline produces a mild symptomatic response. An advantage is the long effect: once it blocks MAO-B, this persists with a 40-day half-life. Although once-daily dosing is conventional, less frequent dosing might still sustain the response.

Rasagiline (Azilect) was discussed in detail in Chapter 9, in relation to a proposed neuroprotective effect. Unfortunately, it probably does not truly slow PD progression. However, like selegiline, it provides mild symptomatic benefit. It also shares the long-lasting MAO-B inhibition with selegiline and is conventionally dosed once daily.

Drugs Blocking Glutamate: Amantadine

Brain cells that release glutamate as the neurotransmitter are widespread in motor control systems. These are called *glutamatergic* neurons. There are intimate interactions of glutamate and dopamine in the basal ganglia, where glutamatergic and dopaminergic projections converge on single neurons. Animal models demonstrate that drugs blocking glutamate improve parkinsonism. However, potent drugs tested for this purpose have limiting side effects, presumably because glutamate is widely distributed in the brain, whereas the drug effects cannot be limited to just basal ganglia.

Amantadine is a weak glutamate-blocking drug that is tolerated. It inhibits only one type of glutamate response, and specifically at the glutamate-NMDA receptor. Amantadine has other pharmacological properties, but the benefits are currently assumed to result from glutamate-NMDA inhibition.

Amantadine was first introduced for PD treatment around the same time as levodopa (over 40 years ago). For years, it was used for treating mild parkinsonism, although with no more than modest benefits. More recently, it was recognized to counter the tendency for levodopa to cause dyskinesias, which are involuntary movements from an excessive levodopa effect. Dyskinesias can always be eliminated by reducing the individual carbidopa/

levodopa doses; however, occasionally the dose reduction is associated with increased parkinsonism. For those who cannot control dyskinesias without losing control of parkinsonism, the addition of amantadine can be quite helpful. This situation is addressed in more detail in Chapter 18.

Another glutamate-NMDA blocking drug, memantine (Namenda), is also available. It should have similar benefits directed at dyskinesias, but because of its expense it is not used for that purpose. Memantine may be used in the treatment of dementia and is discussed further in Chapter 23.

Anticholinergic Medications

We would be remiss to not discuss anticholinergic medications. They were the primary treatment option before levodopa was introduced decades ago. However, their anti-parkinsonian benefit is modest and they have a myriad of side effects. Most neurologists no longer prescribe this class of medications for PD.

Acetylcholine is a neurotransmitter within the striatum; cells that release acetylcholine are called *cholinergic* neurons. Blocking acetylcholine receptors with anticholinergic drugs improves some of the symptoms of PD—primarily tremor, dystonia, and stiffness (rigidity). However, the benefits are small and nearly always overshadowed by adverse effects.

Anticholinergic side effects are substantial and include memory impairment; they have the opposite effect as drugs used to enhance memory in people with dementia. They also cause constipation, slowed stomach emptying, dry mouth and eyes, visual blurring, and slowed urination.

Anticholinergic drugs previously used for treatment of PD included trihexyphenidyl (Artane) and benztropine (Cogentin). Note that other drugs also have anticholinergic properties, most notably drugs for urinary urgency and frequency. Thus the bladder medications, such as oxybutynin (Ditropan) or tolterodine (Detrol), have these same side effects but are not so potent as to have anti-parkinsonian properties. Drugs for urinary symptoms are discussed in Chapter 27.

11

♦ ♦ ♦

Starting Medical Treatment of Parkinson's Disease Movement Problems

When is a good time to start a medication? Which drug should be used, and why? The previous chapters should provide a good background for what we are going to discuss here.

Who Needs to be Treated?

Just because someone has Parkinson's disease (PD) does not mean they must be started on a medication. If we had drugs that slowed the progression of PD, then starting them at the first sign of parkinsonism would be appropriate; unfortunately, we have no such drugs. We do have good drugs to treat the symptoms of PD. It is the *symptoms* that determine when to start a medication for PD. If the symptoms don't bother you, medications can be deferred. Sooner or later, a medication will become necessary, but this can be put off until the symptoms get in the way.

When to start medical therapy and how aggressively to treat symptoms depends on the individual circumstances; there is no one-size-fits-all approach. Treatment decisions should be based on the following premise:

The goal of medical treatment is to keep those with PD within the mainstream of their lives.

Occupational, social, and recreational pursuits are each important and should factor into the decision. A second consideration is the capacity and inclination to engage in exercise. Recall from Chapter 9 that considerable evidence suggests that ongoing aerobic exercise may slow PD progression. Thus, if slowness, stiffness, or gait problems prevent exercise, that is a good reason to start a medication.

As stated earlier, individual circumstances influence medication decisions. Consider two people, each with the same problem: parkinsonism primarily limited to a resting tremor in one hand.

- Mrs. Jones is a trial lawyer. She is concerned that juries are focusing on that tremor, distracting them from her arguments. She is worried that they interpret this as a sign of nervousness and insecurity.

- Mr. Smith is a semi-retired farmer (it seems that farmers never completely retire). His farm work is not compromised. He meets his buddies at the town coffee shop each morning, where they discuss farm politics; his tremor is ignored.

Mrs. Jones deserves treatment; she is worried about her law practice. Mr. Smith, with the same symptoms, is not bothered and treatment can appropriately be deferred. On the other hand, if Mr. Smith were becoming self-conscious about his tremor, staying home, and not socializing and going for coffee, treatment would be appropriate.

Should We Save the Best Drugs for Later?

Medications are most effective during the first several years of PD. This is not to say that they are ineffective later on. They often can maintain people in the mainstream of life for many years. However, after a number of years, the effect is typically not as complete. Moreover, dyskinesias and motor fluctuations may develop, which we discussed in the previous two chapters. Even then, the wheels do not fall off the wagon. Although the management becomes more complicated, the medication strategies often reverse many of these setbacks, which is the focus of subsequent chapters.

Why are the medications less completely and consistently effective after many years? As we discussed in Chapter 10, this is primarily due to disease progression, rather than a function of the number of years someone has taken these drugs:

- Levodopa fluctuations and dyskinesias developing after several years primarily reflect the progressive loss of *dopaminergic* neurons; the residual cells that are left to convert levodopa to dopamine are unable to maintain stable concentrations at dopaminergic synapses.

- Incomplete levodopa responses relate to the Lewy neurodegenerative process subsequently involving *nondopaminergic* neurons within basal ganglia circuits; obviously, levodopa treatment will not replenish other neurotransmitters.

Some older guidelines for treating PD advised that the best drugs, especially carbidopa/levodopa, should be deferred until absolutely necessary. However, there is now increasing recognition that the slow progression of PD continues, regardless of whether we treat conservatively or aggressively early in the disease course. If one chooses to suffer now, hoping to capture the best responses later, this practice may be for naught; this represents a lost opportunity.

More on Dyskinesias and Motor Fluctuations

Further insight into the risks and implications of unstable levodopa responses needs to be discussed here to put carbidopa/levodopa treatment into perspective. To reiterate, these are problems that occur years later, with subsequent changes in the levodopa response, manifesting in two possible ways:

1. The levodopa benefit becomes time-locked to each dose, lasting for only a few hours after carbidopa/levodopa administration and requiring shorter dosing intervals; this may result in response fluctuations.

2. Dyskinesias, representing excessive movement of the body, are a consequence of each levodopa dose being too high; these resolve with levodopa dose reductions. However, occasional people then experience recurrence of parkinsonism with lower levodopa doses.

Often overlooked is the fact that these are treatable problems. That is one important focus of this book, and these issues are specifically addressed in Chapters 17 and 18.

The published reports of frequencies of dyskinesias and motor fluctuations often overstate the problem. When these are tabulated, mild cases of dyskinesias and fluctuations are lumped with the more troublesome problems. Often dyskinesias are limited or barely perceptible; levodopa response fluctuations are often modest. Moreover, simple levodopa dose adjustments effectively treat many of these problems.

Rarely discussed is the fact that the risk of unstable levodopa responses is related to age. At one end of the age spectrum, nearly all of those with PD onset before age 40 years (categorized as young-onset PD) will experience at least mild dyskinesias and motor fluctuations by 5 years of levodopa treatment. At the other extreme, those with PD onset after age 70 years have a less than 20% risk of dyskinesias after 5 years of carbidopa/levodopa. There appears to be an intermediate risk for these problems between age 40 and 70 years. Among all ages combined, the 5-year risk of these problems is approximately 40%.

The notoriety given to dyskinesias and motor fluctuations tends to be overblown. These symptoms can be troubling, but not for everyone, even after many years of carbidopa/levodopa treatment. Recent long-term studies have indicated that these are not the major sources of disability affecting seniors with advanced PD.

Starting a Medication

The drugs for parkinsonism have quite different efficacies. Should we start with a minimally effective drug and work toward a more potent one? This was the common practice when I was in training years ago. If we start with a more potent medication, should we begin with a dopamine agonist? That has been a frequent recommendation. If carbidopa/levodopa is started, should the dose be kept low? That is often advised. Let us consider these different avenues of what I would regard as overly cautious advice.

Start with a mildly efficacious medication. Drugs such as rasagiline, selegiline, or amantadine are occasionally selected by clinicians for first treatment. They are easy to use but not very efficacious. While this is acceptable, why start a drug that you know will not be very effective? Seniors' medication lists are often lengthy; adding a drug with limited efficacy and additional expense may not be sensible.

Start with a dopamine agonist. Pramipexole, ropinirole, and rotigotine have been advocated for initial treatment of PD. They are not nearly as beneficial as carbidopa/levodopa. Some formulations are expensive and they all have unique side effects, discussed earlier in this chapter. In their defense, the dopamine agonist drug levels persist longer in the body (i.e., have longer half-lives) and hence tend to produce more stable responses. However, levodopa response instability is not a problem during the early treatment years. When PD progression later translates into potential for levodopa response instability, the agonist responses will clearly be insufficient. Perhaps an argument can be made for initial dopamine agonist use in those with young-onset PD. In this group, unstable levodopa responses usually develop within the first few years; this is addressed further later in this chapter.

Start with carbidopa/levodopa but keep the dose low. Recall that the goal of PD medical therapy is to keep people active, engaged, and exercising. Arbitrarily restricting the dose could easily sabotage those goals. Moreover, there is no evidence that very conservative levodopa dosing will confer later benefits. Similar to the directive to defer carbidopa/levodopa altogether, this may result in lost opportunities.

Physicians' Choices for Initial Treatment

The available drugs for initial symptomatic treatment of PD are listed in Table 11.1. Clinicians have quite different views on which drug to start. Some are inclined to accept the argument that rasagiline may slow the progression of PD and choose that drug for initial therapy. However, the symptomatic

Table 11.1.   Initial Symptomatic Treatment of Parkinson's Disease (Available Drugs)

Drug Class and Generic Name	Brand Name	Effectiveness Against Parkinsonism	Duration Required to Escalate to Therapeutic Dose
Levodopa			
Carbidopa/levodopa*	Sinemet	Marked	3–5 weeks
Dopamine agonist			
Pramipexole	Mirapex	Moderate	4–8 weeks
Ropinirole	Requip	Moderate	4–8 weeks
Rotigotine	Neupro	Moderate	4–8 weeks
Glutamate blocker			
Amantadine	—	Mild	Within a few days to weeks
MAO-B blocker			
Selegiline	Eldepryl	Mild	Within a few days
Rasagiline	Azilect	Mild	Within a few days

*Benserazide/levodopa in Europe.

effect will be modest and should not be the sole drug for those whose par-kinsonism interferes with activities. Other clinicians believe that carbidopa/ levodopa should be saved for later and treatment should be started with a dopamine agonist. Although this is contrary to my view, this is acceptable if the agonist is tolerated and sufficiently beneficial to allow a relatively normal life. Still other clinicians argue that with very mild symptoms, a drug that is very simple to use is preferred—hence selegiline, rasagiline, or amantadine is selected. My own view is that if the problems are trivial, I prefer to not start a medication. While all these differing perspectives may be defended, they should not override the decision to start carbidopa/levodopa if parkinson-ism is substantial and prominently compromising life.

In the first edition of this book, I allowed for a variety of views relating to drug selection, even though I personally favored initial carbidopa/levodopa treatment. Another 10 years in the clinic has reinforced my simple view of treat-ment: carbidopa/levodopa is the single drug that is absolutely crucial to the care of those with PD. In my view, if you are doing well on no PD drugs, it is OK to continue without medications. Once PD starts to interfere with life's pleasures and activities, I favor going directly to carbidopa/levodopa. The exception is those with young-onset PD, who are at a greater risk of early levodopa instabil-ity (fluctuations, dyskinesias). I may advise starting with a dopamine agonist, but even then will often choose carbidopa/levodopa if the disability is marked and threatening the ability to work and carry on with activities.

Those considering starting with a dopamine agonist may wish to com-pare the advantages and disadvantages with those of carbidopa/levodopa. A summary is presented in Table 11.2.

Carbidopa/Levodopa: Regular Formulation versus Sustained-Release

Carbidopa/levodopa comes in two main formulations, regular pills and sustained-release pills. The sustained-release pills are also termed controlled-release (CR) and often are referred to as Sinemet CR (the original brand name was Sinemet). Note that the regular formulation of carbidopa/ levodopa is also called *immediate-release* carbidopa/levodopa.

There are no advantages to starting with the sustained-release formulation, and there are some disadvantages compared to regular carbidopa/levodopa:

- Incomplete passage into the circulation with the sustained-release pills (i.e., reduced bioavailability)

- The sustained-release pills have complex interactions with meals (CR levodopa enters the circulation more readily when taken with meals, but dietary protein products inhibit levodopa passage across the blood-brain barrier).

**Table 11.2.   Comparative Advantages: Carbidopa/Levodopa
versus a Dopamine Agonist**

Advantages of Carbidopa/Levodopa	Advantages of Dopamine Agonist (Pramipexole, Ropinirole, Rotigotine)
• Substantially more efficacious • Simpler to use • Usually much cheaper • Lower risk of hallucinations • Lower risk of daytime sleepiness • Minimal risk of pathological behaviors (e.g., gambling, sexual ideation) • No risk of edema	• Substantially lower risk of dyskinesias* • Substantially lower likelihood of motor fluctuations*

* The much lower risks of dyskinesias and fluctuations relate to administration of the dopamine agonist alone, without carbidopa/levodopa. Once carbidopa/levodopa is added, the dyskinesia and fluctuation risk markedly increases.

These shortcomings make it difficult to be certain whether the full benefit of levodopa is achieved with the sustained-release pills. Later in the course of PD, the sustained-release formulation may have a limited role; this is discussed in Chapter 17.

Regular (immediate-release) carbidopa/levodopa should also be distinguished from the *orally disintegrating tablet* (ODT) of carbidopa/levodopa, which is dissolved in the mouth and swallowed with saliva. This ODT formulation does not have a substantial role in the initial treatment of PD.

A combination of regular (immediate-release) and sustained-release carbidopa/levodopa has recently been approved, with the brand name Rytary. The role for this combination capsule is in the treatment of motor fluctuations developing in later PD, rather than as initial therapy. It is substantially more expensive than regular carbidopa/levodopa.

To summarize, when carbidopa/levodopa is chosen as the initial therapy for PD, the regular (immediate-release) formulation is preferable. Note also that there is no advantage to brand name Sinemet; generic carbidopa/levodopa is appropriate.

Pramipexole versus Ropinirole versus Rotigotine

If a dopamine agonist is chosen for treatment, which is preferable? The three available agonists have similar pharmacologies; that is, they all have relatively selective affinity for the dopamine D3 receptor. There is not a mg-to-mg correspondence between the pramipexole and ropinirole pills, and allowing for dosing differences, they seem to have very similar efficacy. Ropinirole and rotigotine do have a similar mg-to-mg potency and appear to have similar efficacy. The recommended dose ceiling for rotigotine (8 mg) is substantially less than that for ropinirole (24 mg) despite the similar mg correspondence; this seems somewhat arbitrary.

Rotigotine is formulated as a skin patch, which is changed once every 24 hours. Pramipexole and ropinirole are formulated as an extended-release pill, also allowing once-daily dosing. This is in addition to the regular formulations or pramipexole and ropinirole, requiring 3 times daily dosing.

The bottom line is that these three dopamine agonists are somewhat interchangeable. Experience has suggested no substantial differences in either efficacy or side effects, when one adjusts for the dosing variations.

Early Side Effects Relating to Dopamine Replenishment

The unique side effects associated with the dopamine agonist drugs were discussed in Chapter 10 (pathological behaviors, hallucinations, daytime sleepiness, edema); these are restricted primarily to this class of medications. Carbidopa/levodopa may induce dyskinesias, but this is unlikely during the early years of PD. Both carbidopa/levodopa and the agonist medications may induce either nausea or low blood pressure (orthostatic hypotension) during initial treatment, and these effects deserve further discussion. The more important adverse effect is the potential for low blood pressure and will be addressed first.

Orthostatic hypotension

The autonomic nervous system controls blood pressure (BP), maintaining a consistent value whether one is lying, sitting, or standing. As discussed in Chapter 3, PD is often associated with autonomic dysfunction, including the potential for the BP to markedly drop when *standing*. Orthostatic hypotension (*orthostatic* = upright; *hypotension* = low BP) implies that the BP is substantially lower when upright. This carries the potential for faints due to low blood pressure. The PD drugs that reestablish brain dopamine tend to exacerbate orthostatic hypotension and in proportion to their anti-parkinsonian potency (i.e., carbidopa/levodopa is more provocative than the dopamine agonists, whereas selegiline, rasagiline, and amantadine are not likely to contribute).

Before any drug is started, remind the clinician to check your blood pressure in the standing position and to repeat this after the medication is started. Note that the lowered BP persists for several hours after a given dose but not beyond that; hence checking the BP many hours after the last dose may miss detection of this.

Blood pressure is conventionally recorded with two numbers, for example, 120/80. The upper number is the systolic BP (e.g., 120) and the lower, the diastolic (e.g., 80). They tend to run in parallel, so to keep things simple in this book, we will focus on the upper number (the systolic) to guide BP assessments and ignore the diastolic number. The unit for these BP values is given in millimeters of mercury (mmHg); this relates to the old BP measuring devices in which a column of mercury connected to a BP cuff provided the reading. To reiterate, in this book we will ignore the units (mmHg) and also the diastolic value so that we deal with just a single number, the systolic reading.

As a general rule of thumb, if the *standing systolic* BP is over 90, people will feel fine. Recognizing that carbidopa/levodopa or a dopamine agonist may lower the blood pressure, a slightly higher reading is desirable before starting on one of these drugs. We need a little wiggle room.

If the standing blood pressure is below 100, then review your medication list with your physician to determine if another prescription drug is contributing and might be discontinued. Perhaps certain medications are no longer needed, such as water pills (diuretics) or antihypertensive medications. Drugs that are common offenders are listed in Chapter 21. If it is still low, increasing dietary salt intake and drinking a lot of fluids (perhaps 6 to 8 tall glasses daily) may modestly raise the BP. If a low BP persists, with standing readings less than 90 systolic, read Chapter 21, which focuses on this issue.

Do not rely solely on your doctor or nurse to check the BP if orthostatic hypotension is present. Purchase a reliable BP device and record the values so that you may show them to your clinicians. For most people with this problem, the lowest reading of the day will be after breakfast; check the standing reading then. If the systolic value is over 90, it is likely to be sufficient for the remainder of the day. Be aware that some BP devices do not display low values and instead show an "error" reading. If in doubt about that, compare readings on your device with those in your doctor's office.

Nausea

Both carbidopa/levodopa and the dopamine agonists may induce nausea, primarily when first started or when raising the dose. This is not dangerous and does not indicate potential for a stomach ulcer. The dopamine agonist pills (pramipexole, ropinirole) may be taken with meals, and this practice may be sufficient to prevent nausea.

Carbidopa/levodopa must be taken on an empty stomach, but eating a non-protein food with each dose may help reduce nausea—this might be a few soda crackers, plain bread, toast without butter, or half a banana. Often

Table 11.3. Comparative Costs of Medications That Might Be Used as Initial Therapy of Parkinson's Disease*

Medication	Formulation and Size	Price per 100 Pills ($)
Carbidopa/levodopa		
	Regular	
	25/100	$29
	10/100	15
	25/250	19
	Sustained-release (SR, CR)	
	25/100	29
	50/200	44
	Orally disintegrating tablet (ODT)	
	25/100	83
Carbidopa/levodopa plus entacapone (Stalevo)		
	Generic, 100 mg levodopa	267
	Generic, 200 mg levodopa	258
	Brand name Stalevo-100 (100 mg levodopa)	477
	Brand name Stalevo-200 (200 mg levodopa)	468
Pramipexole		
	Regular formulation, generic	
	0.125, 0.25, 0.50, 1.0, 1.5 mg	9–10
	Sustained-release as brand name Mirapex ER	
	0.375 mg	1225
	0.75, 1.5, 3.0	1307–1309
Ropinirole		
	Regular formulation, generic	
	0.5, 1, 2, 3, 4, 5 mg	11–13

(continued)

Table 11.3. Continued

Medication	Formulation and Size	Price per 100 Pills ($)
	Extended-release, generic	
	2 mg	169
	4 mg	330
	6 mg	490
	8 mg	452
	12 mg	757
	Brand name Requip XL	
	2 mg	263
	4 mg	523
	8 mg	787
Rotigotine		
	Neupro patch	
	1 mg, 2 mg	1595
	8 mg	1579
Selegiline		
	5 mg capsules	137
	5 mg tablets	214
Rasagiline (Azilect)		
	1 mg	1562
Amantadine		
	100 mg	140

*Pharmacy drug pricing is from www.medicaid.gov (June 2014).

nausea resolves with continued dosing. Raising doses more slowly may also prove helpful. More specific strategies for dealing with this problem are addressed in subsequent chapters.

Side Effects Unique to the Minor PD Drugs

Amantadine is generally well tolerated but commonly causes a purplish fish-net pattern of discoloration on the legs. This is usually subtle and is termed *livido reticularis*. It is not of any concern beyond a cosmetic one. Selegiline may cause insomnia; thus it should be taken in the morning rather than later in the day. Rasagiline less frequently causes insomnia but is taken as a morning dose nonetheless.

The FDA lists potentially serious drug interactions when selegiline or rasagiline are combined with one of several classes of drugs, including most antidepressants, narcotics, tramadol, cyclobenzaprine, dextromethorphan, amphetamines, phenylephrine, ephedrine, or St. John's wort. These appear to be extremely rare interactions when selegiline and rasagiline are used in the recommended doses. Finally, if the selegiline or rasagiline doses are raised beyond those recommended, these drugs may then block both MAO-A and MAO-B. A special diet is then required and many medications avoided, to prevent life-threatening conditions.

Expense

The cost of medications should not be ignored. If two drugs have similar efficacy and side effects, expense may be a deciding factor. Table 11.3 lists the comparative drug costs for medications discussed in this chapter. This information was taken from the federal website www.medicaid.gov, relating to pharmacy drug pricing (National Average Drug Acquisition Cost) in June 2014. These values may differ from what you pay at the pharmacy, but they do allow comparisons. The following website provides medication cost comparisons within cities or by zip code: www.goodrx.com.

PART SIX

◆ ◆ ◆

Beginning Treatment of Parkinson's Disease: Medication Guidelines

12

♦ ♦ ♦

Starting Levodopa Treatment

In the previous chapter, the different options for initial symptomatic therapy of Parkinson's disease (PD) were discussed. Obviously, I favor carbidopa/levodopa for most people. If you are about to start levodopa therapy, expect to be very pleasantly surprised. The improvement is often striking. Carbidopa/levodopa is relatively easy to use and is typically well tolerated. No monitoring of blood tests is necessary, since carbidopa/levodopa does not damage internal organs, such as the liver or kidneys. The only potentially serious side effect is orthostatic hypotension, which we discussed in the last chapter; however, only a minority of people are at risk for this. Moreover, it is treatable once recognized.

There is no "one size fits all" carbidopa/levodopa dose. Treatment begins with a low dose, which is slowly raised, guided by the response. In this chapter, we will learn exactly how to do this, what to look for, and the rationale for what we do. First, we need to address certain background issues.

Carbidopa

To recap, the carbidopa in carbidopa/levodopa prevents the premature conversion to levodopa to dopamine outside the brain. This prevents nausea and allows much lower doses of levodopa to be used. Carbidopa/levodopa used in the United States is essentially interchangeable with benserazide/

levodopa, which is used in Europe and other countries outside the United States. If nausea is not experienced, then the amount of carbidopa (or benserazide) can be ignored; progressively higher doses of carbidopa do not increase potency. In fact, the potency of carbidopa/levodopa relates to levodopa and not to carbidopa. Carbidopa appears to have no side effects, even in very high doses.

Regular (Immediate-Release) Carbidopa/ Levodopa Is Preferred over the Sustained-Release Formulation

As we discussed in Chapter 11, carbidopa/levodopa should be started using the regular (immediate-release) formulation. The sustained-release formulation (also termed controlled-release, or CR) is acceptable but not advisable. Whereas the regular formulation easily passes into the circulation (99% of the administered levodopa is detected in the bloodstream after a dose), levodopa in the sustained-release formulation is partially lost in the stool (about 70% enters the bloodstream). Sustained-release carbidopa/levodopa also has complex interactions with meals. Thus, if a suboptimal response is experienced while using the sustained-release formulation, it may be unclear whether the slow-release properties are the limiting factor. In this book, we will keep things simple by advising that carbidopa/levodopa be administered as the regular formulation.

Be aware that even though the dose numbers may appear the same in these two formulations (e.g., 25/100), the sustained-release tablet is not interchangeable with the regular formulation. In other words, there is not a mg-to-mg correspondence of sustained-release (Sinemet CR) to regular carbidopa/levodopa.

The sustained-release (CR) formulation has been available for over 20 years and there has been considerable clinical experience with this. The duration of levodopa in the circulation is only modestly prolonged, by about 90–120 minutes. Hence dosing at least two times daily is still necessary. It takes twice as long to enter the circulation, which can be problematic later in PD when short-duration responses surface. Thus, sustained-release carbidopa/levodopa has a limited role in treatment and will be discussed later in this book.

The dosing scheme for initiating carbidopa/levodopa provided later in this chapter relates to the regular formulation and is not appropriate for sustained-release pills. Rarely, a prescription is inadvertently filled with the sustained-release pills when the regular carbidopa/levodopa was intended. This may result in a suboptimal response. It can be recognized by pill color—the regular carbidopa/levodopa pills discussed in this chapter are uniquely *yellow* (both generic and brand name). If you are uncertain, ask your pharmacist.

Rytary is a new formulation of sustained-release and regular carbidopa/levodopa combined in a single capsule. It had just became available at the time of this book's publication and I have had no experience with it to date. This combination capsule kicks in more quickly than the currently available sustained-release carbidopa/levodopa tablets but with a longer response than that of regular carbidopa/levodopa. It is considerably more expensive than regular carbidopa/levodopa. It does not appear to have a role as initial therapy for PD. This drug is appropriate to consider later in the course of PD if fluctuations due to short-duration levodopa responses become problematic.

Other Formulations of Regular Carbidopa/Levodopa

Regular (immediate-release) carbidopa/levodopa also comes in 10/100 and 25/250 sizes. The 10/100 size could be used for starting treatment using the schedule in this chapter; it has the same amount of levodopa as in the 25/100 size. However, because of a lesser amount of carbidopa in each pill, it is more likely to provoke nausea. It is slightly less expensive (see Table 11.3 in Chapter 11).

The 25/250 formulation is equivalent in potency to two and a half of the 25/100 pills (i.e., same amounts of levodopa). With proportionately less carbidopa, it also is more likely to cause nausea. The levodopa content is too high to use when starting carbidopa/levodopa.

I favor the 25/100 carbidopa/levodopa pills, for two reasons. First, they are less likely to provoke nausea (more carbidopa per pill). Second, using the same type of pill throughout the course of PD keeps things simple and reduces confusion. When expense is a substantial issue, use of the carbidopa/levodopa pills with less carbidopa (10/100, 25/250) is acceptable as long as nausea is not a problem; however, the cost differences are relatively small.

Generic versus Brand Name Carbidopa/Levodopa

Currently, prescriptions for regular carbidopa/levodopa are nearly always filled with generic carbidopa/levodopa, and that is very reasonable. There appears to be no advantage to brand name Sinemet, which is more expensive. It is unclear whether sustained-release carbidopa/levodopa is preferable from a single source (e.g., brand name Sinemet CR). It is usually is filled as a generic; I have not found that this is problematic.

Orally Disintegrating Carbidopa/ Levodopa (Parcopa)

This tablet, with the brand name Parcopa, dissolves in the mouth and is swallowed with saliva; it is not absorbed through the tongue or mouth. It behaves similarly to immediate-release carbidopa/levodopa, except it enters the circulation slightly quicker. The advantage is that water is not necessary when taking this, so it is more convenient.

Parcopa comes in the same concentrations, colors, and carbidopa-levodopa ratios as regular carbidopa/levodopa. As shown in Table 11.3 (Chapter 11), this formulation is much more expensive. For dosing purposes, it is interchangeable with the regular formulations. It has a limited role in PD treatment and will not be addressed here further.

My Recommendation: Start Carbidopa/Levodopa with the Regular (Immediate-Release) 25/100 Formulation

In the first edition of this book, I tried to be fair and balanced in discussing choices for initial treatment, recognizing that other clinicians may view this differently. Now, 10 years later, I have chosen to be more selective. In Chapter 11, I provided the rationale for selecting carbidopa/levodopa as the starting drug for PD. In this chapter, I am simplifying this further by declaring that the 25/100 immediate-release (regular) formulation is my choice of treatment. I advocate not only starting with the 25/100 regular carbidopa/ levodopa pills but also using that formulation throughout the course of PD. An uncomplicated approach is important to laypeople who may not be comfortable with all the different and confusing medication and formulation options.

DOSING SEPARATE FROM MEALS

Recall from previous chapters that dietary protein products (amino acids) compete with levodopa for transport across the blood-brain barrier. Any protein meal or snack may inhibit levodopa from entering the brain. This includes milk and milk products. Diet does not need to be changed, but the carbidopa/levodopa doses must be separated from meals. Each carbidopa/ levodopa dose should be taken

- At least 1 hour before meals
- At least 2 hours after the end of meals

Taking a dose with a meal may negate the effect of that dose.

BEGINNING CARBIDOPA/LEVODOPA

The dosing scheme for initiating carbidopa/levodopa treatment is shown in Table 12.1; it may be reproduced. This starts with a single 25/100 immediate-release carbidopa/levodopa tablet three times daily. Increments are made weekly since it takes approximately that long for the cumulative effect to develop. The starting dose of one 25/100 tablet three times daily may be too low to produce a benefit; however, beginning with a low dose allows better tolerability. In fact, some physicians advise starting with a half-tablet three times daily. In my experience, most people tolerate full-tablet starting doses, which shortens the dose escalation scheme. The only exception is the person who experiences nausea, which we discuss later in this chapter.

Table 12.1 stipulates that each week, a half-tablet is added to all three doses. It is appropriate to progress more slowly if nausea. This dose escalation scheme advances to two and one-half of the 25/100 carbidopa/levodopa tablets three times daily over the course of several weeks. For most people with PD, doses of 2 ½ tablets capture the full benefit. However, some people find the best response with 3 tablets each dose. I have not encountered anyone who needed more than 3 tablets at a time, provided that they are using the 25/100 immediate-release (regular) formulation and taking their pills on an empty stomach. That is the reason the dosing scheme stops at 3 tablets each dose. Conceptually, the dopamine tank is filled with the 3 tablets each dose.

The goal is to restore normal functioning. Hence continued dose escalation is appropriate until this is achieved, up to 3 tablets each dose. There is no good reason to arbitrarily settle on a low dose unless you are doing very well. Once you have advanced through the scheme, a dose must be selected for maintenance. The rules that apply may be summarized:

- Choose the dose that works the best.

- If several doses work equally well, settle on the lowest of those equipotent doses.

We are not locked into the highest or last dose, and can return to a lower dose. We are looking for the dose that fills the dopamine tank, no more and no less. In my experience, once the ideal individual dose is determined, it remains much the same indefinitely. This contrasts with certain other drugs such as narcotic pain relievers, where higher and higher doses are required. Years later in PD, more doses per day are usually needed to avoid gaps in coverage; however, the number of pills per dose stays much the same.

Note that when starting carbidopa/levodopa, the doses do not need to be equally spaced over the course of the day; for example, they do not need to be taken every 8 hours. In early PD, the only important timing factor is to keep the doses separate from meals. After a number of years, the time between doses may be crucial, but not in the beginning.

Table 12.1. Initiating Carbidopa/Levodopa 25/100 Regular (Immediate-Release) Tablets

Start with the low dose shown below for week 1, and increase
 weekly. It takes about a week to develop the full cumulative effect.
 Carbidopa/levodopa should be taken on an empty stomach:
> **at least 1 hour before meals;**
> **at least 2 hours after the end of meals.**

If you skip a meal, take that dose whenever convenient. You do not
 need to have a fixed interval between doses but take them no less than
 3–4 hours apart.

Most people will capture the full effect by week 4 (2 ½ tablets each dose).
 However, if there is an insufficient response, raise the dose to 3 tablets three
 times daily. Higher individual doses are unlikely to provide further benefit.

The purpose of this scheme is to find the appropriate dose to continue.
 When you have gone through the scheme, settle on the dose that works
 best. If several doses provide the same benefit, remain on the lowest of
 those equipotent doses.

Years later, you will likely need more than 3 doses daily, but the number of
 pills per dose usually does not substantially change over time.

If you feel faint, check your standing blood pressure. If the standing systolic
 blood pressure is less than 90, then this needs attention.

Week #1. Start with one 25/100 carbidopa/levodopa tablet three times daily.
Week #2. Increase the doses to one and one-half (1 $^1/_2$) tablets three
 times daily.
Week #3. Increase to 2 tablets three times daily.
Week #4. Increase to two and one-half (2½) tablets three times daily. For
 most people this dose is at the point of diminishing returns.
Week #5 (optional). If there is suboptimal benefit, try one more increment
 to 3 tablets three times per day.
**After completing this dose escalation scheme, settle on the dose that
 works best.**
If there is no improvement on any of the doses, you may taper off over
 7–10 days. However, there are not good alternatives if you fail carbidopa/
 levodopa treatment.

I DON'T EAT THREE MEALS A DAY

For those eating two meals daily, a carbidopa/levodopa dose can be taken
an hour before each of those two meals. The remaining dose can be taken at
any time it is convenient. As long as 3–4 hours elapse between doses, there
should be no overlap of the effects.

For those who eat many small meals throughout the day, this becomes a little more complicated. Two of the doses should easily be workable. Thus the first dose can be taken upon awakening; you can have this laid out on your nightstand with a glass of water. Another dose can be taken at bedtime, provided that at least 2 hours elapse after your last evening snack. The remaining dose can be worked in at any time during the 24-hour cycle when you have not recently eaten or are going to eat; this could even be in the middle of the night if you awaken to go to the washroom.

MAY I TAKE CARBIDOPA/LEVODOPA WITH MY OTHER MEDICINES?

Yes, except for iron pills. Iron can bind levodopa and prevent it from being absorbed. Hence, don't take it with vitamin pills if they also contain iron.

WHAT LIQUIDS ARE OK TO WASH DOWN MY CARBIDOPA/LEVODOPA PILLS?

Most fluids are OK to drink when taking your carbidopa/levodopa pills. The exception is milk and milk products (proteins).

Theoretically, products containing the artificial sweetener aspartame should be avoided when taking carbidopa/levodopa. *Aspartame* is metabolized into phenylalanine, which competes with levodopa for transport into the brain. Aspartame is a common sweetener in diet soda pop and sometimes in juices. It is also used to sweeten coffee and tea (NutraSweet, Equal) and is an ingredient is many sugar-free chewing gums. Aspartame in small amounts may not be problematic, but if you are not doing well, check the labels of the liquids you are drinking. Note that aspartame is OK as long as it is not ingested at the same times as you take your carbidopa/levodopa doses.

WHAT IF I EXPERIENCE NO BENEFIT, DESPITE RAISING THE DOSES?

If there is absolutely no benefit, despite going up to 3, or even 3½ tablets three times daily, double-check three things:

1. Are you taking this on an empty stomach, at least 1 hour before meals (not 15 minutes before) and at least 2 hours after the end of meals?

2. Are your carbidopa/levodopa pills yellow? All of the 25/100 immediate-release carbidopa/levodopa tablets are yellow, whether generic or brand name. The Sinemet CR tablets are not yellow and are not interchangeable with regular carbidopa/levodopa.

3. Are you taking any medications that might block the effects of levodopa? Review Chapter 6 for a list of drugs that might do this and avoid taking it with iron pills.

If none of these explains the lack of effect, we may be out of luck. Furthermore, this strongly suggests that the problem is not PD but another parkinsonian disorder (see Chapter 6). This problem is further addressed near the end of this chapter.

CAN I HAVE MY BLOOD LEVELS OF LEVODOPA CHECKED?

Levodopa can be measured in the bloodstream, but this is not done on a routine basis and there are no reference values for determining the ideal dose. The decisions about whether the levodopa dose is adequate must be based on your response.

HOW DO I KNOW IF I AM GETTING TOO MUCH?

The side effects from levodopa are all up front and apparent. There is no potential for any serious liver or kidney toxicity, as can occur with some other drugs. As we discussed, no blood monitoring is necessary to assess toxicity. More is said about potential side effects later in this chapter.

CARBIDOPA/LEVODOPA MAKES ME NAUSEATED

Mild nausea from levodopa therapy usually dissipates with continued use. For a small minority of patients, however, nausea is more troublesome, sometimes with vomiting. For this group of people, other measures are necessary. There are several relatively simple things to try or consider:

1. Carbidopa/levodopa may be taken with non-protein food. Although the nausea does not originate from the stomach (it is due to stimulation of the brain nausea center), food in the stomach may be helpful. Dry bread, toast without butter (or peanut butter), soda crackers, or half of a banana may be tried.

2. Extra carbidopa may be administered. Plain carbidopa without levodopa is available by prescription. It comes in only one size, 25 mg tablets, and goes by the brand name Lodosyn. Take 1 to 2 Lodosyn tablets with or before each dose of carbidopa/levodopa. Unfortunately, Lodosyn is very expensive. Lodosyn can later be reduced or stopped if the nausea abates.

3. Carbidopa/levodopa may be started in even lower doses and increased very slowly. You may start with one-quarter of a 25/100 carbidopa/

levodopa tablet three times daily. It can be increased weekly by raising all three doses by one-quarter tablet increments. The brain nausea center tends to habituate to the levodopa when it is introduced
in tiny amounts and only slowly escalated. The downside of this
scheme is that it may take about 2 to 3 months to arrive at the optimal
levodopa dose.

4. Take other medications separate from carbidopa/levodopa.
   Medications that may be taken with food can be taken after meals.

5. Supplementary PD medications, such as selegiline, rasagiline, or entacapone, enhance levodopa effects, including nausea. Selegiline, rasagiline, and entacapone may be abruptly stopped.

6. If nausea preceded carbidopa/levodopa, your clinician may explore
   whether there is a primary gastrointestinal problem.

A strategy for initiating regular carbidopa/levodopa when nausea is a problem is outlined in Table 12.2. This involves very slow dose escalation, starting with one-quarter tablet doses.

WHY NOT SIMPLY USE ONE OF THE ANTI-NAUSEA DRUGS?

The prescription drugs for reducing nausea most commonly used in
the United States are metoclopramide (Reglan) and prochlorperazine
(Compazine). Unfortunately, they enter the brain and block striatal dopamine receptors, which will potentially worsen parkinsonism and prevent
levodopa from working. Two other anti-nausea drugs also block dopamine
and should also be avoided: promethazine (Phenergan) and thiethylperazine
(Torecan).

Anti-nausea drugs that may be tried for levodopa-induced nausea are
trimethobenzamide (Tigan) and ondansetron (Zofran). Unfortunately, neither is very effective for this purpose, but at least they do not block brain
dopamine or worsen parkinsonism. Trimethobenzamide may be administered as a 250 mg tablet or 300 mg oral capsule taken an hour before each
carbidopa/levodopa dose; alternatively, the 200 mg rectal suppository can
be tried. Ondansetron is an anti-nausea drug often used during cancer che-
motherapy. It typically is administered in a dose of one 8 mg pill two to
three times daily. It has a theoretical potential to prolong the QT interval
on the electrocardiogram, which is a very rare occurrence but with serious
consequences. Hence, it would be judicious to check an electrocardiogram
just after starting ondansetron.

Outside the United States, the potent anti-nausea medication domperidone (Motilium) is available by prescription. This drug blocks dopamine
but does not cross the blood-brain barrier and is thus is well tolerated.
Outside the United States, it is routinely used to treat nausea in those with

Table 12.2.   If Nausea: Initiating Carbidopa/Levodopa 25/100 Regular (Immediate-Release) Tablets*

If there is prominent nausea, start with ¼ carbidopa/levodopa tablet three times daily; increase weekly by adding another ¼ tablet to all three doses. You may increase more slowly if necessary to minimize nausea. Carbidopa/levodopa should be taken at least 1 hour before meals and at least 2 hours after the end of meals. However, take these doses with non-protein products such as soda crackers, half a banana, plain bread or toast to help reduce the nausea. You do not need to have a fixed interval between doses, but take them no less than 3–4 hours apart.

The purpose of this scheme is to find the appropriate dose to continue. When you have gone through the scheme, settle on the dose that works best. If several doses provide the same benefit, remain on the lowest of those equipotent doses. Substantial benefit may require 2 to 2½ tablets three times daily; hopefully, this will be tolerated.

Years later, you will likely need more than three doses daily but the number of pills per dose usually does not substantially change over time. If you feel faint when standing, check your standing blood pressure. If the systolic blood pressure is less than 90, then this needs attention.

Week #1. Start with one-fourth (¼) 25/100 carbidopa/levodopa tablet three times daily.

Week #2. Raise to one-half (½) tablet three times daily.

Week #3. Increase to ¾ tablet three times daily

Week #4. Raise to a full tablet three times per day.

Week #5. Raise to 1 ¼ tablets three times daily.

Week #6 and so on. Continue to raise all three carbidopa/levodopa doses by ¼ tablet, up to 2 ½ tablets three times daily, as tolerated.

After completing this dose escalation scheme, settle on the dose that works best. If there is no improvement on any of the doses, you may taper off over 7–10 days.

*Additional carbidopa (Lodosyn; 25 mg tablets) may be added to each carbidopa/levodopa dose to further reduce nausea. Take 1–2 Lodosyn tablets with or before each carbidopa/levodopa dose. For unclear reasons, plain carbidopa tablets (Lodosyn) are extremely expensive, so for some people this may not be a good alternative.

PD (typically 10–20 mg three times daily). It also may prolong the electrocardiogram QT interval, and this should be checked just after starting this drug or raising the dose.

SINEMET CR FOR INTRACTABLE NAUSEA

Occasionally, the sustained-release formulation of carbidopa/levodopa is tolerated when the regular pills provoke nausea. This is the single situation in which the sustained-release tablets is indicated for initial treatment. Table 12.3 shows the dosing scheme for use of sustained-release carbidopa/levodopa to minimize nausea. Because it does not completely enter the bloodstream, larger levodopa amounts are necessary to equate with

Table 12.3.   Alternative Strategy for More Severe Nausea: Sustained-Release Carbidopa/Levodopa (25/100 Sinemet CR Tablets or Generic)*

If there is prominent nausea, start with ½ of a sustained-release 25/100 carbidopa/levodopa tablet three times daily; increase weekly by adding another ½ tablet to all three doses. You may increase more slowly if necessary to minimize nausea.

Take these pills at least 1 hour before meals and at least 2 hours after the end of meals. However, use non-protein products to help counter the nausea, such as soda crackers, half of a banana, plain bread or toast. You do not need to have a fixed interval between doses, but take them no less than 3–4 hours apart.

The purpose of this scheme is to find the appropriate dose to continue. When you have gone through the scheme, settle on the dose that works best. If several doses provide the same benefit, remain on the lowest of those equipotent doses.

Years later, you will likely need more than three doses daily but the number of pills per dose usually does not substantially change over time.

If you feel faint when standing, check your standing blood pressure. If the systolic blood pressure is less than 90, then this needs attention.

Week #1. Start with one-half (½) 25/100 sustained-release carbidopa/levodopa tablets three times daily.

Week #2. Raise to 1 tablet three times daily.

Week #3. Raise to 1 ½ tablets three times daily.

Week #4. Raise to 2 tablets three times per day.

Week #5. Raise to 2 ½ tablets three times daily.

Week #6. Raise to 2 ½ tablets three times daily.

Week #7. Raise to 3 tablets three times daily.

If tolerated, you may subsequently raise the sustained-release carbidopa/levodopa to 3½, then 4 tablets three times daily.

After completing this dose escalation scheme, settle on the dose that works best.

If there is no improvement on any of the doses, you may taper off over 7–10 days.

*Additional carbidopa (Lodosyn; 25 mg tablets) may be added to each carbidopa/levodopa dose to further reduce nausea. Take 1–2 Lodosyn tablets with or before each carbidopa/levodopa dose. For unclear reasons, plain carbidopa tablets (Lodosyn) are extremely expensive, so for some people this may not be a good alternative.

regular carbidopa/levodopa; hence the reason for raising the dose as high as 300–400 mg of levodopa three times daily.

IF I'M NAUSEATED FROM LEVODOPA, WHY NOT SWITCH TO A DOPAMINE AGONIST DRUG?

Unfortunately, dopamine agonists (pramipexole, ropinirole, rotigotine) also cause nausea because they similarly stimulate dopamine receptors in the brainstem. They may be tolerated in very low doses in those prone to nausea, but when raised to levels sufficient to improve parkinsonism, they also provoke nausea in susceptible people. Moreover, use of an agonist is a stop-gap measure; after a few years, nearly everyone with PD will need carbidopa/levodopa.

WILL CARBIDOPA/LEVODOPA HELP NON-MOVEMENT PROBLEMS?

Not all PD symptoms relate to movement, walking or tremor. A variety of non-movement problems also have a dopamine substrate and may benefit from carbidopa/levodopa treatment. This includes insomnia, anxiety, restlessness, and sometimes depression. These are discussed in subsequent chapters, including Chapters 19, 20, and 22.

Side Effects from Levodopa Therapy

Carbidopa/levodopa is generally well tolerated. The nausea that we discussed is problematic in only a small minority of people. Carbidopa/levodopa has no potential for internal organ toxicity (i.e., it will not damage the liver, kidneys, heart, or lungs). The only serious side effect that may occur early in levodopa treatment is orthostatic hypotension, which may result in fainting or near-fainting. This problem can be anticipated in susceptible people and is treatable. This was discussed in Chapter 11, but a few points deserve further discussion.

LOW BLOOD PRESSURE WHEN UPRIGHT (ORTHOSTATIC HYPOTENSION)

Chapter 11 provided principles for assessing the potential for clinically important orthostatic hypotension. These may be summarized:

- Focus on the systolic value of the blood pressure (BP), which is the upper number in BP readings (i.e., the "120" in a reading of 120/80).

- People susceptible to this problem will tend to have a normal BP when sitting but a low value when standing or walking.

- The lowest BP readings of the day are typically after breakfast, which is a good time to assess this.

- Before starting carbidopa/levodopa, we want the standing systolic BP to be at least 100. (Recall that BP units are given in millimeters of mercury, which we are ignoring here for simplicity's sake).

- While taking carbidopa/levodopa, we want the standing systolic BP to remain above 90; if it drops below that, additional measures need to be taken.

- Low BP values should trigger a review of medications plus limited blood tests to be certain no medical conditions (e.g., anemia) are contributing.

- Fluid losses such as vomiting or diarrhea will exacerbate low BP values.

- Salt and fluid intake help maintain BP levels.

- Chapter 21 focuses on this problem with specific treatment advice. Medications that may cause a low BP are listed in that chapter.

DYSKINESIAS

If you read about PD online, you may encounter admonitions about the use of carbidopa/levodopa as it may cause dyskinesias. Levodopa therapy certainly can provoke dyskinesias, but this is very rare during the early years except in very young people with PD (e.g., PD onset before age 40 years). Moreover, such levodopa dyskinesias can always be eliminated by reducing the levodopa dose. Among seniors over age 70 years, the risk of dyskinesias after 5 years of carbidopa/levodopa treatment is estimated at 16%. Thus, the concern about levodopa dyskinesias is often extremely overstated.

Dyskinesias from levodopa are often confused with certain of the motor problems of PD. Dystonia such as cramping of the toes or feet (e.g., toe curling or foot inversion) are symptoms of PD and nearly always represent a dopamine deficiency, not excess; these respond to more, not less levodopa. Inner restlessness is another levodopa-responsive symptom of PD (akathisia) that should not be misinterpreted as levodopa dyskinesias. Finally, the tremor of PD is sometimes misconstrued as dyskinesias, but it can easily be recognized by the repetitive, rhythmic movements that typify tremor.

Dyskinesias and how to recognize and treat them are covered in detail in Chapter 17. Read that chapter if you think they are occurring when starting on carbidopa/levodopa; there may be another explanation.

HALLUCINATIONS

Hallucinations imply seeing something that is not there. They may be provoked by levodopa treatment, but this is uncommon unless certain other drugs are also being administered. Even among those with advanced PD, carbidopa/levodopa is not highly likely to provoke hallucinations unless other drugs that enter the brain are administered. Any of the lesser drugs for treating PD (e.g., selegiline, rasagiline) may provoke hallucinations when used concurrently with carbidopa/levodopa. Thus if hallucinations develop when starting carbidopa/levodopa, review your list of drugs and consult Chapter 24.

Carbidopa/Levodopa Failures

If you experience no benefit from taking carbidopa/levodopa, despite adhering to these guidelines (i.e., correct formulation; escalated doses taken on an empty stomach), you probably do not have PD but may have one of the conditions discussed in Chapter 6. Before reaching that conclusion, however, review your medication list for any of the parkinsonism-inducing drugs listed in Chapter 6.

If there is absolutely no improvement with carbidopa/levodopa, there is no purpose in continuing it. It may be slowly tapered off over 7–10 days; you may use the dose escalation scheme shown in Table 12.1 in reverse, but lowering the dosage every day or every other day instead of weekly. This tapered dose reduction allows you to assess any possible benefit one last time. As the dosage is lowered, you may recognize deterioration, which would suggest that it has been beneficial.

Will Any Other Drugs Help If There Is No Levodopa Benefit?

If you did everything according to the guidelines in this book, and if there is no response to adequate doses of carbidopa/levodopa, the options are very limited. The dopamine agonist medications (pramipexole, ropinirole, and rotigotine) also work through brain dopamine systems. If the most potent dopamine drug, carbidopa/levodopa, failed, there is no good reason that a dopamine agonist would work.

Amantadine has mild anti-parkinsonian effects that are primarily mediated via non-dopamine mechanisms. It may be tried if carbidopa/levodopa failed, but the benefit will be modest at best. It is helpful in treating dyskinesias that complicate levodopa therapy (discussed in Chapter 18), but that is a different topic. The usual amantadine starting dose is a single 100 mg tablet twice daily. After a week it can be raised to three times daily and could be escalated as high as 5 tablets a day. It commonly causes a reversible fishnet pattern of skin discoloration of the legs, which is not worrisome. Occasionally, it will cause confusion or hallucinations.

If tremor is a problem and has not responded to carbidopa/levodopa, medication strategies outlined in Chapter 14 can be used. Very troublesome tremor responds well to deep brain stimulation (DBS), discussed in Chapter 33. Unfortunately, other aspects of levodopa-unresponsive parkinsonism besides tremor do not benefit from DBS.

Adding Carbidopa/Levodopa to Dopamine Agonist Therapy

Although I favor carbidopa/levodopa as the initial drug choice for treating PD, not all clinicians agree with this choice. Certain physicians may choose a dopamine agonist—pramipexole, ropinirole, or rotigotine. Chapter 13 provides guidelines for starting a dopamine agonist as the first drug; this allows readers of this book to still work with their clinicians even if the treatment perspective differs from mine. However, the dopamine agonists will not be adequate indefinitely, even in high doses. At some point, carbidopa/levodopa will be necessary. Hence, a strategy is necessary for those taking a dopamine agonist but with increasing parkinsonism.

For those on a dopamine agonist that is not adequately treating parkinsonism, one choice is to increase the agonist dose. The next chapter puts this into perspective. Low agonist doses can be raised toward the target dose of the agonist. However, if the dopamine agonist is close to the target dose but there is still substantial parkinsonism, the addition of carbidopa/levodopa is likely necessary. What to do with the agonist at that juncture depends on the overall response:

- If the dopamine agonist is causing substantial side effects, it may be necessary to taper it off before starting carbidopa/levodopa. Remember to change only one medication at a time.

- If the agonist is beneficial but insufficient, it can be maintained in the current dose and carbidopa/levodopa then added.

The guidelines for initiating carbidopa/levodopa provided earlier in this chapter are also appropriate for those already taking a dopamine agonist drug (Table 12.1). However, with the concurrent dopamine agonist, you may not need to raise the carbidopa/levodopa dose as high. If you achieve good control of the parkinsonism, you don't need to elevate the levodopa dose to the maximum.

Although carbidopa/levodopa should be taken on an empty stomach, the dopamine agonist medication is usually taken with meals; however, if you are not nauseated, you may take the agonist drug at the same time as your carbidopa/levodopa, about 1 hour before meals. Follow through with the weekly escalation schedule shown in Table 12.1. Advance the carbidopa/levodopa dose until you capture the optimum benefit.

If the combination of agonist drug and carbidopa/levodopa results in dyskinesias, then reduce the carbidopa/levodopa dose by small decrements to capture the effect that works best. Note that the combination of carbidopa/levodopa and the dopamine agonist may provoke side effects that may not occur if taking carbidopa/levodopa alone. Thus hallucinations might develop as you add carbidopa/levodopa to a stable agonist dose. In that case, it would usually be wise to reduce or taper off the agonist. Restated, reduce your levodopa doses to counter dyskinesias, but reduce or eliminate the dopamine agonist to counter hallucinations.

13

◆ ◆ ◆

Starting Dopamine
Agonist Treatment

The dopamine agonists pramipexole, ropinirole, and rotigotine behave like synthetic forms of dopamine. They are not nearly as efficacious as carbidopa/levodopa but have longer durations in the circulation. They are used to treat Parkinson's disease (PD) in two situations:

1. As the initial PD medication, and

2. Added to carbidopa/levodopa later in the course to help counter motor fluctuations.

In Chapter 11, I provided my rationale for selecting carbidopa/levodopa as initial treatment for PD, but recognize that other physicians may disagree. In my practice, the primary exception is among those with young-onset PD (onset before age 40 years), who notoriously tend to be very prone to unstable levodopa responses. Hence, I may start with a dopamine agonist in that age group. If PD starts in middle age and beyond, I nearly always start carbidopa/levodopa. The other indication for a dopamine agonist is among those already on levodopa and experiencing unstable responses, which may surface after a number of years. The dopamine agonists have longer durations of effect and may be added to attenuate the levodopa "off" states.

The strategies for starting and escalating the dopamine agonists are similar whether used as the first PD drug or later in the course for control of levodopa fluctuations. The specific dosing guidelines are provided in this chapter. Further details pertaining to the use of agonists when added to help control levodopa fluctuations are found in Chapter 18.

Background

Dopamine agonist medications directly stimulate brain dopamine receptors. The three agonists that are available in the United States for chronic use are:

Pramipexole (Mirapex) available in regular and sustained-release tablets

Ropinirole (Requip) available in regular and sustained-release tablets

Rotigotine (Neupro) skin patch

Their affinity for brain dopamine receptors is predominantly restricted to the D3 class; these drugs have substantially less binding affinity for the other four classes of dopamine receptors.

Another dopamine agonist, apomorphine, is available as "rescue therapy" for levodopa-off states. This has broad-spectrum affinity for all the dopamine receptors, with efficacy similar to carbidopa/levodopa. However, it is available only for subcutaneous injection, with an effect that lasts 60–90 minutes. This will be discussed further in Chapter 18 and will not be addressed further in this chapter.

Characteristics of the three dopamine agonist medications that are used for chronic treatment are shown in Table 13.1. Note differences in the mg-potency. Whereas ropinirole and rotigotine have approximately the same mg-to-mg correspondence, pramipexole is about 3 times more potent in terms of mg. However, when adjusted for the differences in mg-potency, these drugs have approximately the same efficacy. Restated, even though pramipexole requires fewer mg for a given benefit, that does not translate into a better effect, allowing for the mg dose adjustments.

When Is a Dopamine Agonist a Poor Choice?

The dopamine agonist drugs are much more likely to cause hallucinations and delusions than the other PD drugs. This problem is unlikely in most people, but those with dementia or previous hallucinations/delusions are at risk and dopamine agonists should not be used. Chapter 24 addresses this in more detail.

As discussed in Chapter 10, pathological compulsive behaviors may be provoked by any of these three dopamine agonists. People who are struggling with bad habits (e.g., gambling, smoking, excessive alcohol use, sexual proclivities) should not be started on one of these agonist drugs.

Table 13.1.   Dopamine Agonist Medications*

Generic Name	Brand Name	Tablet, Capsule, Patch Sizes	Typical Daily Target Dose (and Maximum Dose)
Pramipexole Regular**	Mirapex	0.125, 0.25, 0.5, 0.75, 1.0, 1.5 mg	3–4.5 mg (6 mg)
Sustained-release	Mirapex ER	0.375, 0.75, 1.50, 2.25, 3.0, 3.75, 4.5 mg	
Ropinirole Regular**	Requip	0.25, 0.5, 1, 2, 3, 4, 5 mg	9–12 mg (24 mg)
Sustained-release	Requip XL	2, 4, 6, 8, 12 mg	
Rotigotine (skin patch)	Neupro	Patch sizes: 1, 2, 3, 4, 6, 8 mg	8 mg ***

* See Chapter 11 for cost comparisons.

** Available as generic.

*** The recommended maximum dose is the same as the target dose for the Neupro patch: 8 mg. In practice, higher doses of rotigotine are sometimes used, but published guidelines are lacking. Note that ropinirole and rotigotine have a mg-to-mg correspondence and theoretically, the rotigotine dosage should be similar to ropinirole.

Finally, the dopamine agonists may induce drowsiness. Among those who are already excessively sleepy, it would be wise to defer starting an agonist until this has been sorted out and treated.

Are the Agonists Expensive?

If the expense of your prescription medications is a concern, review Table 11.3, which shows the costs. The cost of the regular formulations of both ropinirole and pramipexole (i.e., not sustained-release) has recently plummeted, since they can be prescribed as generic (they have gone off patent). However, the sustained-release formulations of the agonists are very expensive (still on patent), and the rotigotine patch (on patent) is even more costly. Comparatively, carbidopa/levodopa is very cheap.

Which Agonist Should We Choose?

Head-to-head studies of these agonist drugs are lacking. However, the general experience suggests similar anti-parkinsonian efficacy when adjusted for dosing (mg-mg) differences. Side effects are also similar when comparable doses are used.

Certain side effects appear less with the rotigotine patch; however, the dosing range advised by the pharmaceutical company is substantially lower for rotigotine than for pramipexole or ropinirole when considering the mg-potency. Note that ropinirole and rotigotine have similar mg-efficacy, yet the conventional dose ceiling for rotigotine is substantially less than that given for ropinirole.

Factors that may affect the choice of agonist are the route of administration (oral versus patch) or once-daily versus three times daily administration (i.e., patch or sustained-release formulations, versus regular pramipexole or ropinirole). Expense may also influence the choice of agonist.

Multiple Steps to the Target Dose

All three agonist drugs require graduated escalation over many weeks to achieve a dose that improves symptoms. The starting doses are too low to provide benefit; hence patience is necessary. Doses are escalated until "target" doses are reached. These target doses are a bit arbitrary but represent approximate amounts that are likely to capture meaningful benefit and yet are tolerated:

Pramipexole: 3–4.5 mg daily

Ropinirole: 9–12 mg daily

Rotigotine: 8 mg daily

Table 13.1 shows not only the target doses but also the maximum doses. Doses beyond these maximum values are substantially more likely to induce side effects. Common sense dictates that if you identify a dose that works very well and is tolerated, you should remain on that dose even if less than the target.

Note that the most common cause of dopamine agonist failure is too low a dose. Typically this occurs when the dose is not raised after the first week or two. The *minimum* daily doses of the agonist drugs likely to achieve perceptible benefit are approximately:

Pramipexole: 2 mg

Ropinirole: 6 mg

Rotigotine: 6 mg

You have probably noted that the rotigotine target dose is only slightly higher than the minimum dose likely to provide benefit. Presumably, this relates to how one defines benefit.

The oral agonists (pramipexole and ropinirole) work equally well if taken with food instead of on an empty stomach. Conventionally, they are taken with meals to minimize nausea.

Side Effects from a Dopamine Agonist Suggesting It Will Not Be Tolerated

Those already experiencing hallucinations should not start a dopamine agonist, and if these begin after the agonist is initiated it should be tapered off. Daytime drowsiness is common in PD and is treatable (see Chapter 20). However, if new drowsiness begins after starting an agonist, this also indicates the need to either reduce or discontinue this drug (unless there is another explanation). In either case, one should not drive until these problems have resolved.

Pathological behaviors (e.g., compulsive gambling, sexual ideation, spending) triggered by dopamine agonists were discussed in Chapter 10. If one of these problems surfaces, the dopamine agonist drug should be tapered off. These are difficult to control until the agonist is out of the system. The spouse, partner, or other family members should be aware of this potential before beginning a dopamine agonist, since the person experiencing this may not have insight to recognize this problem.

Dosing Schemes for Dopamine Agonist Medications

Pramipexole and ropinirole each have two formulations, regular and sustained-release. The dose escalation schemes for these two formulations are obviously different. Rotigotine is only offered as a skin patch, hence there is only one schedule for that drug. There are multiple ways that these drugs may be raised from very low doses into therapeutic ranges. The provided schedules are slightly arbitrary; departures are acceptable as long as the starting dose is low and escalated over weeks. The goal for initial treatment is the same as for carbidopa/levodopa: reverse parkinsonism sufficiently for people to remain active and fully engaged in their life. The goal for the addition of a dopamine agonist to carbidopa/levodopa later in the course is specifically to smooth fluctuations, that is, to counter levodopa short-duration responses that result in frequent off states; this is discussed in detail in Chapter 18.

Multiple pill (or patch) sizes are necessary for dose escalation and care must be taken to not confuse the different pills. Following are five schemes corresponding to each of the drugs and the respective formulations. They are directed at escalating up to the so-called target doses. However, if a lower dose is providing excellent benefit, that dose should be maintained. As with any drug, if several doses are equally effective, settle on the lowest of those equipotent doses.

PRAMIPEXOLE (MIRAPEX), REGULAR FORMULATION (IMMEDIATE-RELEASE)

When pramipexole was first introduced, the target dose was 4.5 mg daily (1.5 mg three times daily). However, clinicians often favor a slightly lower target dose of 3 mg daily (1 mg three times daily). The schedule shown in Table 13.2 allows for either target dose. Perceptible benefits should start around week 4.

Table 13.2 shows a scheme for escalating regular pramipexole into the therapeutic range, utilizing only two pill sizes, 0.25 mg and 1 mg. These pills are usually scored and can be broken in half. Ultimately, a 1.5 mg pill can be substituted if settling on the 4.5 mg daily dose (i.e., 1.5 mg three times daily).

PRAMIPEXOLE SUSTAINED-RELEASE FORMULATION (MIRAPEX ER)

The sustained-release formulation of pramipexole is easier to use in one sense—it is given in once-daily doses; however, it requires multiple different pill sizes: 0.375, 0.75, 1.50, 2.25, 3.0, 3.75, and 4.5 mg. The pills are very expensive—much more expensive than the generic regular formulation (see Table 11.3). Furthermore, they are priced so that administering two pills to make a higher dose approximately doubles the expense (e.g., two of the 0.375 mg tablets to make 0.75 mg). Thus, if the target dose is 4.5 mg daily, seven prescriptions are necessary; if the target dose is 3 mg daily, then five prescriptions are needed. If that is acceptable, then the scheme is simple:

Week 1: 0.375 mg once daily

Week 2: 0.75 mg once daily

Week 3: 1.5 mg once daily

Week 4: 2.25 mg once daily

Week 5: 3 mg once daily

Week 6: 3.75 mg once daily

Week 7: 4.5 mg once daily

As with regular pramipexole, perceptible benefit should first be recognized around week 4.

Table 13.2.   Pramipexole (Mirapex) Regular (Immediate-Release) Formulation

Week	Tablet(s), Milligrams (mg)	Take Each Dose 3 Times Daily (with Food to Minimize Nausea)	Total Number of Tablets per Day	Amount Each Dose (mg)	Total Daily Dose (mg)
1	0.25 mg	½ tablet	1 ½	0.125	0.375 mg
2	0.25 mg	1 tablet	3	0.25	0.75 mg
3	1 mg	½ tablet	1 ½	0.5	1.5 mg
4	0.25 mg and 1 mg	One-half 1 mg tablet and one 0.25 mg tablet	1 ½ of the 1 mg tablets and 3 of the 0.25 mg tablets	0.75	2.25 mg
5	1 mg	1 tablet	3	1	3 mg
6	0.25 mg and 1 mg	One 1 mg tablet and one 0.25 mg tablet	3 of both the 1 mg and 0.25 mg tablets	1.25	3.75 mg
7	0.25 mg and 1 mg	One 1 mg tablet and two 0.25 mg tablets	3 of the 1 mg tablets and 6 of the 0.25 mg tablets	1.5	4.5 mg*

*You may substitute one 1.5 mg tablet, three times daily, to make the same dose; do this if 4.5 mg daily is going to be maintained. The maximum advisable dose is 6 mg daily.

General comments relating to this scheme:

- Each dose is taken three times daily. Escalate the total daily doses up to 3 mg to 4.5 mg. If there is an excellent result on a lower dose, you may remain on that.
- Do not increase the dose if excessive drowsiness or hallucinations occur (also do not drive a car).
- Check your standing blood pressure occasionally to make certain it is not low. We want your standing systolic blood pressures to be over 90.
- You will need prescriptions for two tablet sizes for this schedule: 0.25 mg and 1 mg. If ultimately settling on 4.5 mg daily, you may substitute 1.5 mg tablets (3 times daily).

This sustained-release tablet may be taken at any time each day, but doses should be about 20–24 hours apart. It may be taken with or without food. The sustained-release drugs depend on the pill being swallowed whole for their slow-release effect. They should not be chewed or crushed, which will prevent the slowed release.

The drowsiness that occurs in a minority of those taking a dopamine agonist is more difficult to recognize with the sustained-release formulation. With immediate-release pramipexole, those susceptible to this side effect experience sleepiness about an hour after each dose. The sustained-release formulation is much slower to kick in and the temporal relationship to the dose may be inapparent.

ROPINIROLE (REQUIP), REGULAR FORMULATION (IMMEDIATE-RELEASE)

For the regular formulation, the ropinirole initiation strategy is similar to that of pramipexole but uses more pill sizes. Ropinirole tablets are not scored in the middle and it is difficult, if not impossible, to break them in half. Our schedule will require four tablet sizes, as shown in Table 13.3.

Perceptible benefits should start around week 6, with the dose of 2 mg three times daily. As with pramipexole, it may not be necessary to push the dose to the target level; if a given dose is working well, stick with that.

ROPINIROLE SUSTAINED-RELEASE FORMULATION (REQUIP XL)

The daily total starting dose that is advised by the pharmaceutical company is a little higher with the sustained-release pills than with the regular formulation. Thus it is begun with a dose of 2 mg once daily. As with sustained-release pramipexole, this formulation of ropinirole should not be chewed or crushed, which will prevent the slow release.

The sustained-release formulation of ropinirole is very costly, and even more so when prescribed as brand name Requip XL (see Table 11.3). If expense is a concern, the regular formulation is clearly preferable. The cost of the smaller size tablets of sustained-release ropinirole is somewhat proportional to the mg amount; however, that is no longer the case with larger pill sizes. Hence, the most cost-effective and efficient strategy for starting this formulation is with a different pill size for each increment. The pharmaceutical company recommends starting with 2 mg once daily and increasing the daily dose by 2 mg every 1–2 weeks. Assuming a target dose of 12 mg daily, this translates into:

Weeks 1–2: 2 mg once daily

Weeks 3–4: 4 mg once daily

Weeks 5–6: 6 mg once daily

Weeks 7–8: 8 mg once daily

Weeks 9–10: 10 mg once daily

Weeks 11–12: 12 mg once daily

Table 13.3.   Ropinirole (Requip), Regular (Immediate-Release) Formulation

Week	Tablet(s) Size, Milligrams (mg)	Take Each Dose 3 Times Daily (with Food to Minimize Nausea)	Amount, Each Dose	Total Daily Dose (mg)
1	0.25 mg	1 tablet	0.25 mg	0.75 mg
2	0.5 mg	1 tablet	0.5 mg	1.5 mg
3	0.25 plus 0.5 mg	1 tablet of each size	0.75 mg	2.25 mg
4	1 mg	1 tablet	1.0 mg	3 mg
5	0.5 and 1 mg	1 tablet of each size	1.5 mg	4.5 mg
6	2 mg	1 tablet	2.0 mg	6 mg
7	0.5 and 2 mg	1 tablet of each size	2.5 mg	7.5 mg
8	1.0 and 2 mg	1 tablet of each size	3.0 mg	9 mg
9	2 mg*	2 tablets	4.0	12 mg**

* If remaining on a dose of 4 mg three times daily, you may substitute a 4 mg tablet for two of the 2 mg tablets.

** Note that a higher dose may be recommended by your physician, up to as high as 8 mg three times daily.

General comments relating to this scheme:

• Each dose is taken three times daily. Escalate the total daily dose to 9 mg to 12 mg. You should remain on a lower dose if there is an excellent response.

• Do not increase the dose if excessive drowsiness or hallucinations occur (also do not drive a car).

• Check your standing blood pressure occasionally to make certain it is not low. We want your standing systolic blood pressures to be over 90.

• You will need prescriptions for four different tablet sizes for this schedule: 0.25 mg, 0.5 mg, 1 mg, and 2 mg. Note that ropinirole also comes in 4 mg and 5 mg sizes.

Thus, if easily tolerated and advancing every week, this target dose could be achieved by 6 weeks. As with sustained-release pramipexole, the pills should be taken at intervals of 20–24 hours. It may be administered at any time during the 24-hour cycle and taken with meals if nausea is a concern. Perceptible benefit should start around 6 mg daily. Be aware that if substantial drowsiness ensues, this might be a side effect of ropinirole, even if not precisely time-locked to the dose. Do not drive if drowsy.

ROTIGOTINE PATCHES (NEUPRO)

In my view, to justify the expense of the Neupro patch, it should cure PD (see Table 11.3); it does not. The symptomatic benefit is similar to ropinirole, mg to mg. Pricing relates to each patch rather than the mg amount. Hence, using two patches per day doubles the price of an already very costly medication; using a patch with more mg is appropriate since it costs about the same as a patch with fewer mg of rotigotine. The pharmaceutical company advises starting with a 2 mg patch placed on the skin once daily. It may be increased weekly by 2 mg. Thus the scheme directed to a target dose of 8 mg may be summarized as follows:

> Week 1: 2 mg patch
>
> Week 2: 4 mg patch
>
> Week 3: 6 mg patch
>
> Week 4: 8 mg patch

Recognizing the similar mg-potency to ropinirole, higher doses should theoretically be more efficacious. However, the pharmaceutical company does not encourage that and their pricing scheme clearly discourages such a practice (i.e., requiring more than one patch daily).

The patch should be applied at approximately the same time each day (i.e., every 20–24 hours). It should be placed on different regions of the body to avoid a rash and should not be returned to the same body location until 2 weeks elapse. It should not be applied to unwashed or hairy regions, or to skin where lotions have been applied; these may inhibit absorption. It is advised to apply pressure over the patch for 30 seconds when first placed. Old patches should be taken off daily. The patch should be removed before undergoing an MRI scan. As with the sustained-release oral agonists, rotigotine may induce sleepiness that may not be recognized because of the insidious onset.

A Common Reason for Dopamine Agonist Failures

The starting doses of the agonists are subtherapeutic. People often become stuck on one of the initial doses of these lengthy dose escalation schedules. The doses employed in the first 2 to 4 weeks are rarely of substantial benefit.

Newly Developing Side Effects While Raising Agonist Doses

As already discussed in Chapter 10, pathological compulsive behaviors may occur after starting one of these dopamine agonists. This is characterized

by excessive engagement in one or more of a variety of inherently rewarding activities, such as gambling, shopping, or eating. Obsessive sexual ideation with inappropriate sexual proclivities may develop. In most cases, these
behaviors are out of character and never surfaced before the dopamine agonist was started. Usually, these develop insidiously, often noted months after
the agonist was initiated and the dose escalated into the therapeutic range.
If these behaviors surface, the agonist nearly always needs to be tapered to
zero. More information regarding this will be provided in Chapter 24.

The three available dopamine agonists also have potential to provoke hallucinations (i.e., seeing imaginary people or objects), as well as delusions
(illogical, inappropriate thoughts, such as paranoia). If these surface, typically the agonist needs to be tapered to zero.

Daytime sleepiness starting after the agonist was initiated typically
requires dose reduction and usually elimination. Note that drowsiness is
common in PD in general and often is due to poor sleep (sometimes sleep
degraded by sleep apnea). However, if prominent sleepiness develops after
starting an agonist and has no other explanation, this typically signals the
need to taper off. Although drowsiness may dissipate on a lower agonist
dose, this reduced dose is often subtherapeutic, with no benefit.

An alternative strategy to tapering off the dopamine agonist if serious
side effects develop (e.g., pathological behaviors, hallucinations, delusions,
or sleep attacks) would be to simply lower the agonist dose. In most cases,
however, dose reduction sufficient to eliminate these problems is too low to
treat parkinsonism, and the low dosage may still provoke these side effects.

Among those taking an agonist for many months to years, tapering off
the drug must be done slowly. Long-term dopamine agonist use may make
it difficult to eliminate this drug, which can be challenging to both the clinician and patient. Hence, if any of the above troublesome conditions surface
early in treatment, it is advisable to taper off sooner rather than later.

Finally, chronic dopamine agonist therapy occasionally causes swelling of
the legs. While this is not dangerous it is sometimes is difficult to treat unless
the agonist is discontinued. Note, however, that there are other reasons for
leg swelling, some serious (e.g., leg vein clot; congestive heart failure). New
development of one tender, swollen leg may signal a blood clot (deep vein
thrombosis), which requires urgent attention. On the benign side, spending
much of the day sitting predisposes to leg swelling.

A few other side effects from the dopamine agonist drugs do not require
discontinuation and should be treatable: nausea, low blood pressure (orthostatic hypotension), and dyskinesias. These deserve discussion here.

> *Nausea* from agonist therapy can sometimes be circumvented by raising
> the doses more slowly than shown in the dosage schedules; people
> tend to acclimate to this side effect. As with levodopa, there is no dan-
> ger of stomach ulcers; the nausea is mediated via brain nausea centers.

Unlike levodopa therapy, dopamine agonist drugs may be taken with food, which helps attenuate nausea.

Orthostatic hypotension may be provoked by the dopamine agonist drugs. This may result in fainting, near-fainting, or chronic lightheadedness. As discussed in Chapter 11, we want the standing systolic blood pressure to be over 90. It is wise to check the standing blood pressure before starting the agonist and then occasionally while the dose is being raised. If readings less than 90 are documented, do not continue to raise the agonist dose. This should be discussed with your physician. General guidelines for treating this are found in Chapter 21.

Dyskinesias are rare when dopamine agonists are taken without carbidopa/levodopa. If they occur in the absence of carbidopa/levodopa, they are usually mild and do not affect functioning or cause embarrassment; nothing needs to be done. Note that other movements are frequently mistaken for dyskinesias. Chapters 17 and 18 define dyskinesias and how to distinguish those from dystonia, tremor, or restlessness (akathisia); these three conditions typically represent inadequate dopamine replenishment, whereas true dyskinesias indicate an excessive dopamine response. You may wish to review the definitions in Chapters 17 and 18 if suspicious of dyskinesias. Movements that are truly dyskinesias will resolve with medication reduction. If you are taking only a dopamine agonist, then lowering the agonist dose should lead to resolution. On the other hand, if you are adding an agonist to carbidopa/levodopa, the appropriate strategy to eliminate dyskinesias is to slightly lower the carbidopa/levodopa dose; typically, a half-tablet carbidopa/levodopa (25/100) reduction for all doses is sufficient. Once symptoms are resolved with levodopa reduction, the dopamine agonist may continue to be escalated, guided by the response. Note that a dopamine agonist may be initiated when someone is already experiencing dyskinesias from carbidopa/levodopa alone. After the carbidopa/levodopa is reduced to eliminate the dyskinesias, the agonist dose can be raised until the dyskinesias worsen, followed by further small reduction of the carbidopa/levodopa doses.

How to Discontinue a Dopamine Agonist Drug

If certain agonist side effects are problematic, such as hallucinations or pathological compulsive behaviors, the agonist may need to be discontinued. As is true for most drugs, it is advisable to taper off the medication rather than stop it abruptly. To do this, you can reverse the steps in the dosing schedules provided earlier; however, you may not need to go as slowly when doing this in reverse. The rapidity of dose reduction depends on the dose and how long it has been taken. In general, if the daily dose is below the therapeutic values cited earlier in the chapter (i.e., 2 mg of pramipexole or 6 mg of either ropinirole or rotigotine), the agonist may be tapered off over 7–14 days. Doses of the oral agonists that are around the target values (i.e., 3–4.5 mg of pramipexole or 9–12 mg of ropinirole daily) should be tapered off over 3–4 weeks or even longer if taking one of those drugs for many months. The rotigotine patch may be tapered off by reducing the daily dose by 2 mg every 3–4 days if at the target dose of 8 mg or less. The tapering schedules are arbitrary and should be guided by the responses; slow down the dose reduction if that seems appropriate.

When the Agonist Proves Insufficient: Adding Carbidopa/Levodopa

If a dopamine agonist was the first and only medication for PD, there will come a time when the benefit is not adequate. Obviously, the agonist dose may first be increased to the target range (if tolerated); however, if prominent parkinsonism remains, carbidopa/levodopa would then be appropriate.

To proceed, the first question is whether to taper off or maintain the dopamine agonist. Unless there are side effects, most clinicians would advise continuing the agonist and adding carbidopa/levodopa. If there is a reason to reduce or eliminate the agonist, that should be done before starting carbidopa/levodopa to avoid changing two medications at the same time.

The strategy for adding carbidopa/levodopa is the same as that outlined in Chapter 12, using the immediate-release 25/100 formulation. The starting carbidopa/levodopa dose is 1 tablet three times daily (on an empty stomach). It is increased by adding a half-tablet to all three doses weekly up to 2 ½ tablets three times daily. Note that less carbidopa/levodopa will likely be necessary if the dopamine agonist is continued; hence the reason for specifying a ceiling dose of 2 ½ tablets (each dose, not per day). Ultimately, settle on the carbidopa/levodopa dose that works best. If several doses all work the same, then settle on the lowest of those equally effective doses.

Certain side effects are due to the combined effect when adding carbidopa/levodopa to dopamine agonist treatment. The most concerning are pathological compulsive behaviors, hallucinations, and delusional thinking; presumably these would not have been provoked by plain carbidopa/levodopa. They require tapering off the dopamine agonist, with a tapering strategy as discussed earlier. During the agonist tapering, the carbidopa/levodopa dose should not be escalated. Once the problematic side effects resolve, carbidopa/levodopa can be raised to therapeutic levels.

When a Dopamine Agonist Is
Added to Carbidopa/Levodopa

As discussed in prior chapters, the response to carbidopa/levodopa becomes less stable after years of PD. Short-duration levodopa responses surface with the beneficial effect lasting hours after each dose and then wearing off. As will be addressed in Chapter 17, the usual first step is adjustment of carbidopa/levodopa dosage (i.e., shortening the carbidopa/levodopa dosing interval to match the response duration; adding extra doses each day as necessary). If that is insufficient, other medications are sometimes added, including dopamine agonists. Because these agonists have very long effects, they help smooth out the fluctuations. Unfortunately, they are not as efficacious as levodopa so they never totally eliminate fluctuations.

Before starting a dopamine agonist in this situation, the carbidopa/levodopa dosing scheme should be optimized. The agonist is then started and escalated using the schemes outlined in this chapter. These specific strategies are discussed in further detail in Chapter 18.

14

♦ ♦ ♦

Refractory Tremor Syndromes: "Medications Don't Help My Tremor!"

Parkinsonian rest tremor often is controlled with carbidopa/levodopa therapy (less commonly with a dopamine agonist). Sometimes, however, it is not completely abolished but is markedly attenuated. With treatment, it may come and go, especially surfacing during times of stress or nervousness.

Note that tremor is conspicuous, unlike bradykinesia and other aspects of parkinsonism, which blend into the background. A mild degree of slowness (bradykinesia) might go unnoticed, unlike tremor.

Excitement sabotages tremor control, seemingly overriding the effect of medications. Both good stress (e.g., an exciting sporting event) and bad stress are equally likely to provoke tremor. During times of major stress, tremor is likely to recur despite otherwise perfect control with carbidopa/levodopa treatment. However, this is transient, time-locked to the stressor.

This chapter focuses on people with prominent tremor that overall is poorly responsive to levodopa. This may occur in one of several settings:

- Inadequate or inappropriate medication administration

- Break-through tremor (tremor comes and goes)

- Only partial tremor control (despite maximum treatment)
- Benign tremulous parkinsonism
- Not PD, but a variant of essential tremor
- Combination of PD and essential tremor

We will discuss each of these settings.

Inadequate Medication Dosing

Dopamine agonists usually do not control the rest tremor of PD nearly as well as levodopa. Thus, if taking only an agonist medication, the strategy is simple: add levodopa therapy (see Chapter 12).

If already taking carbidopa/levodopa, consider whether you have followed all the guidelines in Chapter 12, including:

- Using the immediate-release 25/100 formulation (the controlled-release is not fully absorbed), and
- Taking it on an empty stomach (dietary protein blocks the effect).

Sometimes higher than the usual doses of carbidopa/levodopa are required to control tremor. If the tremor isn't responding to more moderate doses, slowly push the dose up to 3 tablets of the 25/100 immediate-release formulation of carbidopa/levodopa three times per day (at least 1 hour before each meal and at least 2 hours after the end of meals). If after a couple of weeks on this dose the tremor persists, then read on.

Break-Through Tremor

Some people report poor control of their tremor when, in fact, this is true only part of the time. In other words, the tremor is indeed quiescent at times, but not persistently. This may be misperceived. When tremor is present, it is seen and felt and can't be easily ignored. Conversely, when it is gone, people tend to take that for granted and have a selective memory for the tremor recurrences. Obviously, there is potential to mislead the physician if tremor control is intermittent but this is not recognized. Thus you need to be a good observer and pay attention to the patterns.

Intermittent tremor control may lend itself to further treatment. There are three treatable possibilities to consider:

- The levodopa dose is not quite high enough to be consistently effective.

- The levodopa effect is wearing off.

- You are experiencing stress-induced exacerbation of tremor.

If the dose of carbidopa/levodopa is on the margins of effectiveness, the parkinsonian symptoms may respond intermittently—that is, sometimes it will be effective and sometimes not (i.e., some doses will be above threshold and others not). In that case, raising the dose slightly higher should treat this. If you suspect this problem, raise all the carbidopa/levodopa doses by a half-tablet; if still inadequately controlled, go up by another half-tablet. If this is indeed the problem, these small increases should be sufficient. Otherwise revert back to the original dose. However, you should not need to raise carbidopa/levodopa beyond 3 tablets each dose, provided that you are using the 25/100 immediate-release formulation and taking it on an empty stomach.

A second explanation for intermittent tremor control is that the levodopa effect is wearing off. In this case, each dose of carbidopa/levodopa controls tremor for a few hours or less, then wears off; the tremor recurs when it is getting near the time for the next carbidopa/levodopa dose. The simplest strategy is to reduce the interval between doses to match the duration of the levodopa response (using the same amount each dose that provides the on-response). As you shorten the interval between doses, you will then need to add an extra dose or two each day. Do not worry about the number of doses or tablets per day. Chapters 17 and 18 discuss treatment of wearing-off of the levodopa effect in more detail.

Tremor of any type worsens under stress. Unfortunately, intermittent loss of tremor control due to stress is nearly impossible to treat with any dose of carbidopa/levodopa. Obviously, minimizing life stressors is advisable, but this is never completely possible. If this is a recurrent problem, a beta-blocker may be added, as will be discussed later in this chapter. Beta-blockers attenuate tremor exacerbations due to stress. However, these drugs also lower blood pressure and should not be added if orthostatic hypotension is potentially present. For most people with PD, stress-induced tremor is not so frequent as to require another medication.

Only Partial Tremor Control, Despite Maximum Treatment

Sometimes PD tremor is not adequately controlled despite maximum levodopa therapy. This is not a case of tremor coming and going, as discussed earlier; rather, the tremor is persistent. For that problem, like frequent stress-induced tremor exacerbations, a beta-blocker may be tried. However, their efficacy is usually incomplete; moreover, marked ongoing tremor will not likely substantially improve. Nonetheless, a beta-blocker may be considered.

Beta-Blockers for Tremor Control

Beta-blockers are a class of prescription medications that inhibit a component of the adrenalin response. They are commonly used to treat hypertension or certain heart conditions. They lower the blood pressure and slow the pulse rate.

Not all beta-blockers reduce tremor. The more commonly used beta-blockers for blood pressure control are atenolol and metoprolol. These block only one type of beta receptor, beta-1. For tremor control, the drug must block beta-2. Hence, atenolol and metoprolol are not useful for tremor. Fortunately, two older beta-blockers that block beta-2 receptors are available, propranolol (Inderal) and nadolol (Corgard). They are termed nonselective beta blockers since they block both types of receptors (beta-1 and beta-2).

Either propranolol or nadolol may be added for tremor control, provided that the following conditions are not present:

- Low blood pressure (orthostatic hypotension)
- Slow heart rate (bradycardia)
- Asthma
- Insulin-treated diabetes mellitus with frequent low blood sugar (hypoglycemic) reactions

Beta-blockers should not be started if the standing systolic blood pressure is less than 100 or the pulse rate is less than 55 beats per minute. They should not be used by those with asthmatic tendencies as they have properties opposite to bronchodilators. Insulin-induced low blood glucose symptoms are blunted with the beta-blockers; that may delay recognition and treatment.

These beta-blockers should be used with the understanding that they are not dramatically effective for PD tremor control. They are commonly used for essential tremor of the hands, where the responses are gratifying if the tremor amplitude is no more than mild to moderate (essential tremor was previously described in Chapter 6 and will be discussed later in this chapter). With the more prominent PD rest tremor (i.e., larger tremor amplitude), these may not be very effective, although they tend to reduce the tremor exacerbations from stress. In practice these are not used very often for PD, but are worth considering for selected people.

If a beta-blocker is to be tried for tremor, the characteristics of propranolol and nadolol should be considered in order to make the proper selection. Nadolol is a once-daily medication with a long-duration response (20- to 24-hour half-life). Regular propranolol has much briefer effects, lasting a few hours (4-hour half-life). The sustained-release formulation of propranolol (Inderal LA) has a longer duration effect, but still only a little more than twice as long as the regular propranolol formulation (i.e., 10-hour half-life). *Half-life* is a pharmacological term relating to the duration in which an administered drug stays in the body or circulation—that is, the time following a drug dose for the blood level to decline by half from the steady-state drug level.

In my practice, I use nadolol for chronic daily treatment and regular propranolol for as-needed administration. *As-needed* implies taking a single dose in anticipation of a stressor that will exacerbate tremor. I tend to not prescribe sustained-release propranolol (Inderal LA) since it does not last nearly as long as nadolol and requires twice-daily administration to have a sustained effect (many clinicians would advise a more persistent, 24-hour effect, if chronic beta-blockade is utilized). If a beta-blocker is started, occasionally check the standing blood pressure and pulse.

Nadolol is typically started in a dose of one 40 mg tablet once daily. It may be increased after perhaps 2 weeks to 2 tablets once daily and a couple of weeks later to 3 tablets once daily (120 mg). That dosing range should capture most of the anti-tremor effect, although it occasionally is raised beyond that. If higher doses add no incremental benefit, return to a lower dose.

If a beta-blocker is to be used intermittently (as needed) in anticipation of tremor, I would start with a 10 to 20 mg tablet of regular propranolol. This will kick in within about an hour and produce an anti-tremor effect that will persist for several hours. It can be repeated later in the day. Higher doses can be used, up to 40 mg each dose.

Finally, bear in mind that just because tremor is present does not mean that it must be treated. If it does not bother you, there is no need to aggressively add medications to control tremor.

Benign Tremulous Parkinsonism

Very little has been published about a parkinsonism variant that is sometimes termed *benign tremulous parkinsonism*. This is a condition marked by the following features:

- Prominent parkinsonian hand tremor, typically both at rest and with sustained posture

- Other aspects of parkinsonism are present but relatively mild, with preserved gait

- Very slow progression, without major deterioration apart from increased tremor

- Usually a partial or no tremor response to carbidopa/levodopa

- Often with a family history of tremor or PD

Those with this disorder tend to remain relatively stable for many years and, apart from tremor, tend to have relatively preserved movement and walking. This condition responds only partially or not much at all to carbidopa/levodopa, and other tremor medications, including the beta-blockers, are not very effective. This tremor-predominant disorder is not truly benign, as the tremor can be quite troublesome. However, it does respond very well to deep brain stimulation, discussed later in the chapter and in Chapter 33.

Not Parkinson's Disease but Essential Tremor

As discussed in Chapter 6, essential tremor may be misdiagnosed as PD. This should not be a problem if head or voice tremor is present, since these are recognized as typical of essential tremor (not PD). However, misdiagnosis occurs more frequently when essential tremor involves the hands, because they are affected in both conditions.

The hallmark features of essential hand tremor can be succinctly summarized as follows.

- Essential tremor is typically absent when the hands are relaxed. It surfaces when the hands are in use (e.g., holding something) or held against gravity (arms outstretched). PD tremor is primarily present when the hands are in a relaxed position, especially at one's side when walking. PD tremor may persist when the hands are outstretched (postured), but it abates when the hand is moving (e.g., bringing a fork to the mouth).

- There are no other neurological signs seen in essential tremor, including no signs of parkinsonism.

Occasional people with essential tremor also have a resting hand tremor, especially if essential tremor is long-standing; however, this is uncommon and, when present, the rest tremor component is mild and intermittent.

Note that as humans approach 80 years of age, they tend to become a little stooped, walking a little more slowly with shorter steps. If these age-related signs are present in conjunction with essential tremor, it could be mistaken for PD.

Essential hand tremor that is mild to moderate usually responds to the beta-blockers just discussed. Other medications are also used for essential tremor, such as primidone or topiramate; however, they have more side effects. Essential head or voice tremor is usually poorly responsive to any medications but typically benefit from botulinum toxin injections. Essential tremor does not respond to carbidopa/levodopa.

Combination of Parkinson's Disease and Essential Tremor

Essential tremor is present in about 5% of the adult population, whereas PD occurs in around 1%; by chance, these occasionally co-occur. If someone has both PD and essential tremor, the parkinsonism should respond to levodopa treatment, whereas the essential tremor component will not.

Note that rare people with PD initially develop a hand tremor identical to essential tremor before developing other symptoms of PD. It may be impossible to diagnose PD at that early point in time. Within a few years, the correct diagnosis becomes apparent; nothing is lost by treating this as essential tremor in the beginning.

Severe and Unresponsive Tremor: Consider Surgery

Tremor of any type (essential tremor, PD tremor, benign tremulous parkinsonism, or other) can typically be controlled with brain surgery, currently offered as deep brain stimulation (DBS). DBS involves implanting a stimulating electrode into a specific brain region. Since it is insulated except for the tip, the electrical stimulation is focused on a precise brain region. When properly placed and stimulating at a very high frequency, it turns off tremor. The targets of this surgery are either the thalamus or subthalamic nucleus; both are illustrated in Figure 2.5 (Chapter 2). This is major brain surgery and is not a trivial endeavor. However, it can be dramatically effective in abolishing or nearly abolishing severe tremor. This is discussed in detail in Chapter 33.

PART SEVEN

◆ ◆ ◆

The Early Years on Medications

15

♦ ♦ ♦

The First Few Years on Carbidopa/Levodopa Treatment

When carbidopa/levodopa is started in the early stages of Parkinson's disease (PD), the brain is able to easily utilize the administered levodopa. Since PD progresses slowly, the levodopa responses typically remain robust and stable for several years or more. These early stages are an important period of time for those with PD; this provides the opportunity to make important life changes directed at long-lasting good health and longevity. This starts with adequate brain dopamine replenishment, typically with carbidopa/levodopa.

Can I Save These Best Responses for Later?

This issue was broached in previous chapters. However, the admonition to save carbidopa/levodopa for later is so commonly voiced that it may be worthwhile to revisit this issue. As we previously discussed, neither carbidopa/levodopa nor dopamine agonist treatment per se is responsible for the less stable or less robust responses after several years. Rather, this reflects the natural progression of PD. Two changes in the levodopa response slowly occur over years, as part of this progression:

1. The levodopa benefits tend to be less complete after 5–10 years, although still very beneficial. This presumably reflects other (nondopaminergic) components of the basal ganglia movement system that are progressively affected by the Lewy neurodegenerative process. Contrary to what is sometimes written in the lay press, levodopa does *not* stop working.

2. The levodopa benefit tends to become less stable years later, due to the development of "short-duration" responses. Thus, the predominant response becomes time-locked to each carbidopa/levodopa dose and the effect wears off several hours after that dose. This is presumably due to progressive loss of the residual nigrostriatal dopaminergic terminals. Thus, in early PD, levodopa is taken up by the surviving nigrostriatal terminals and converted to dopamine; see Figure 15.1. During these early years of PD, surviving dopaminergic terminals are sufficient to compensate and are able to restore nearly normal dopamine concentrations in most regions of the striatum. Over several years, the progressive loss of these residual dopaminergic terminals translates into unstable responses. At that time other (nondopaminergic) neurons as well as glia (brain supporting cells) take over but are unable to maintain consistent dopamine concentrations at the synapses, resulting in the short-duration effects. By a similar mechanism, dyskinesias tend to be provoked, reflecting excessive dopamine levels.

Restated, progression of the Lewy neurodegenerative process is responsible for later alterations in the levodopa responses. This is not caused by levodopa

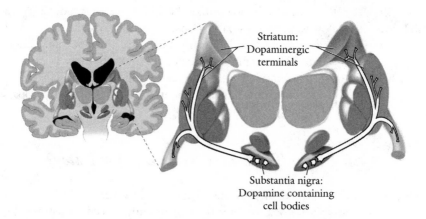

Striatum:
Dopaminergic
terminals

Substantia nigra:
Dopamine containing
cell bodies

15.1 Normally, continuous dopamine release by nigrostriatal terminals produces stable dopamine levels in the striatum; this translates into stable movement patterns.
In early PD, the surviving nigrostriatal terminals are still able to take up administered levodopa, convert it to dopamine, and maintain stable movement patterns.
After a number of years, these surviving dopaminergic terminals decline further. At that time, other (nondopaminergic) neurons and supporting cells (glia) are responsible for taking up levodopa, converting it to dopamine and releasing it into the synapse. These cells are much less able to maintain constant synaptic dopamine levels, resulting in unstable responses.

therapy but by the natural history of PD. Thus the best levodopa responses cannot be saved by deferring carbidopa/levodopa in early PD.

Opportunities

With the diagnosis of PD, there is a tendency for some people to give in and scale back their life. Compounding this is the fact that many middle-aged and early senior people have had poor life habits with weight gain, sedentary inclinations, and deconditioning. Unfortunately, this is the product of our culture, where 21st-century innovations tend to make us couch potatoes, munching on chips as we watch TV or surf the Internet; driving has replaced walking. Rather, the diagnosis of PD should be viewed as a wake-up call and an opportunity to mobilize resources to attack this head-on. Chapter 9 summarized the benefits of ongoing exercise and these cannot be underestimated. The early years of PD should be the time when we take stock of our lives, readdress priorities, and use this time to establish good life habits. Of course, this is difficult if one is deferring carbidopa/levodopa or using it very conservatively; carbidopa/levodopa needs to be optimized to effectively fight PD. Once a commitment is made to attack rather than give in to PD, it is important to set goals to remain active and engaged: schedule and maintain regular exercise routines and avoid the weight gain that is so common in middle age and beyond. These habits should then translate into not only better quality of life but also longevity. These goals are the same as advocated by your primary care doctor, internist, or cardiologist for overall health.

Treatable Problems That May Surface During Early Years of Parkinson's Disease after Starting Carbidopa/Levodopa

If the guidelines in Chapter 12 have been followed and an optimal dose of carbidopa/levodopa determined, major dosing changes should not be necessary for several years. Unlike narcotics, where the doses must be progressively raised for pain control, the optimum individual carbidopa/levodopa doses initially established are appropriate indefinitely. Years later, more doses per day will likely be necessary, but usually about the same amount for each dose (i.e., same dose but more doses per day).

Several problems that may occur during the early carbidopa/levodopa treatment years deserve discussion. A few illustrative examples follow.

"My parkinsonism was easy to control with only a single carbidopa/levodopa tablet three times a day, but no longer."

Problem: Low-dose therapy or mealtime dosing

An exception to the statement that the individual doses tend to remain stable over years is illustrated by this case. If only a low carbidopa/levodopa dose has been used, a larger dose may be necessary after several months to years. This dose may need to raised, using the general scheme outlined in Chapter 12.

The second possibility is that this person became careless and started taking the carbidopa/levodopa doses with meals. Remember that carbidopa/levodopa must be taken at least an hour before meals and 2 hours after the end of meals. Most snacks count as meals (i.e., snacks with protein content).

"My symptoms were initially controlled all day long; now they come and go."

Problem: Wearing-off of the levodopa effect

Short-duration levodopa responses are suggested by this problem. The first step in treating this is to recognize what is happening. The true short-duration levodopa response pattern is often easiest to discern after awakening in the morning. If prominent parkinsonism is present after rising from sleep, only to improve an hour after the first carbidopa/levodopa dose, a short-duration response is suggested; that is, the beneficial effect becomes time-locked to each dose.

During the first several years of typical PD, the levodopa benefit is around the clock; skipping a dose goes unnoticed unless many doses are skipped. Short-duration levodopa responses usually do not develop until several years later. However, a small minority of people experience this pattern during the first couple of years.

If the fluctuations are minimal, nothing further needs to be done. If they are more troublesome, then it may be necessary to shorten the interval between doses to match the response duration and add more doses to avoid gaps in coverage. Although published directives sometimes advise taking a lesser amount of levodopa when adding doses, that is incorrect. The dose that works best should be maintained each time carbidopa/levodopa is taken, regardless of the number of doses per day. This is discussed in more detail in Chapter 17.

"I have twitchy movements of my head" (or hand, foot, trunk).

Problem: Levodopa-induced dyskinesias

Like short-duration levodopa responses, dyskinesias are uncommon during the early years of PD. They represent an excessive levodopa response; they are transiently provoked by each dose of carbidopa/levodopa. They develop about an hour after taking carbidopa/levodopa and then resolve in a few hours or so. The strategy for treating these is to lower each dose of levodopa by a small amount.

Correct recognition of dyskinesias is crucial. They appear as dancing, chaotic movements of some portion of the body. They are fundamentally different from certain other symptoms with which they are frequently confused; it is important to distinguish them from the following:

1. Dystonia, for example, toes curling, foot torsion, cramps

2. Akathisia, where subjective restlessness is experienced in the absence of visible involuntary movements

3. Tremor, which is a repetitive movement typical of untreated PD

These three symptoms represent inadequate levodopa coverage; they require more, not less, levodopa or more frequent carbidopa/levodopa. These important distinctions and appropriate treatment strategies are addressed in detail in Chapter 17.

> "My carbidopa/levodopa works well during the daytime, but I can't get to sleep."
>
> *Problem*: A bedtime dose of carbidopa/levodopa is probably needed for sleep.

Often, insomnia is experienced when PD is not well controlled; the restlessness and discomfort of parkinsonism are incompatible with the relaxation necessary for sleep. For those taking three carbidopa/levodopa doses daily, the long interval from the last dose before supper until bedtime may be the cause. Adding a fourth full dose about an hour before bedtime usually solves this problem. Note that the dose should be the same as that used during the daytime. Restated, this should be the carbidopa/levodopa dose identified as optimal; the sleep benefit requires a full dose. Another dose may be taken upon awakening in the middle of the night, if necessary to sustain sleep. More details and advice on sleep-related issues are found in Chapter 20.

> "I get cramps at night"
>
> *Problem:* Inadequate levodopa coverage

In the setting of PD, frequent cramps usually signal loss or absence of the levodopa effect and tend to be more common at night. Parkinsonian cramps may be typical "charley horses" with painful contraction of calf muscles. They frequently involve the toes, which may painfully curl or point up. Cramps may also develop during the day, reflective of the levodopa effect wearing off.

Rather than adding an antispasmodic drug to treat cramps, these are appropriately treated by adjusting the dosage of carbidopa/levodopa. This might entail shortening the interval between doses if cramps appear to represent wearing off of the levodopa response. Alternatively, they may represent inadequate levodopa, requiring higher individual doses.

Note that cramps are common in the general population and may have other causes. Among those who do not have PD, carbidopa/levodopa does not treat cramps.

"I was doing great and suddenly my parkinsonism has deteriorated"

Problem: There's something else going on.

PD progresses very slowly, over years. Prominent deterioration that occurs over hours, days, or weeks suggests some other cause. This might include the following:

- Inadvertent changes in the carbidopa/levodopa dose or timing (such as mealtime dosing)

- A new medication (notoriously known to cause or worsen parkinsonism are drugs that block dopamine, listed in Table 6.1, Chapter 6)

- Another illness or medical condition (e.g., pneumonia, urinary tract infection)

Do not assume that any rapidly developing problem reflects progression of PD. Your primary care doctor should review your general health and your medication list.

"I never had problems with carbidopa/levodopa until recently. Now I have pain in my stomach and I'm nauseated."

Problem: Something other than carbidopa/levodopa

Nausea is not uncommon with carbidopa/levodopa therapy, but when it occurs, this is early in the treatment or after raising the dose. In rare individuals, it may persist. However, if a stable dose of carbidopa/levodopa has been maintained for months without gastrointestinal symptoms, then newly developing nausea likely has another source.

Be aware that the carbidopa component of carbidopa/levodopa is the agent that prevents nausea. Switching from the 25/100 formulation to pills with less carbidopa (e.g., 10/100 or 25/250) may be responsible for newly developing nausea.

Carbidopa/levodopa does not cause abdominal pain, only nausea. If your abdomen hurts, this should not be from carbidopa/levodopa. Note, however, that occasional people with PD experience abdominal cramp-like pain from PD, responsive to carbidopa/levodopa.

16

♦ ♦ ♦

The Early Years of Parkinson's Disease If Started on Other Drugs

I suspect that numerous people reading this book have been started on a PD medication other than carbidopa/levodopa; this might include the following:

Rasagiline (Azilect)

Selegiline

Amantadine

Pramipexole (Mirapex)

Ropinirole (Requip)

Rotigotine (Neupro patch)

If one is doing well and has no substantial side effects, simply remaining on one of these medications is reasonable. Recall the goals of symptomatic treatment of PD: keeping people in the mainstream of their lives, staying both socially and physically active, and engaging in regular exercise. If these goals are met then there is no need to change.

If one is not doing well on these medications, questions arise: Take a higher dose? Start another drug from the above choices? Start carbidopa/levodopa? Stop the current drug? Taper off rather than stop abruptly? This chapter is for people on one or more of these medications who are having problems. Since the options differ depending on the current drug, these medications will be considered one by one. The common side effects associated with these drugs and their cost were discussed in Chapters 10 and 11.

Rasagiline (Azilect), Selegiline

These two drugs irreversibly inhibit the brain dopamine-degrading enzyme MAO-B (monoamine oxidase, type B). They have almost identical efficacy and side effects. They have a very long duration of action (half-life, 40 days) and can be abruptly stopped without the need for tapering off. They have a mild symptomatic effect on parkinsonism. They are taken once daily and the usual doses, 5 mg selegiline or 1 mg rasagiline, capture the full benefit; there is no reason to try higher doses. If raised substantially higher, these drugs may then block both the A- and B-forms of MAO, which may have serious consequences. Specifically, drugs that inhibit both forms of MAO require a special diet to avoid a life-threatening hypertensive crisis.

These drugs should be taken in the morning to avoid insomnia. As shown in Table 11.3, rasagiline is more than 10 times more expensive than selegiline capsules.

If one is taking selegiline or rasagiline but experiencing increasing symptoms of parkinsonism, it would be appropriate to add carbidopa/levodopa (see Chapter 12). Rarely, the combination of these two drugs (rasagiline or selegiline plus carbidopa/levodopa) provokes hallucinations or psychosis. In that event, the selegiline/rasagiline should be abruptly stopped and the carbidopa/levodopa held until the hallucinations resolve. After several days to a few weeks, the carbidopa/levodopa may then be restarted (but without selegiline or rasagiline).

Amantadine

Occasionally, amantadine is prescribed as the initial drug for PD when the symptoms are very mild. The primary role for amantadine in the current era is to reduce levodopa dyskinesias, which is addressed in Chapter 18; however, some physicians choose to start this medication when the parkinsonism is minimal. It comes in one size of tablets: 100 mg.

Amantadine is the only drug listed here that does not work through dopamine. It blocks glutamate NMDA receptors. Admittedly, it does have slight dopamine-enhancing properties, but these are not thought to be responsible for the benefit.

There is a dose-related effect from amantadine, up to about 5 tablets daily (divided doses). However, doses beyond 3 tablets daily are reserved for dyskinesia treatment. If this is the sole drug for PD and if parkinsonism is worsening, the dose could be raised to 3 of the 100 mg tablets daily; however, do not expect a dramatic response. If there is more than minimal parkinsonism, it would then be appropriate to consider carbidopa/levodopa.

Amantadine side effects are usually not problematic. Common is mild discoloration of the skin (primarily legs), with a purple fishnet pattern (livido reticularis). This is not dangerous and is only a cosmetic issue. Uncommonly, it may provoke hallucinations; if these occur, it should be discontinued. Note that amantadine is pharmacologically very similar to memantine (Namenda), which is used for cognitive impairment (discussed in Chapter 23). It seems advisable to not use amantadine and memantine concurrently because of their similarity.

Pramipexole (Mirapex), Ropinirole (Requip)

These two drugs have similar properties, although the mg-doses are quite different. They do have anti-parkinsonian efficacy that is substantially greater than that of the other drugs discussed here but also substantially less than that of carbidopa/levodopa.

Chapter 13 provided dose escalation schedules for these two drugs. Poor efficacy with these agonists often relates to insufficient doses. In Chapter 13, the minimally effective total daily doses were specified: pramipexole, 2 mg, and ropinirole, 6 mg. If you are not doing well on lower doses but have no side effects, it would be appropriate to raise the dosage to the target doses (also specified in Chapter 13). If still not doing well, then consider carbidopa/levodopa.

If carbidopa/levodopa is to be added, and if pramipexole/ropinirole is tolerated, it is reasonable to maintain the dopamine agonist in the current dose to avoid changing two medications at the same time. Often an agonist and carbidopa/levodopa are taken together indefinitely. If the preference is to use only one drug for PD (i.e., carbidopa/levodopa), maintain the dopamine agonist at the current dose until the carbidopa/levodopa dose is stabilized. Then the agonist can be tapered off. Chapter 13 provides general guidelines for tapering off these agonists.

If the expense of the agonists is an issue, note that the regular generic formulations of these two drugs are inexpensive, whereas the sustained-release forms are costly; see Table 11.3 in Chapter 11 for comparative pricing. If you are taking the sustained-release form and expense is of concern, consider simply switching to the regular formulation. The total mg per day is equivalent between the sustained-release and regular formulations. For example, if you are taking a 4.5 mg tablet of extended-release pramipexole (Mirapex ER) once daily, simply take 1.5 mg of regular pramipexole three times daily. Similarly, if taking a 6 mg tablet of sustained-release ropinirole (Requip XL) once daily, switch to a 2 mg tablet of regular ropinirole three times daily. This switch can be done overnight (i.e., take the extended-release dose in the morning, and the following day substitute the regular formulation in the comparable dosage).

Side effects from pramipexole and ropinirole were discussed in Chapters 10 and 11. Certain of these—pathological compulsive behaviors (e.g., gambling, sexual ideation); sleep attacks; massive leg swelling; hallucinations or delusional thinking (e.g., paranoia)—require elimination of the agonist using a tapering schedule. With serious side effects, it is generally advisable to completely taper off the agonist well before starting carbidopa/levodopa to avoid overlap and uncertainty about which drug is causing these problems.

If sleepiness is a suspected side effect, consider also whether there is some other cause, most notably poor nighttime sleep or sleep apnea. If excessive drowsiness started shortly after beginning a dopamine agonist and there is no other explanation, it will probably be necessary to at least substantially lower the dose and often taper off. Driving while sleepy is dangerous.

Rotigotine Patch (Neupro)

All of the previous discussion regarding pramipexole and ropinirole is appropriate for the rotigotine patch. Rotigotine and ropinirole are very similar in potency and side effects. However, several things are specifically worth noting about rotigotine.

First, the Neupro patch is very expensive, currently priced at around $16 per patch (as of June 2014), regardless of the dose. If you are paying some or all of this expense and are not wealthy, this may not be the best drug for you. If this is of concern, there are two options for switching to another drug. Often the simplest and most efficacious strategy is to taper off the rotigotine (guidelines for tapering off are found in Chapter 13) and then start carbidopa/levodopa (Chapter 12). Alternatively, if you wish to remain on a dopamine agonist, an overnight switch to ropinirole is easy, recognizing that the mg-amount per day is interchangeable between rotigotine and ropinirole. Thus, if using the 6 mg Neupro (rotigotine) patch daily, substitute regular ropinirole in the same dose of 6 mg daily, taken as 2 mg three times per day. The medication in the patch will decline after 24 hours to sufficiently low levels to allow starting ropinirole the following day.

Trihexyphenidyl (Artane), Benztropine (Cogentin)

The anticholinergic medications, trihexyphenidyl and benztropine, were not listed at the beginning of this chapter as drugs that may be continued if one is doing well. Anticholinergic drugs date back to the pre-levodopa era of 50-plus years ago. They have mild efficacy, primarily for tremor and rigidity. Unfortunately, their side effects often overshadow the benefits. They cross the blood-brain barrier and potentially impair memory; their pharmacological properties are opposite those of the memory-enhancing drugs (e.g., donepezil) that will be discussed in Chapter 23. Hallucinations and psychosis may be provoked by anticholinergic drugs. They also have many peripheral side effects, including dry eyes, dry mouth, visual blurring, constipation, and slowed stomach emptying. These non-brain side effects are similar to those of drugs used for a hyperactive bladder, discussed in Chapter 27. Hence it is unwise to use these two classes of anticholinergic drugs concurrently.

Since we have so many better drugs for treating the symptoms of PD, in my view there is no role for anticholinergic drugs in the present era. I typically advise tapering off anticholinergic PD drugs (but not at the same time as adjusting other medications). Usually, these anticholinergic drugs can be slowly reduced to zero over about 2 weeks. However, if maintained for many months or years, tapering must be more prolonged, perhaps over a month or more.

Sudden Deterioration of Parkinsonism

As discussed in Chapter 15, PD does not progress rapidly. If there is a sudden decline over a few days to a few weeks, consider other causes. Occasionally, such simple things as a urinary tract infection may transiently worsen parkinsonism. Certain drugs, such as the dopamine-blocking medications for nausea (metoclopramide or prochlorperazine), notoriously worsen parkinsonism. If there is an unexplained and rapid deterioration, your primary care physician should review the medication list and address general health issues.

PART EIGHT

◆ ◆ ◆

Later Medication Inconsistency: Motor Fluctuations and Dyskinesias

17

◆ ◆ ◆

Later Developing Movement Problems: Motor Fluctuations and Dyskinesias Treated with Levodopa Adjustments

Instability of the levodopa response may surface after several years of Parkinson's disease (PD). This takes two forms:

1. Fluctuations of parkinsonism due to short-duration levodopa responses; and

2. Involuntary movements, termed *dyskinesias*, which represent an excessive levodopa effect.

These problems develop to variable extents and are minimal in some people, even after many years. Young people are the most prone to dyskinesias and fluctuating responses. These problems typically can be controlled with adjustments of carbidopa/levodopa dose, provided that the condition is correctly diagnosed. Hence we will first discuss recognition of these problems, starting with fluctuations of parkinsonism.

Levodopa Fluctuations

The first several years of PD and carbidopa/levodopa treatment are typically characterized by very stable medication responses, the long-duration levodopa response. This long-duration levodopa response builds up over about a week when a consistent carbidopa/levodopa dose is administered.

Over years, the progression of the PD neurodegenerative process leads to fewer and fewer dopaminergic neurons. Other cells take their place but are not as efficient at storing and releasing dopamine. This increasing loss of dopaminergic terminals translates into declining capacity to maintain continuous dopamine levels in the striatum. With fluctuating striatal dopamine concentrations, the levodopa responses become time-locked to each dose. Thus the levodopa control of parkinsonism increasingly tends to mirror the levodopa levels in the circulation. In effect, the system behaves as if dopamine can no longer be stored beyond a few hours. Dopamine levels fluctuate in the synapse and the corresponding response fluctuations are magnified by sensitized dopamine receptors. Although this is not simply a dopamine storage issue, the responses behave like that. With these "short-duration" levodopa responses, the benefit is tied to each carbidopa/levodopa dose, with the effect lasting for a few hours, then tailing off. PD control then becomes analogous to driving a car with a 5 gallon fuel tank: you need to stop frequently to fill the tank. The long-duration effect is not lost completely but fades into the background; we almost never see it because carbidopa/levodopa is rarely stopped long enough for this to become apparent.

LEVODOPA FLUCTUATIONS OFTEN ARE UNRECOGNIZED

Those with PD often fail to recognize the fluctuating pattern of this levodopa response. Humans tend to have a selective memory for bad times and may simply report to their doctor that they no longer respond to carbidopa/levodopa. In fact, they continue to respond, except that the good times are repeatedly interrupted by levodopa off-states; the off-states tend to be remembered and the on-states overlooked.

Recognition of off-states is crucial, as they can be treated with levodopa adjustments. Clues to this pattern are often apparent in the morning when no carbidopa/levodopa has been taken overnight. At that time, people may experience difficulty walking, slowness, or tremor before the first carbidopa/levodopa dose of the day but marked improvement an hour later (when the effect has kicked in). The levodopa response then persists for several hours but wears off, with recurrence of parkinsonian symptoms. Another dose replicates this scenario.

For some people with PD, the morning is their best time due to a restorative effect from a night's sleep (even though they've had no carbidopa/levodopa overnight). In that case, other clues may point to fluctuations. Questions to ask yourself include the following:

- Am I a lot better during certain times of the day than others?

- Am I better an hour or two after my levodopa doses?

- Are my problems primarily when it is close to the time for my next dose?

- Do toe or foot cramps come and go?

- Do my typical PD symptoms vary dramatically?

These questions address whether there is substantial variability in your day. Answering yes to these questions suggests that you are experiencing fluctuations in your levodopa response, likely reflecting development of a short-duration levodopa response. To get a handle on this, construct in your mind the full levodopa response over time. How am I doing before I take the carbidopa/levodopa dose? How long does it take to kick in? How long does this effect last, and when does the effect wear off after each dose? If you can answer these questions, you can then envision the full levodopa cycle, as illustrated in Figure 17.1.

Keep in mind that the response to a dose of carbidopa/levodopa is not immediate and takes up to 1 hour to kick in (up to 2 hours with sustained-release carbidopa/levodopa). This occasionally is a source of confusion when the dosing interval is just a little too long; in that case, the benefit from the last dose wears off right *after* the next dose is taken and before this new dose has time to kick in. This may give the incorrect impression that this new dose caused the benefit to subside.

TREATMENT OF LEVODOPA SHORT-DURATION RESPONSES

Wearing-off is the term applied to the loss of benefit several hours after the last dose. This indicates a short-duration levodopa response. If your fluctuating benefit follows the simple pattern we have just described, the medication adjustments are straightforward. Let's break this down into the two critical components of this levodopa cycle, which are illustrated in Figure 17.1:

1. Peak effect of the dose

2. Duration of the response

To effectively treat a short-duration levodopa response, we need to separately consider each of these two components.

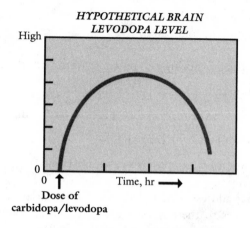

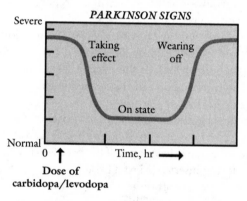

17.1 The short-duration levodopa response is triggered by each dose of carbidopa/ levodopa, lasting a few hours and then wearing off. One might think of this as paralleling the hypothetical brain level of levodopa (although it is not quite that simple).

The Peak Effect of the Levodopa Dose: Sufficient Response?

The maximum effect is fully developed about 60–90 minutes after each dose of carbidopa/levodopa (or, in the case of Sinemet CR, 2 hours after the dose). Focus on how you are doing at that time. If doing well, then we have the correct dose. On the other hand, if you are experiencing substantial parkinsonism when the levodopa dose is peaking, a larger dose may be necessary. The carbidopa/levodopa dose (25/100 immediate-release tablets) can be raised by half-tablet increments until you find the dose that works best, up to 3 tablets each dose. Recall that individual doses higher than 3 tablets confer no further benefit (provided taken on an empty stomach). Be aware that while trying to find the best dose, it is important to maintain the doses sufficiently far apart so that the effects do not overlap. Once we have that sorted out, we will then focus on how often to take it.

Duration of the Levodopa Response

Once you have determined the optimal amount of carbidopa/levodopa to be taken each dose, focus on how long the effect lasts. The general rule for those with wearing-off may be simply stated:

Match the interval between doses to the duration of the response.

In other words, when you have established the dose, observe how long it takes each dose to kick in and how long that effect lasts. Then reduce the interval between doses so that the effects slightly overlap. The strategy is to have the current dose kick in just before the effect from the last dose has worn off. Remember that the response is not immediate following any given dose; it takes 30 to 60 minutes for immediate-release carbidopa/levodopa to start working. You need to allow for this when determining the interval between doses.

WHY DON'T I SIMPLY TAKE LARGER DOSES OF CARBIDOPA/LEVODOPA TO MAKE THE EFFECT LAST LONGER?

This is a sensible idea, but it doesn't work. Taking a larger dose may last slightly longer, but usually does not substantially lengthen the response. Instead, you will likely just add to side effects, especially dyskinesias.

The only exception to this rule relates to people who have been taking a very small dose of carbidopa/levodopa. If you are taking a dose that is right on the margins of a response (e.g., a half to one 25/100 tablet), a larger dose may lengthen the response. If a half to 1 tablet increment doesn't extend the response, you can revert back to the previous dose and follow through with the strategies we have outlined.

HOW MANY DOSES MAY I TAKE EACH DAY?

If you shorten the interval between your carbidopa/levodopa doses, you will need to add extra doses to continue the effect going through bedtime. There are no limits to the number of doses, provided that they fit your needs. Guided by these principles, take as many doses as you need to provide continuous coverage.

SOME PEOPLE HAVE A VERY BRIEF LEVODOPA RESPONSE

The duration of the levodopa response varies among people with fluctuations. For most, the effect lasts a few hours; however, for a few, it may be as brief as 2 hours or, in rare cases, about 1 hour. Over years of PD, the duration of the levodopa response tends to shorten. Presumably, this relates to the progressive loss of the dopaminergic neurons in the brain, with the need for other brain cells to substitute, functioning in a role for which they were not designed.

WHAT IS THE MAXIMUM AMOUNT OF LEVODOPA PER DAY?

For those with fluctuations in their levodopa response, we have focused on the size of the individual doses and ignored the total daily dose. There is no arbitrary ceiling on how much you can take per day as long as you follow the principles just outlined.

DOES CARBIDOPA PLAY ANY ROLE IN THESE LONG- AND SHORT-DURATION RESPONSES?

As you raise or lower levodopa to manage your responses, you will, of necessity, also be changing your *carbidopa* dose. However, this is of no practical consequence and you may ignore it. It is only important if you are bothered by nausea from levodopa. In that case, you need sufficient carbidopa, as we discussed in Chapter 12.

WILL I NEED TO ADJUST MY LEVODOPA DOSES AGAIN IN THE FUTURE?

Once you have determined the dose that produces the optimum "on" response, this typically will not change substantially over subsequent years. In other words, if two 25/100 tablets works well, you won't need 3 tablets per dose in 2 years, 4 tablets in 5 years, and so on. Some minor adjustments of the size of each dose may be necessary, but you will not experience an ever-increasing requirement for higher and higher doses.

Although the optimum size of each carbidopa/levodopa dose typically doesn't change substantially over time, the optimum dosing interval tends to slowly diminish over many years. If you adjust the interval between levodopa doses to match the response duration, then more doses per day will be required. Consequently, the total daily dose of carbidopa/levodopa tends to increase over the years. This is not a sign of medication tolerance or addiction; this is not due to the body "getting used to" carbidopa/levodopa. More frequent dosing is primarily reflective of the natural progression of PD and not due to drug tolerance.

TO SUMMARIZE

For those with fluctuating responses, there are two principles that are basic to using carbidopa/levodopa:

1. Adjust the size of the individual doses to produce the optimum response.

2. Shorten the interval between doses to match the response duration, and take as many doses per day as necessary to provide continuous coverage.

Don't worry about the number of doses per day, or the total daily levodopa dosage, as long as your parkinsonism is well controlled.

Adjustment of the levodopa dosing scheme is not the only strategy for managing these levodopa complications. It is, however, the most effective approach and should be done first if fluctuations ensue. Although supplemental drugs may have a role in treating unstable levodopa responses, levodopa adjustments are quicker, cheaper, and often sufficient. Supplemental drug use will be discussed in Chapter 18.

WOULD SWITCHING TO SUSTAINED-RELEASE CARBIDOPA/LEVODOPA (SINEMET CR) CONTROL SHORT-DURATION RESPONSES?

The rationale for developing a sustained-release carbidopa/levodopa formulation was to extend the effect and counter short-duration levodopa responses. Such a pill has been available for many years, initially marketed as Sinemet CR. This sustained-release tablet contains an adherent matrix that more tightly binds the active ingredients (carbidopa and levodopa), holding them longer to provide a more sustained release. Intuitively, this made excellent sense. In practice, this was not so simple, with the following limitations of the currently available sustained-release carbidopa/levodopa tablets:

- The response is delayed—twice as long as regular carbidopa/levodopa.

- Release is incomplete and somewhat erratic (only 70% enters the circulation, as compared to 99% with regular carbidopa/levodopa).

- The pills release the ingredients poorly when the stomach is empty (but an empty stomach is necessary to avoid dietary amino acids from preventing levodopa from crossing into the brain).

- The prolongation of the levodopa response is only 60–90 minutes (perhaps up to 2 hours at night).

If you need a quick return to your levodopa "on" state, the delay of the sustained-release response can be a frustration. Also, because release of levodopa from the matrix is not as consistent as with the immediate-release tablet, the results are less predictable. The rather modest increase in the response duration of only 60–90 minutes typically fails to offset the downside of the sustained-release formulation.

Because of these shortcomings, a complete switch to sustained-release carbidopa/levodopa (Sinemet CR) usually confers no major benefits and sometimes leads to more complications. For those with very short levodopa responses (e.g., 2-hour durations), transitioning to sustained-release carbidopa/levodopa causes even more upheaval and cannot be recommended. I no longer switch fluctuating PD patients from regular to sustained-release carbidopa/levodopa. I do occasionally add a low dose of the sustained-release formulation to the regular carbidopa/levodopa to prolong the effect (discussed later in this chapter).

THE DOSE OF IMMEDIATE-RELEASE CARBIDOPA/ LEVODOPA IS NOT INTERCHANGEABLE WITH THE SUSTAINED-RELEASE FORMULATION

If you are considering switching or adding sustained-release carbidopa/levodopa, it is crucial to recognize that there is not a mg-to-mg correspondence between these two formulations. Because of incomplete release of levodopa (70%) plus the different dynamics of the release, a larger dose of levodopa is necessary when trying to equate the effect of the sustained-release with regular (immediate-release) carbidopa/levodopa.

For those who choose to transition from regular (immediate-release) to sustained-release carbidopa/levodopa, a simple strategy will hopefully allow this to be done seamlessly. Assuming that you have determined the optimum immediate-release carbidopa/levodopa dosing schedule, use the following rules to switch to sustained-release carbidopa/levodopa:

1. The individual sustained-release doses of levodopa should be 50% higher than the regular formulation (this might be slightly more than necessary in a minority of cases).

2. The interval between doses should be prolonged by 60–90 minutes (you can start with the longer increment, 90 minutes, and then reduce it, once you have determined how long it lasts).

Note that if you are using sustained-release carbidopa/levodopa in the morning for your first dose of the day, it often will not kick in reliably, and the levodopa may need to be 50–100 mg higher than subsequent doses (or take ½ to 1 immediate-release 25/100 tablet with that first dose).

EXAMPLE OF SWITCHING FROM IMMEDIATE-RELEASE TO SUSTAINED-RELEASE CARBIDOPA/LEVODOPA

Consider the person taking 2 ½ of the 25/100 immediate-release tablets four times daily, at 3-hour intervals, and experiencing a predictable response. The intent of the transition to the sustained-release formulation would be to take it less frequently. If we were going to completely transition this person to sustained-release carbidopa/levodopa, we first need to recognize that the current dose of 2 ½ of the 25/100 tablets represents 250 mg of levodopa. The following steps illustrate the levodopa arithmetic for making this switch:

1. Increase the levodopa content by 50%. The new sustained-release dose should be 150% of the current levodopa dose. Thus, 150% of 250 mg is 375 mg. We can round out the dose to fit with the available pill sizes. The sustained-release formulation comes in 25/100 and 50/200 sizes. Thus two of the 50/200 tablets could be used to make 400 mg of levodopa, which is close to the targeted 375 mg.

2. The interval between doses can be increased by 90 minutes. We can go from doses at 3-hour intervals to 4 or 4 ½ hours. If that proves too long, it can subsequently be shortened.

If we have done the arithmetic correctly, the total daily levodopa dose should be slightly higher with the sustained-release formulation (i.e., more levodopa per dose but fewer doses per day).

This can become a bit complicated. Because of that, plus the limited advantages of switching completely to sustained-release carbidopa/levodopa, this is often not advisable. However, adding a small dose of sustained-release carbidopa/levodopa to regular carbidopa/levodopa may occasionally be helpful, discussed next.

ADDING SUSTAINED-RELEASE CARBIDOPA/LEVODOPA TO IMMEDIATE-RELEASE FORMULATION

Combining the two carbidopa/levodopa formulations may allow a longer dosing interval plus avoid the delayed response. The strategy typically starts by establishing the optimum dose of regular (immediate-release) carbidopa/levodopa and then adding a small dose of sustained-release carbidopa/levodopa. The immediate-release component allows a quicker kick-in (sustained-release takes twice as long), whereas the sustained-release dose will hopefully add an hour or slightly more to the end of the response. Note that this is the rationale for the new drug Rytary, which is a combination capsule of sustained-release and regular carbidopa/levodopa, briefly discussed later in this chapter.

To use this strategy of both sustained-release and immediate-release carbidopa/levodopa, first determine the dose of regular 25/100 carbidopa/levodopa that produces the best response, then note the duration of the effect. Then add a 25/100 sustained-release carbidopa/levodopa tablet to each dose. This combination may result in an excessive effect, often experienced as dyskinesias (involuntary movements); these will be discussed in detail later in this chapter. The excessive effect can be treated by reducing the regular (immediate-release) component by a half-tablet.

For example, if taking 2 ½ of the regular carbidopa/levodopa tablets at 3-hour intervals, the addition of sustained-release carbidopa/levodopa may allow a 4-hour dosing interval. If adding a 25/100 sustained-release tablet to each dose causes dyskinesias, reduce the number of regular carbidopa/levodopa tablets from 2 ½ to 2.

Further adjustments can be made by systematic experimentation with the doses of these two carbidopa/levodopa formulations.

SLEEP, CARBIDOPA/LEVODOPA, AND THE SUSTAINED-RELEASE FORMULATION

Insomnia is common in PD and often relates to an inadequate levodopa effect at night or during the night. As discussed in more detail in Chapter 20, a full dose of regular carbidopa/levodopa in the late evening, near bedtime, often allows natural sleep. Thus, if you are unable to initiate sleep, consider when you last took carbidopa/levodopa. If the last dose was before supper, many hours before bedtime, simply add a full dose of regular carbidopa/levodopa an hour before bedtime.

Although this bedtime dose typically helps to initiate sleep, occasional people will experience further awakening and insomnia in the middle of the night. The simplest strategy for treating this is to take another full dose of regular carbidopa/levodopa when you awaken later in the night. As long as 3–4 hours have elapsed between the bedtime dose and the one taken in the middle of the night, there should not be substantial overlap.

Note that a "full dose" of carbidopa/levodopa has been stipulated. Intuitively, a lower dose might be expected as sufficient at night, since sleep should not require as much levodopa. However, that is not correct. To use carbidopa/levodopa for sleep, the full dose established for daytime use is also necessary at night.

A slightly more complex strategy for sustaining sleep involves use of the sustained-release formulation. This formulation is not used to initiate sleep, since the slow effect is problematic. However, the delayed effect of the sustained-release pills allows them to kick in around 2 hours into sleep if taken just as your head hits the pillow. In other words, this is a two-step process: use a late-evening dose of regular carbidopa/levodopa to get to sleep and just as you are ready to fall asleep, take a dose of sustained-release carbidopa/levodopa. If these two formulations are taken an hour apart or more, the effects should not substantially overlap. Note that the sustained-release carbidopa/levodopa dose will need to be adjusted so that it is comparable to the regular (immediate-release) carbidopa/levodopa dose, as outlined earlier in this chapter.

As an example of how the two formulations might be used in the same night, consider the person who takes two 25/100 regular carbidopa/ levodopa tablets an hour before each of three meals and complains of insomnia—unable to get to sleep. The first step would be to add a full dose of two of the regular tablets an hour before bedtime. If that person now experiences good initial sleep but awakening in the middle of the night, one might then add a dose of sustained-release carbidopa/levodopa just before going to sleep. This should be about an hour after the last evening dose of regular carbidopa/levodopa. Sleep requires a "full dose" of levodopa, so the sustained-release levodopa dose should be about 50% more than the dose of regular carbidopa/levodopa (as discussed earlier). For this person taking two 25/100 immediate-release tablets for the daytime doses, the appropriate sustained-release dose would be 300 mg, or three of the 25/100 sustained-release tablets. If this does not allow sleeping through the night, the sustained-release dose could be raised to 400 mg (two of the 50/200 tablets) to ensure a supra-threshold amount of levodopa. Levodopa for sleep tends to respond all-or-none, as if there were a threshold amount necessary for sleep; hence the reason for trying a slightly higher dose.

RYTARY

Rytary is the brand name of a combination of sustained-release and immediate-release carbidopa/levodopa in a single capsule. It had just reached the market as this book went to press, thus I have no personal experience with it. It is unclear if it has major advantages over using the two carbidopa/ levodopa formulations together as just discussed. Dosage conversions from regular carbidopa/levodopa to Rytary may require trial-and-error adjustments. Rytary is priced substantially higher than the generic formulations of regular and sustained-release carbidopa/levodopa.

ADVANCING PD, SHORT-DURATION LEVODOPA RESPONSES, AND MEALS

Recall our rule of carbidopa/levodopa administration: take at least an hour before meals and at least 2 hours after the end of meals. This may become problematic later in the course of PD if dosing intervals decline to less than 4 hours. With much shorter intervals, some doses necessarily will be too close to meals, recognizing that it takes about a half-hour to eat.

As discussed in previous chapters, meal protein is the culprit. Proteins are critical to good nutrition, but are problematic when consumed around the time of carbidopa/levodopa doses. Recall that proteins consist of strings of amino acids and digestion releases these amino acids into the bloodstream. Levodopa is an amino acid; it competes with circulating dietary amino acids for binding sites on the blood-brain barrier transporter that carries these amino acids into the brain. If carbidopa/levodopa is taken close to meals, it is easily outnumbered by dietary amino acids and cannot enter the brain (i.e., the transporter does not have enough binding sites). Thus protein-containing meals tend to inhibit the levodopa response.

Clearance of dietary amino acids from the circulation after a meal typically takes 2 hours; hence the rule to wait 2 hours after the end of a meal before taking the next dose of carbidopa/levodopa. The "1-hour before" rule includes the time it takes for the carbidopa/levodopa pill to dissolve and enter the circulation; for some people, the levodopa response is much quicker, but others require a full hour to ensure that it kicks in. Unfortunately for those who experience 2- to 3-hour levodopa responses, these rules conflict with the advice to adjust the dosing interval to match the response duration. Such 2- to 3-hour levodopa responses rarely occur *early* in Parkinson's disease, but are much more common after many years of PD.

One might think that certain food products would have sufficient levodopa content to shift the balance and overshadow the other amino acids. Unfortunately, this is not the case, and almost no foods have enough levodopa to make a difference. The single exception is fava beans, which have very high levodopa concentrations and are a staple of some Mediterranean diets. However, regularly eating fava beans is a very impractical treatment of PD, especially considering the difficulty in ascertaining a consistent and adequate levodopa dose.

SPECIAL STRATEGIES TO OVERCOME MEAL EFFECTS

In longer-standing PD, meals and snacks are the most common reason for otherwise unexplained failure of carbidopa/levodopa doses. Among those with advancing PD and short-duration levodopa responses, the levodopa effect tends to occur all-or-none, as if there were a threshold for the "on" response. Dietary amino acids typically reduce the levodopa influx into the brain just enough to lower the dose below the on-threshold. This phenomenon has been termed the *skipped dose effect*, or *dose failure*.

This relationship to meals is often not recognized. People report to their physician that some of their carbidopa/levodopa doses fail to work, oblivious to the association with time of eating.

SIMPLE THINGS TO COUNTER MEAL EFFECTS ON CARBIDOPA/LEVODOPA

For those who take carbidopa/levodopa at short intervals, simply avoiding high-protein foods should theoretically be helpful. However, adequate dietary protein is important for good nutrition and general health; a certain amount of daily protein intake is essential.

One strategy is to shift the times of meals to match your social and occupational schedule. If you have an important engagement that may be sabotaged by a meal, avoid eating before or during that event. For example, if you are attending a family wedding in the early afternoon, defer lunch and avoid protein-containing foods at the wedding reception (wedding cake should be OK, but not the meat or cheese sandwiches). Change mealtimes to match the day's activities.

The meal content also makes a difference. If having a luncheon or dinner with friends, you might order a salad. Remember, however, that some ingredients used to top off salads are high in protein, such as grilled meats, chicken, cheese, cottage cheese, and nuts and seeds. You might push some of these aside if they appear on your salad.

Foods high in protein are shown in Table 17.1. You should not avoid these altogether, but you may choose to consume these in moderation, especially during times of the day when you need carbidopa/levodopa to work well.

Bear in mind that protein snacks are often as problematic as regular meals. A big bowl of ice cream in the mid-afternoon may translate into a late-afternoon off-state. Snack if you like, but recognize the potential relationship to your levodopa responses.

Another strategy for countering meal inhibition of the levodopa response involves redistributing the protein content of meals: limited protein is consumed with breakfast and lunch, with the evening meal supplying most of the daily protein requirement. When doing this, be careful to consume enough protein to meet your daily needs; a dietician can supply advice regarding daily protein requirement. This might be most appropriate for those with a daytime work schedule who need to be "on" during the working day but would tolerate levodopa off-states in the evening. This is a reasonable fit with our typical American diet, with the largest meal of the day being at supper.

Table 17.1. Protein Foods

• Milk products (including ice cream, yogurt, butter, cheese, cottage cheese)	• Dietary supplements, such as Ensure or Slim-Fast
• Eggs and egg substitutes	• Nuts (including peanut butter, sunflower seeds)
• Meats of all types	• Beans, peas
• Poultry (including chicken, turkey)	• Soybeans (including tofu, which is soybean curd)
• Fish of all types (including shellfish)	• Puddings, custards

However, you may choose to make lunch or even breakfast the high-protein meal if that fits better with your needs.

To ensure that you will not become malnourished, it is wise to seek advice from a dietitian or nutrition specialist before embarking on one of these protein redistribution diets. They can advise exactly which foods to avoid and which to substitute to make palatable meals. Theoretically, such daily protein redistribution should be a very effective strategy. In my experience it helps, but works inconsistently.

ANOTHER STRATEGY FOR WORKING AROUND MEALS: MORE LEVODOPA

Levodopa inhibition by dietary protein reflects a numbers game. Dietary amino acids compete with levodopa for binding sites on the blood-brain barrier transporter. Providing additional levodopa during mealtimes can provide more of a competitive advantage. Thus one might take larger doses of carbidopa/levodopa when close to meals.

Our rules have stipulated that carbidopa/levodopa doses taken within an hour before or within 2 hours from the end of meals will tend to be inhibited by dietary protein. For doses falling within this meal time-frame, a slightly larger dose would be more likely to work. However, we should also be careful to avoid an excessive levodopa effect causing dyskinesias. Hence, I usually advise the following:

> Take a larger carbidopa/levodopa dose if within 20 minutes before a meal, during a meal, or within 2 hours after completion of a meal.

This strategy translates into two different doses throughout the day: one dose is for when your stomach is empty; the other, larger dose is for around mealtimes.

How do we determine these two different doses? Generally, we have already established the carbidopa/levodopa dose that works when the stomach is empty. With that dose as a reference point, raise the mealtime doses by half-tablet increments (i.e., half of a regular 25/100 tablet). After a few days, if it appears that these doses still fail to kick in, they may be raised by another half-tablet. I typically do not have people raise the mealtime doses higher than an extra 1 ½ tablets each dose.

With this scheme, you need to ask yourself when due for another carbidopa/levodopa dose: Does this fall into the critical meal interval? If yes, take the larger dose; if not, take the smaller. Although this makes sense, the results tend to be somewhat inconsistent, but worth trying.

I CAN TAKE MY CARBIDOPA/LEVODOPA WITH MEALS AND IT STILL SEEMS TO WORK

If that is the case, don't worry about it. If your parkinsonism is well controlled, don't change anything.

SWEETS AND THE LEVODOPA RESPONSE

High-sugar foods devoid of protein may slightly enhance the levodopa response. For example, a large candy bar without nuts (nuts contain proteins) may induce a more potent effect from your dose of carbidopa/levodopa. Presumably, this is because the sugar (glucose) triggers your body to release insulin. Insulin is known to increase the exit of amino acids from the bloodstream into cells. Without the competition from other amino acids, administered levodopa can cross the blood-brain barrier more readily.

Regularly taking carbidopa/levodopa with candy bars is not a good general strategy, however. Sugars contain empty calories (not nutritious) and tend to facilitate obesity and cause tooth cavities.

MY CARBIDOPA/LEVODOPA TAKES
A LONG TIME TO KICK IN

If you lapse into a levodopa "off" state, you want a quick response from your next dose of carbidopa/levodopa. With immediate-release carbidopa/levodopa, this should take about 60 minutes, although rarely up to 2 hours. A minority of people with PD report responses within 20–30 minutes.

One impediment to a quick response relates to the carbidopa/levodopa pills sitting undissolved in the stomach. To enter the bloodstream, the pill must first dissolve and then the fluid containing the carbidopa/levodopa is released into the small intestine. Absorption into the bloodstream takes place exclusively in the small intestine (none from the stomach). This process is illustrated in Figure 17.2.

One simple strategy to facilitate the carbidopa/levodopa response is to wash the pills down with adequate fluids. Besides providing a medium to dissolve the pills, the fluid volume may promote release of the stomach contents into the small intestine. Any fluids will be appropriate as long as it is not a milk product or protein drink.

Occasional people chew their carbidopa/levodopa pills. It that works for you, that is OK, but often, some of the pill contents are left on the teeth.

EXERCISE AND FLUCTUATIONS
IN THE LEVODOPA RESPONSE

Exercise is an important component of PD management, as discussed in detail in Chapter 9. Those with fluctuations in their levodopa response need to be aware that physical exercise tends to use up the levodopa faster. The short-duration levodopa response usually does not last as long during exercise. If you become aware of this, you may take your next carbidopa/levodopa dose early, to avoid this premature off-response. Once the exercise is over, you can revert back to your usual dosing intervals. Don't worry about

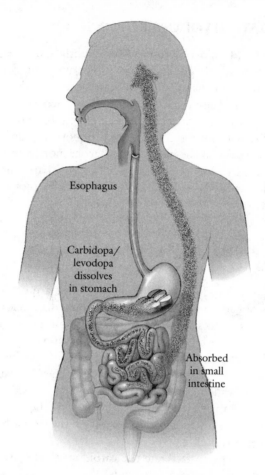

Esophagus

Carbidopa/
levodopa
dissolves
in stomach

Absorbed
in small
intestine

17.2 The carbidopa/levodopa pills must first dissolve in the fluids within the stomach. The fluid solution then passes into the small intestine (jejunum) where levodopa passes across the intestinal wall into the circulation. From the bloodstream, it is transported across the blood-brain barrier.

how many doses you take per day. If you burn the fuel faster, you simply need to fill the tank a little more often.

FLEXIBILITY WITH THE CARBIDOPA/LEVODOPA DOSING INTERVAL

The previous advice about taking a dose early during exercise is also appropriate for other times of the day. If you recognize that your carbidopa/levodopa is wearing off before the usually scheduled next dose, you may take that dose early. You will then need to move the subsequent doses up in time to avoid gaps in coverage.

Most people with these problems recognize certain symptoms that signal that their levodopa response is being lost. This might be toe-curling, tremor, recurrence of walking problems, or slowness. Sometimes the clues are more subjective, such as anxiety, restlessness, or even shortness of breath.

If you need to take a dose early, you should take your full dose, rather than a partial dose. When the tank is empty, you want to fill it full, not half-full. Don't worry about the number of carbidopa/levodopa doses per day.

Bear in mind that we are talking about taking a dose a little early. This implies that the levodopa effect has occurred and is starting to wear off prematurely. This is different from a dose failing to work, which requires a different strategy (see discussion later in this chapter).

MOST OF MY DOSES WEAR OFF EARLY

If this is your problem, the interval between doses is too long. Shorten the interval to match the duration of the typical response. Take as many doses each day as necessary to maintain an "on" response.

SHOULD I BE COMPULSIVE ABOUT TREATING THESE WEARING-OFF SYMPTOMS?

You do not need to shorten the dosing interval if the wearing-off symptoms are not a problem for you. Some people experience a mild decline in their levodopa effect each dose cycle, but without any compromise in function. If this pattern is not troublesome, stick with your current dosing schedule, rather than trying to compulsively adjust your medication doses. You are better off living with mild wearing-off effects than becoming obsessed with tightly regulating your dosing schedule. Moreover, longer dosing intervals make it easier to work around meals.

I OFTEN FORGET TO TAKE MY PILLS AND THEN LAPSE INTO AN OFF-STATE.

A frequent need for scheduled medication doses is challenging. The solution may be a pillbox timer. Most medical supply stores and many pharmacies carry these timers. The most user-friendly models allow you to set the dosing interval and then run the timer from a separate button. Once you have set this dosing interval, you don't need to set the timer again. Smartphones also may be programmed to ring at fixed intervals.

MY LEVODOPA DIDN'T KICK IN!

Failed carbidopa/levodopa doses can be very troubling, especially if this occurs when important engagements are pending. Failed doses have two likely causes. The most common one is a meal or snack inhibiting the levodopa response. Less commonly, occasional people are slightly underdosed and need a higher levodopa dose to surpass the on-threshold (e.g., another half-pill of 25/100 carbidopa/levodopa each dose).

What should one do if a carbidopa/levodopa response fails and a quick fix is necessary? Things you could try include the following:

- Take another full dose of carbidopa/levodopa now (i.e., 60 to 90 minutes after the dose that failed). This probably will kick in, but you may experience an excessive effect, such as dyskinesias, which we will address later in this chapter.

- Take a fraction of your usual dose now (i.e., 60 to 90 minutes after the dose that failed). This partial dose might be a half or one 25/100 immediate-release carbidopa/levodopa tablet. This may allow you to lapse into an on-state, but sometimes partial doses fail to kick in.

- Wait until it is closer to the time for your next dose and then take your full carbidopa/levodopa dose. Obviously, this will likely kick in, but the wait may be frustrating.

These are all reasonable but imperfect options. Rescue therapy is often needed!

RESCUE THERAPY WITH LIQUID SINEMET

Imagine you are playing golf and suddenly your levodopa effect wears off. It is hard to walk, much less hit a golf ball. How can you quickly reverse this off-state so that you can finish the round of golf? Liquefying your full dose carbidopa/levodopa is the simplest solution. You do this by crushing your tablets (the full dose) and dissolving this in soda pop or some other liquid. For example, if your usual daily dose is 2 of the 25/100 carbidopa/levodopa tablets four times daily, use 2 tablets as the rescue dose; crush 2 of these tablets, dissolve, and drink the solution. This will start to work in about 20 minutes, but with an effect that only lasts an hour; however, this buys you time.

Carbonated beverages seem to work well for this purpose, perhaps because carbonation tends to stimulate gastric emptying. Juice or water is also fine, as long as it is palatable. Obviously, do not mix it in milk or other protein drinks. In general, about 4 to 6 ounces of fluid is appropriate. Note that the entire contents of your mixture must be drunk to receive the full dose.

If the need for rescue therapy is a frequent occurrence, you might premix this solution. As long as it does not become heated (e.g., in the hot sun), it should be stable for many hours. It can be kept in a sealed sports-drink container. When ready to drink, shake the contents to make sure the carbidopa/levodopa is fully dissolved.

Note that if you take the liquid carbidopa/levodopa soon after taking your carbidopa/levodopa pills, the doses will summate and may cause dyskinesias (see discussion later in this chapter). If dyskinesias are a major concern, you may need to subsequently dissolve a lesser amount of carbidopa/levodopa to make this solution. Even if dyskinesias develop, they will be over in perhaps 60 to 90 minutes with the liquid formulation. If you take too little, then the rescue dose won't work.

I'VE TAKEN THE LIQUID SINEMET AND I'M FEELING BETTER—NOW WHAT?

Anticipate that the response to liquifying carbidopa/levodopa will last only about an hour. You will need to take your carbidopa/levodopa pills shortly after the liquid Sinemet kicks in. Since it takes up to an hour for the carbidopa/levodopa tablets to work, you will need to take them right after you recognize that the liquid rescue dose is starting to kick in. Don't forget to do this or you will lapse into another off-state.

There is no limit to how often you may add extra doses of liquid Sinemet. However, if you frequently need this strategy, you should consider whether there are other means of preventing off-states, such as those discussed earlier and in the next chapter.

ANOTHER RESCUE TREATMENT: APOMORPHINE

An injectable drug, apomorphine (Apokyn), is very effective for relieving levodopa off-states. This dopamine agonist produces responses similar to those from carbidopa/levodopa, unlike the more modest effects of other dopamine agonist pills or patches. After an injection, an on-state develops in about 10 minutes and lasts 60–90 minutes. Identification of the optimal dose requires monitoring in the clinician's office. Since apomorphine tends to provoke orthostatic hypotension, the clinician will need to check standing blood pressure values during the initial dose-finding assessment in the office. This drug is discussed in more detail in Chapter 18.

ORALLY DISINTEGRATING CARBIDOPA/LEVODOPA (PARCOPA)

An orally disintegrating formulation of carbidopa/levodopa pills is available, with the brand name Parcopa. It dissolves in the mouth and is swallowed with your saliva. It is not absorbed in the mouth. Data available from the pharmaceutical company suggest that it kicks in at about the same time as conventional, immediate-release carbidopa/levodopa, although some patients have reported to me that it works faster. It is advantageous when water or other liquid isn't available or when socially conspicuous (e.g., at a party). It is more expensive than regular carbidopa/levodopa.

LIQUID SINEMET FOR CHRONIC USE

About 20 years ago, liquifying carbidopa/levodopa and taking an hourly dose was in vogue for PD treatment. The short-hand term for this was *liquid Sinemet*. This strategy turned out to be too complicated and cumbersome for most people. Still, there are rare individuals who might benefit from its use. If one is able to stay on time with the hourly doses, a more consistent and predictable benefit may be achieved. It is also easier to make nuanced dose adjustments. This is not a useful strategy for those who are experiencing at least a 3-hour response to carbidopa/levodopa pills. For the few people whose levodopa effect spans less than 2 hours, this may prove helpful (if you can tolerate the inconveniences of this strategy).

There is no commercial form of liquid Sinemet. Using liquid Sinemet for every dose requires mixing this in a large volume ahead of time. Crushing and dissolving the pills every hour is far too cumbersome to be tolerated. The standard recipe for mixing a large volume of carbidopa/levodopa solution ahead of time yields 1 mg (milligram) of levodopa for every mL (milliliter); this allows the dose to be determined with a mL measuring container; thus 1 mg = 1 mL.

A liter of solution that provides 1 mg of levodopa for every mL is made by dissolving 10 of the 25/100 carbidopa/levodopa pills in 1,000 mL (1 liter) of liquid. The liquid can be whatever you find most palatable, such as juice, Kool-Aid, soda pop. Note that the carbidopa content can be ignored; the levodopa amount is the crucial component. If a liter seems too cumbersome, cut this recipe in half and dissolve 5 pills in a half-liter (500 mL). Each dose is determined by the mL. If you have been taking 2 of the 25/100 immediate-release tablets each dose, then your levodopa dose is 200 mg and the volume of liquid Sinemet is 200 mL. If you decide that the response is slightly excessive, you can easily adjust the dose by taking a lesser volume; for example, 175 mL provides 175 mg of levodopa (25 mg less than 200 mg). Note the response is quick, kicking in within about 20 minutes.

The turnover of levodopa is much quicker with the liquid formulation. You will be taking the same amount, but at shorter intervals. The daily amount of carbidopa and levodopa will be substantially greater, but this is not of concern.

This strategy requires that you prepare the liquid Sinemet each morning and carry the liquid container all day. You will need some type of milliliter measuring cup (note that cubic centimeters, cc, and mL are interchangeable). You will likely need a timer, since the effect typically lasts about an hour.

If you decide to try liquid Sinemet, you can transition overnight, starting the new day with the liquid form rather than pills. If you don't like it after a day, week, or month, just switch back to the pills.

USING LIQUID SINEMET

If you transition to liquid Sinemet, there are two guidelines, assuming that the mixture concentration is 1 mg per each mL:

1. Each dose of liquid Sinemet is now measured in mL. If you previously took one 25/100 carbidopa/levodopa pill each dose, take 100 mL of liquid Sinemet.

2. Start with dosing intervals a little longer than an hour, perhaps 90 minutes. This will allow you to appreciate the duration of the response, as it kicks in and wears off. You can reduce this interval to match the response duration.

To stay on schedule, use a pillbox timer or a smartphone set to ring at a fixed interval. You will want such a timer that allows you to initially set the dosing interval, without the need to reset it every time.

Once you have made this transition, you are then in a position to fine-tune your levodopa response. For example, if you are taking 200 mL of liquid Sinemet (i.e., 200 mg levodopa) and experience excessive responses (e.g., dyskinesias, discussed later in this chapter) you can lower the doses by 20–50 mL (20–50 mg) decrements. Find the dose providing the best balance between over- and underdosage effects.

Liquid Sinemet prepared as described here should be good for the entire waking day, but it may not remain stable beyond that. Refrigeration helps maintain stability—at the very least, avoid very hot temperatures. If the solution turns dark, that is a clue that the levodopa is becoming degraded and may not work.

If you wish to prepare liquid Sinemet a day or two in advance, you may add vitamin C (ascorbic acid), which is an antioxidant preservative. The conventional amount is 2 mg of ascorbic acid for every mL of solution and every 1 mg of levodopa. This should remain stable for 2 full days and up to 3 days if refrigerated when not in use.

INTESTINAL ADMINISTRATION OF CARBIDOPA/ LEVODOPA WITH DUODOPA

The U.S. Food and Drug Administration (FDA) recently approved a gel formulation of carbidopa/levodopa that is continuously administered via an infusion pump directly into the upper small intestine (jejunum). It is

indicated for better treatment of levodopa fluctuations. Surgical implantation of the infusion tube via the abdominal wall is necessary; this is a minor
procedure. The tube exiting from the skin of the abdomen is not apparent
when one is wearing a shirt or blouse. The carbidopa/levodopa suspension,
with the brand name Duodopa, bypasses the stomach and allows for more
consistent responses; delivery of carbidopa/levodopa is not impeded by
delayed emptying of the stomach contents. However, the levodopa responses
will still be subject to the effects of dietary proteins, since these compete
with levodopa downstream at the blood-brain barrier.

This product is too new to allow conclusions about its general usefulness,
and I have not had firsthand experience with it. Hence, I will not comment
further on this strategy in this book. Hopefully, it will provide an option for
PD patients with levodopa fluctuations who are not able to undergo deep
brain stimulation surgery (discussed in Chapter 33) or are not interested in it.

No Fluctuations, Just Doing Poorly

The focus of the chapter to this point has been on fluctuations and instability of the levodopa response. What if your PD does not follow this pattern
and the initial levodopa benefit during the early months and years is not
sustained and without fluctuations?

If you truly have Parkinson's disease, there should not be loss of the
levodopa response a few months or years later. Although there might be a
mild decline in the levodopa effect, this should be minimal. This assumes
that carbidopa/levodopa has been optimized using the guidelines in
Chapter 12. If there is a major drop-off of the levodopa response within the
first few years, and if not simply the fluctuations just described, there are
several possibilities that should be considered.

- You have continued on a very low dose of carbidopa/levodopa and are
  underdosed.

- You have started a drug that is blocking the levodopa effect.

- You have inadvertently changed your levodopa formulation or dosing
  strategy.

- New PD symptoms do not have a substrate in dopamine systems (e.g.,
  urinary or bowel symptoms; orthostatic hypotension).

- New problems have developed that are independent from PD.

- Age is the problem: brain aging affecting gait and balance tends to
  become problematic around 80 years of age.

- You do not have Parkinson's disease.

Let's consider each of these in detail.

Occasional people with early and mild PD initially do well on a very small dose of carbidopa/levodopa (e.g., one 25/100 tablet three times daily). After a few months or years, this low dose may prove insufficient (i.e., it does not fill the "dopamine tank"). If your carbidopa/levodopa dose is low and you are now doing poorly, revisit Chapter 12 and consider appropriate dose escalation.

Dopamine receptors can be blocked with certain drugs, specifically medications to treat nausea (e.g., metoclopramide, prochlorperazine) or drugs for psychosis. These drugs were listed in Chapter 6.

The dosing scheme in Chapter 6 stipulates taking carbidopa/levodopa on an empty stomach at least 1 hour before meals and at least 2 hours after the end of meals. People sometimes begin to cheat and take their carbidopa/levodopa doses with meals. Also, protein snacks may be forgotten. If the levodopa response starts to fail, consider these issues.

Rarely, a carbidopa/levodopa prescription will be filled with the sustained-release formulation of carbidopa/levodopa. This formulation has different properties from those of regular (immediate-release) carbidopa/levodopa, and the dosing scheme in Chapter 12 is not appropriate for that formulation. How can you tell? Immediate-release carbidopa/levodopa pills, generic or brand name, are yellow. The controlled-release pills are another color (gray-blue if generic; tan or rose-colored if brand name Sinemet CR).

Not all PD symptoms are due to dopamine deficiency. PD does affect bowel and bladder function, and these problems require treatment other than dopamine replacement. Low blood pressure (orthostatic hypotension) may compromise walking and thinking but is not treated with carbidopa/levodopa (levodopa exacerbates these problems); see Chapter 21 if feeling faint is the problem. Thinking and memory problems may surface in PD, either due to the Lewy neurodegenerative process or some secondary cause. For those problems, read Chapter 23.

As we reach middle age, a variety of medical problems tend to surface, unrelated to PD. And, of course, PD does not protect people from other medical disorders.

Normal brain aging impairs walking and balance. In fact, normal aging often takes on the pattern of PD, with a stooped posture and slowness. As a rule of thumb, mobility among those over 80 years of age is increasingly problematic. Although some seniors are still athletic and active well beyond age 80, it is at around that time that motor function becomes more impaired. Among those over 80, the levodopa response is less complete. Note that age 80 is a crude cutoff; for some, the decline starts a little earlier and for others, normal gait and balance persist for years beyond. Carbidopa/levodopa will not benefit the gait problems and slowness of normal aging.

Those with PD should experience robust carbidopa/levodopa responses, and these tend to persist for years or indefinitely. If after a few months or years the levodopa benefit is lost and if this is not explained by the issues just outlined, the diagnosis may not be PD. Disorders such as multiple system atrophy (MSA) or progressive supranuclear palsy (PSP) sometimes masquerade as PD for a few years before the true diagnosis declares itself. Chapter 6 addresses these other parkinsonian disorders.

If carbidopa/levodopa is failing to provide benefit, other PD drugs working through dopamine mechanisms are unlikely to help. The dopamine agonists and rasagiline/selegiline also facilitate dopamine neurotransmission, but they do this with a much less robust response than that of carbidopa/levodopa. Hence, there is no good reason to expect them to work if carbidopa/levodopa fails.

Dyskinesias

The term *dyskinesias* in the context of PD implies involuntary exaggerated movements from an excessive levodopa effect. Not all excessive movements seen in PD are dyskinesias. For example, tremor is an involuntary movement but should not be considered a dyskinesia. Literally, *dyskinesia* translates as "abnormal movements"; however, it has a very specific connotation in PD. In this context it refers to *chorea* (the adjective is *choreiform*). Chorea implies involuntary, flowing, dancing-like movements. When we use the term *dyskinesias* in this book, we are using it in this strict sense to refer to these choreiform movements provoked by levodopa. Although the other PD drugs that facilitate brain dopamine may provoke or enhance dyskinesias, levodopa is the primary cause in most cases.

Levodopa-induced dyskinesias are on the opposite end of the spectrum from PD-related bradykinesia. Bradykinesia connotes the slowness of PD (*brady* = slow; *kinesia* = movement). On a "kinesia" continuum, too little brain dopamine translates into too little movement, or bradykinesia. Conversely, excessive brain dopamine causes too much movement, which might more appropriately be termed hyperkinesia. However, the term *dyskinesia* is embedded in the PD vernacular.

These dancing, choreiform dyskinetic movements from an excessive levodopa dose give the appearance of chaotic motion. It typically waxes and wanes. Dyskinesias may be present in only one area of the body, such as a hand or arm. Or, they may involve half the body, such as affecting the arm and leg on one side. They may affect the entire body, or perhaps just the head and neck. A dyskinetic foot may wiggle while someone is seated. Head and neck dyskinesias give the appearance that the head is bouncing back and forth. Often the person who has these dyskinesias is unaware of them. They are painless and, if not severe, do not interfere with most activities.

Most people with dyskinesias can control these with simple medication adjustments. However, if mild, they may be so inconsequential that nothing needs to be done (e.g., a wiggly foot). Restated, it is not necessary to treat dyskinesias if they are not getting in the way.

Levodopa dyskinesias rarely develop early in the course of PD treatment but may surface after several years. By 5 years of levodopa therapy, about 40% of PD patients will experience at least some dyskinesias. When they occur, simply reducing the levodopa dose (or the dose of another dopamine medication) will abolish these. However, it is not always that simple. There is a small minority of people who have a narrow therapeutic window between optimal control of parkinsonism and dyskinesias. Lowering the dose sufficiently to stop dyskinesias results in poor control of parkinsonism. It appears that such hard-to-control dyskinesias ultimately surface in a little more than 10% of those with PD.

Medication-induced dyskinesias are most common among young people with PD. PD uncommonly develops before age 40 years, but when it does, dyskinesias (and motor fluctuations) become apparent in nearly all by 5 years of levodopa treatment.

Since levodopa is the most potent of the anti-parkinsonian drugs, these dyskinetic movements are largely levodopa induced. Other drugs that work through dopamine (dopamine agonists, MAO-B inhibitors, COMT inhibitors) are rarely the primary cause of dyskinesias. However, when added to carbidopa/levodopa, they may facilitate dyskinesias, by virtue of enhancing dopamine neurotransmission.

The cause of dyskinesias especially relates to the increasing loss of dopaminergic terminals in the striatum. These striatal dopaminergic terminals, shown in Figure 17.3, not only store and release dopamine but also regulate the dopamine levels in the synapse. This is done by "reuptake," which implies that the dopamine is sucked back into the terminal. This prevents excessive stimulation of dopamine receptors. Early in PD, when there are sufficient dopaminergic terminals to control synaptic dopamine concentrations, excessive dopamine stimulation (i.e., dyskinesias) does not occur. With progression of PD and loss of these dopaminergic terminals, other cells substitute. Unfortunately, these other cells are not very good at regulating the dopamine concentrations in the synapse and dopamine receptors then can be excessively stimulated; dyskinesias result.

Why are dyskinesias limited to only certain areas of the body? Presumably, this relates to the uneven loss of dopaminergic terminals in the striatum. Intuitively, one would expect that the PD neurodegenerative process would affect these neurons uniformly. However, the loss is somewhat haphazard, with certain areas of the striatum more devoid of surviving dopaminergic terminals than other regions.

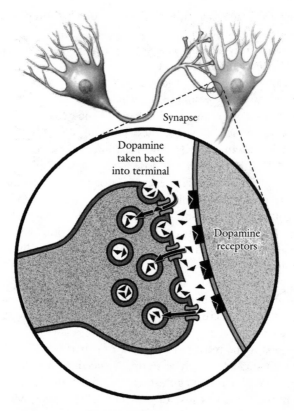

17.3 Dopaminergic terminals tightly regulate the concentration of dopamine in the synapse. If this regulatory effect is lost, excessive synaptic dopamine levels can easily overstimulate the receptors, provoking dyskinesias (excessive movement). This tends to occur after years of PD when few dopaminergic terminals remain. The other (nondopaminergic) cells that substitute are unable to optimally regulate synaptic dopamine concentrations.

Distinguishing Levodopa Dyskinesias from Other Involuntary Movements

Treatment of levodopa dyskinesias requires correct identification. Other involuntary movements also occur in PD, especially dystonia and tremor, both due to PD itself. PD also frequently causes an inner restlessness, termed *akathisia*, which should not be mistaken for levodopa-induced dyskinesias. Dystonia, tremor, and akathisia typically require levodopa therapy and are not due to excess levodopa. Restated, they represent an opposite set of problems and deserve further discussion.

DYSTONIA

Dystonia implies an abnormal muscle contraction state resulting in an abnormal posture. This muscle contraction or tightness may be painful, like a muscle cramp. Dystonia is a frequent symptom of PD and usually responds well to carbidopa/levodopa. Hence, one should not inappropriately attribute dystonia to carbidopa/levodopa, since this drug is the treatment rather than the cause in most cases.

Typical dystonias of PD include toe curling or toe extension. Leg cramps are common in general, but if frequent in someone with PD, these may represent dystonia, often with foot inversion. Leg cramps in the general population are usually due to muscle conditions, such as excessive muscle demand from very vigorous exercise. In PD, what seems like muscle cramps are actually mediated at the brain level.

Whereas dystonias of the limbs typically respond to carbidopa/levodopa, they may not respond if the dystonia involves the axis of the body, that is, the trunk or neck. For example, neck dystonia in PD is uncommon, but when a tilted or twisted dystonic neck does occur, carbidopa/levodopa often fails to help. Trunk dystonia may cause involuntary tilting or flexion of the trunk, which also usually fails carbidopa/levodopa treatment.

Botulinum toxin injection is often used to treat dystonia. It is primarily effective when the dystonia involves a limited area of musculature, such as the neck. There is a maximum amount of botulinum toxin that can be safely administered. Thus, a major tilt of the trunk from dystonia typically involves too much of the musculature to allow treatment with botulinum toxin.

Occasionally, dystonia is attributed to carbidopa/levodopa, even though it is not likely the cause. To assess this issue, the easiest strategy is to observe what happens after going overnight without carbidopa/levodopa. If the dystonia is present in the morning before carbidopa/levodopa is taken, then levodopa should not be the culprit. If carbidopa/levodopa is the cause of involuntary movements, these are time-locked to the last dose, starting around an hour after a dose and resolving several hours later. Once many hours have elapsed, the side-effect potential of levodopa is gone.

Occasionally, true levodopa dyskinesias also include a component of dystonia. A typical example would be a dancing, choreiform arm from levodopa, but with the arm postured backwards. It would be correct to conclude that the arm posturing is dystonia, but the dancing movements would indicate that the predominant feature is chorea and, hence, due to carbidopa/levodopa. Thus in the context of PD, chorea plus an element of dystonia is almost certainly due to carbidopa/levodopa; pure dystonia is likely due to PD. Pure dystonias typically respond to carbidopa/levodopa, whereas chorea plus dystonia requires less levodopa.

PD-related dystonia should not be confused with levodopa dyskinesias since the treatment for one is the opposite of the treatment of the other. Table 17.2 summarizes differences between levodopa-provoked dyskinesias and PD-related dystonia.

Very rarely, pure dystonia may be provoked by carbidopa/levodopa. The cause for the dystonia can be identified by considering the time course. Recall that involuntary movements provoked by carbidopa/levodopa

Table 17.2. Levodopa-Induced Dyskinesias versus Parkinson's Disease–Related Dystonia

	Levodopa-Induced Dyskinesias *	PD-Dystonia
Appearance	Predominantly chorea: rapidly flowing, dancing, chaotic involuntary movements	Sustained muscle contraction causing twisting, turning or contortion (e.g., toes curled or turned up; foot turned in)
Relationship to levodopa	Caused by this	Relieved by this
Relation to timing of levodopa	Starts 30–60 minutes after a dose (twice that long after sustained-release carbidopa/levodopa); resolves within a few hours	Starts several hours after last levodopa dose (wearing-off effect, but if insufficient levodopa, may be present continuously)
Morning, before medications	Absent, unless levodopa during the night	Often present if no levodopa during the night
Subjective sensation	Dyskinetic limbs do not feel tense	Cramp-like, or tense feeling in muscle. May feel restless, but does not appear restless to onlookers
Pain	No	Often
Treatment	Lower each levodopa dose	Optimize the carbidopa/levodopa

* Supplemental drugs that work through dopamine (e.g., dopamine agonists, entacapone) potentially increase dyskinesia severity.

develop around an hour after a dose and resolve several hours later. This time-locked relationship should allow this to be sorted out. For example, if the dystonia is absent first thing in the morning after going overnight with carbidopa/levodopa, but develops an hour after the first morning dose, the cause should be apparent.

The term *dystonia*, in the context of PD, relates to one particular symptom that is part of the entire PD complex. In that sense, it parallels the term *tremor*, which is another symptom of PD. Note, however, that the term *dystonia* is also used in a different context to connote neurological conditions in which the dystonia is the only problem; these are separate from PD and not related. Conditions such as torticollis (cervical dystonia) or writer's cramp (writer's dystonia) fall into the category of primary dystonias. In these primary dystonias, there are no other neurological manifestations besides the dystonia. These primary dystonias are not associated with Lewy body changes in the brain.

RESTLESSNESS: AKATHISIA

An inner restlessness is a common symptom of untreated PD. The medical term for this is *akathisia*. Although the person with akathisia feels restless, they appear just the opposite, slow and stiff. Ironically, those with levodopa-dyskinesias do not feel restless, even when dyskinesias are so prominent that they can't sit still. In fact, this is when they often feel the most relaxed. These conditions should not be confused, as this could result in the wrong treatment. Restated:

- "I feel restless" = parkinsonism
- Moving constantly but not feeling restless = dyskinesias

Dyskinesia and akathisia are on opposite ends of the spectrum.

TREMOR

Tremor is occasionally confused with dyskinesias, but the distinction should be obvious, once the characteristics are defined. Tremors are rhythmic, to and fro, always with the same recurring pattern, in contrast to the chaotic, choreiform movements of levodopa dyskinesias. These stereotyped, pendulum-like movements of tremor may come and go. Among people with PD, tremor most often affects the hand(s), but it may also affect one or both legs. While seated, a knee involuntarily going up and down with a regular rhythm represents tremor. The chin is another common area of parkinsonian tremor.

Unlike this recurring, stereotyped, back-and-forth tremor pattern, chorea, by definition, is NOT stereotyped; that is, it has no ongoing pattern of movements. The chorea of levodopa-induced dyskinesias makes that part of the body look fidgety. However, these movements are without a recurring pattern and are not rhythmic.

CAUSE OF DYSKINESIAS: EXCESSIVE DOPAMINE STIMULATION

Carbidopa/levodopa is the most efficacious way to replenish brain dopamine, so it makes sense that this is also the primary cause of excessive dopamine stimulation. The other drugs that work through dopamine may also contribute, but much less so than carbidopa/levodopa. Thus, if levodopa-induced dyskinesias are present and entacapone (Comtan) is added, this will exacerbate the dyskinesias. Recall that entacapone makes the levodopa response more potent. By the same token, adding a dopamine agonist to carbidopa/levodopa will have a similar impact.

REDUCING CARBIDOPA/LEVODOPA TO REDUCE ELIMINATE DYSKINESIAS

Levodopa-induced dyskinesias are due to an excessive effect from the most recent dose. Thus, the dyskinesias start when the levodopa response reaches the peak effect and lasts as long as this is maintained. With regular (immediate-release) carbidopa/levodopa, these peak-dose dyskinesias begin about an hour after a dose and last 2–4 hours. This temporal pattern is illustrated in Figure 17.4. A more complicated pattern of dyskinesias, termed *biphasic dyskinesias*, develops in no more than 1% of PD patients and is discussed near the end of this chapter.

On a simplistic level, peak-dose dyskinesias might be conceptualized as brain dopamine concentrations exceeding a hypothetical threshold. As previously discussed, the benefit from levodopa often seems to occur all-or-none. Thus, it appears that low doses do nothing, and even slightly more than low doses are ineffective. Once the levodopa dose seemingly surpasses a hypothetical threshold, the on-response develops. In this scheme, when the brain levodopa (and dopamine) concentrations not only exceed the on-threshold but further exceed the dyskinesia threshold, then these involuntary movements occur. One might think of this as two thresholds with the goal of selecting a dose that exceeds only the improvement threshold. This is illustrated in Figure 17.5.

Implicit in Figure 17.5 is the concept that levodopa dyskinesias can always be eliminated by a reduction of the individual carbidopa/levodopa doses. As long as the two thresholds shown in Figure 17.5 are substantially separate, a dose of carbidopa/levodopa can be used that surpasses the improvement threshold, but short of the dyskinesia threshold. In this scenario, a small reduction sufficient to result in a peak levodopa level between these two thresholds will eliminate the involuntary movements without loss of parkinsonism control. Unfortunately, sometimes the two thresholds are close to one another; then a carbidopa/levodopa dose reduction that eliminates dyskinesias also translates into reduced parkinsonism control.

One point worth noting is that PD websites sometimes imply that once dyskinesias begin, they cannot be eliminated. This is terribly incorrect; they can always be terminated with lower levodopa doses. The problem for occasional people is that this comes at the expense of worsening parkinsonism control with dose reduction. An important characteristic of levodopa dyskinesias deserves special emphasis:

> *Levodopa dyskinesias relate to the last dose of carbidopa/levodopa and not to the total daily dose of levodopa.*

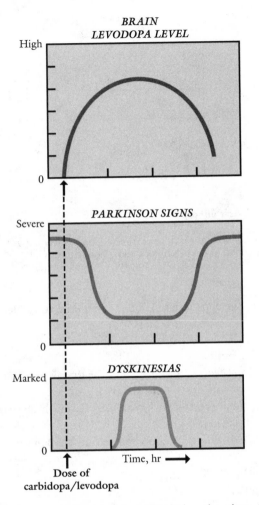

17.4 Peak-dose dyskinesias. Following a dose of carbidopa/levodopa, improvement in PD symptoms occurs as the brain levodopa/dopamine level rises. Those prone to such dyskinesias will experience these excessive movements at the same time, when the brain levodopa (dopamine) level is maximum.

Restated, these dyskinesias are time-locked to each dose of carbidopa/levodopa. Thus, they follow a short-duration pattern; there is no long-duration dyskinesia effect. Once dyskinesias are provoked, they span only the 2–4 hours, corresponding to the peak levodopa levels. There is no buildup of the dyskinesia effect over the day as long as the doses do not overlap—that is, are not too close to each other. Typically, there should be no overlap if the doses are at least 3–4 hours apart.

An example may give more insight into treatment. If choreiform movements are recurring with each carbidopa/levodopa dose, this means these doses should be reduced. If the dosing scheme is 2 ½ tablets of carbidopa/levodopa

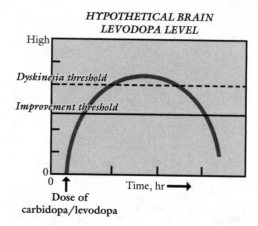

**HYPOTHETICAL BRAIN
LEVODOPA LEVEL**

17.5   The goal of carbidopa/levodopa dose selection is a levodopa dose that exceeds only the improvement threshold and not the dyskinesia threshold. Unfortunately, some people have these two thresholds close together, making this difficult.

four times daily, the appropriate strategy would be to reduce each dose by a half-tablet, that is, down to 2 tablets four times daily. If dyskinesias are still problematic, then another half-tablet reduction is indicated, down to 1 ½ tablets four times daily.

If the reduction of levodopa eliminates the dyskinesias, but at the expense of control of parkinsonism, we are left with a dilemma: accept the dyskinesias or live with the increased parkinsonism. Given these two options, most people choose dyskinesias, although with doses adjusted to keep these as minimal as possible. There are, however, other strategies to consider:

1. Capitalize on the levodopa long-duration response to capture a better anti-parkinsonian effect without exacerbating dyskinesias.

2. Add amantadine while keeping the carbidopa/levodopa adequate to capture a satisfactory levodopa response.

The use of amantadine to attenuate dyskinesias is discussed in the next chapter. Optimizing the carbidopa/levodopa dosing scheme is typically done first.

WHEN LOW-DOSE LEVODOPA PROVOKES DYSKINESIAS

What if dyskinesias are provoked by relatively low doses of carbidopa/levodopa? For example, suppose that doses as low as 1 ½ tablets of 25/100 carbidopa/levodopa provoke dyskinesias. That would potentially limit the individual doses to only 1 tablet. Taking 1 tablet three times daily is often too low to provide substantial benefit. We do have a strategy for working around this problem, recognizing the differing dynamics of levodopa responses: short duration and long duration.

Dyskinesias obey short-duration response patterns. In other words, these involuntary movements occur an hour or so after each carbidopa/levodopa dose, then resolve a few hours later. Although levodopa dyskinesias exclusively have such a pattern, the benefit from carbidopa/levodopa always includes a long-duration effect (i.e., builds over a week of stable dosing). Whereas the short-duration benefit from levodopa is responsible for the fluctuations addressed in the first half of this chapter, the long-duration effect can be utilized to minimize dyskinesias and still capture benefit. This long-duration response relates to the total daily levodopa amount that is maintained over a week or more. The full long-duration benefit from levodopa builds up over at least a week to reach a plateau, reflecting stable daily carbidopa/levodopa doses.

How much levodopa per day is necessary to capture the full long-duration effect? No clinical trial evidence has been published on this subject. However, my own sense, based on experience in the clinic, is that the full long-duration levodopa benefit requires approximately 600–800 mg of levodopa daily. In other words, the full long-duration effect should be established if someone takes 6 to 8 of the 25/100 regular carbidopa/levodopa tablets per 24 hours, daily for more than a week, on an empty stomach.

If one is taking only low doses of carbidopa/levodopa because of dyskinesias (e.g., one 25/100 tablet three times daily), the long-duration benefit will not be achieved. However, it is possible to work around these issues. The strategy is to spread the low carbidopa/levodopa doses over the entire 24 hours of each day. This is especially workable if the levodopa benefit is not linked to each dose, that is, not short-duration (recall the short-duration responses typically do not surface for several years).

Returning to our example of 1 ½ tablets of carbidopa/levodopa causing dyskinesias, we could reduce the doses to 1 tablet; presumably this would be below the dyskinesia threshold. Instead of taking only three doses daily, 1 tablet could be taken six to eight times daily, including at bedtime and during the night. As long as these doses are at least 3–4 hours apart, they should not overlap and should be tolerated. Note that if taken too close together, the doses would then summate and cause dyskinesias (which is not dangerous but undesirable). Note that the bedtime dose might be tolerated even if more than 1 tablet, since dyskinesias do not occur during sleep. The goal would be to take as many 25/100 tablets per 24 hours as tolerated, up to 6–8 per day. After a week or more on this higher total daily dose, the benefit should be substantially greater than with the lower dosage, but without dyskinesias.

CARBIDOPA/LEVODOPA SIDE EFFECTS ALL HAVE SHORT-DURATION DYNAMICS

This strategy for working around dyskinesias actually works for nearly every carbidopa/levodopa side effect. The side effects from carbidopa/levodopa all obey the short-duration rule. Any side effect that prevents more than small doses of carbidopa/levodopa should be considered for this strategy, with the focus being on the long-duration benefit (typically requiring 6–8 tablets of 25/100 carbidopa/levodopa per 24 hours). For example, nausea may be tolerated if low carbidopa/levodopa doses are taken around the clock, including at night when one might easily sleep through mild nausea. For the rare person who experiences sleepiness from carbidopa/levodopa, taking the entire dose of carbidopa/levodopa at bedtime and during the night should allow the long-duration benefit. In that case, higher doses could be used, since induced sleepiness at bedtime is not problematic. For example, even doses as high as 2 ½ tablets might be tolerated if one dose was taken before bedtime and the other two were taken when awakening during the night.

A Rare Dyskinesia Pattern: Biphasic Dyskinesias

Biphasic dyskinesias occur in no more than 1% of the people with PD, but often go unrecognized. The dyskinesias begin just as the levodopa dose is *starting* to kick in, which then subside and recur later as the levodopa effect is wearing off. Hence the term *biphasic*, implying two phases of dyskinesias, one at the beginning and another at the end of the levodopa response cycle. It is usually the dyskinesias at the end of the cycle that are problematic; those at the beginning are typically brief or minimal. The dyskinesias typically manifest as chorea, with the chaotic, dancing movements described earlier in this chapter. This pattern can be hard to recognize and hard to treat.

RECOGNITION OF BIPHASIC DYSKINESIAS

The common form of levodopa-induced dyskinesias is easy to recognize, the peak-dose dyskinesias illustrated in Figures 17.4 and 17.5. In contrast, biphasic dyskinesias are primarily characterized by prominent choreiform movements 3 or more hours after a dose, that is, as the levodopa effect is terminating. Often the brief period of dyskinesias at the beginning of this levodopa cycle is overlooked, since it tends to be mild and last only a few minutes. The end-of-cycle dyskinesias are the problem. This is illustrated in Figure 17.6.

Note that the distinction between these two dyskinesia patterns (peak-dose and biphasic) is made over hours of observation. It may be obscured if carbidopa/levodopa doses are too close together. If uncertain about the pattern of your dyskinesias, set aside a few hours in the morning to observe. This can start before the first carbidopa/levodopa dose of the day, taking none during the night so that the period of observation begins in a levodopa off-state. Pay attention to your walking, movement, and involuntary motion just before a full dose of carbidopa/levodopa dose. You can then serially observe for the next several hours after a usual carbidopa/levodopa dose. You should be able to recognize the levodopa on-state and also when it

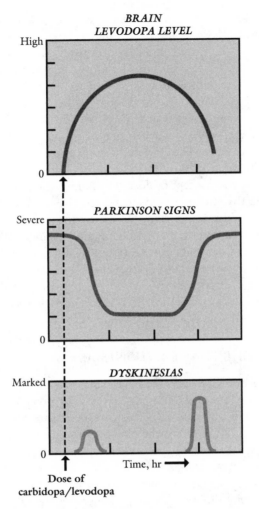

17.6 Biphasic dyskinesia pattern, following a single dose of carbidopa/levodopa. Mild dyskinesias briefly develop at the beginning of a levodopa cycle but quickly resolve. More severe dyskinesias recur as the dose is wearing off.

begins to wear off. Observation through a full cycle should allow confirmation of the dyskinesia pattern.

This period of observation should also enable recognition of other involuntary movements that might be confused with choreiform dyskinesias. Thus, choreiform dyskinesias should not be confused with *dystonia* occurring exclusively at the end of a levodopa dose cycle. This is common, occurring as the levodopa effect is wearing off, signaling loss of the levodopa effect. This is sometimes called *end-of-dose dystonia*. Often this is experienced as cramps of the leg or toes (e.g., toe curling or extension). Cramp-like sensations among those with PD typically represent dystonia and are a symptom of PD, rather than a medication effect. Dystonia at the end of dose cycles suggests the interval between carbidopa/levodopa doses is too long and a short dosing interval might be considered. Brief tremor just as the carbidopa/levodopa is starting to kick in should also not be interpreted as biphasic dyskinesias; not uncommonly, parkinsonian tremor surfaces about 20–30 minutes after a dose of carbidopa/levodopa, but dissipates after 5–15 minutes. Typically, no specific treatment is needed since this is so brief.

Biphasic dyskinesias are somewhat paradoxical and, intuitively, the mechanism is not very obvious. These are sufficiently uncommon that little discussion of these is found in the PD medical literature. My understanding of these is based on the concept of dose thresholds. The response to levodopa manifests when the two thresholds in Figure 17.5 are reversed, that is, the dyskinesia threshold is lower than the improvement threshold. Thus, lower carbidopa/levodopa doses that surpass only the dyskinesia threshold but not the improvement threshold provoke only dyskinesias. When the levodopa dose is raised, then both thresholds are surpassed and the full biphasic pattern becomes apparent. It appears that when the improvement threshold is surpassed, this seems to override the dyskinesias. The dyskinesias only recur with declining concentrations of brain dopamine, at the end of the levodopa cycle.

TREATMENT OF BIPHASIC DYSKINESIAS

Inherent in the behavior of these biphasic dyskinesias is that lower doses of carbidopa/levodopa provoke only dyskinesias. In other words, after a low dose, dyskinesias begin as soon as the dyskinesia threshold is reached and persist for several hours or so; the anti-parkinsonism response is minimal with only a low dose. Only higher doses capture substantial benefit, albeit with the biphasic dyskinetic pattern. Because low carbidopa/levodopa doses are problematic, it has proven impractical to take many low doses per day to capture the long-duration levodopa benefit. Although tiny carbidopa/levodopa doses (e.g., half-tablet) could be taken many times per 24 hours, this has not proven workable (the dosing interval needs to be at least 3 hours so the dose effects do not summate). By the same token, considerable experience with the less potent dopamine agonists (pramipexole, ropinirole) has not worked out. None of the alternative drugs used for PD treatment has been helpful in this setting. Thus, we must deal with the dynamics of this biphasic response using carbidopa/levodopa.

With typical biphasic levodopa responses, experience has taught me several rules regarding the use of carbidopa/levodopa:

1. Low levodopa doses simply provoke dyskinesias.

2. Sufficiently high doses of carbidopa/levodopa are necessary to override the dyskinesias but with a transient anti-parkinsonian effect, perhaps lasting 2 hours.

3. Overlapping the carbidopa/levodopa doses (e.g., administered every two hours) can defer the end-of-dose dyskinesias, but this is not feasible around the clock.

4. Overlapping more than a few doses (e.g., 3–4) usually translates into a severe end-of-dose dyskinesia episode—that is, the dyskinesias are more pronounced and last longer.

With these rules in mind, the dosing strategy is trial-and-error, requiring systematic experimentation with the carbidopa/levodopa doses and intervals. The carbidopa/levodopa dose that is sufficient to surpass the improvement threshold and suppress the dyskinesias is typically 1 ½ to 2 ½ tablets (25/100 immediate-release carbidopa/levodopa). Usually three and sometimes four doses can be overlapped at about 2-hour intervals (i.e., an interval sufficient to avoid the end-of-dose dyskinesias). This then translates into a total daily dose of 6–8 carbidopa/levodopa tablets daily, which should capture the long-duration benefit. This also results in about 6–8 hours of on time without dyskinesias when these doses are overlapped. This strategy is illustrated in Figure 17.7.

The figure shows three doses being overlapped. One could try overlapping four doses to determine the response, that is, a trial-and-error approach.

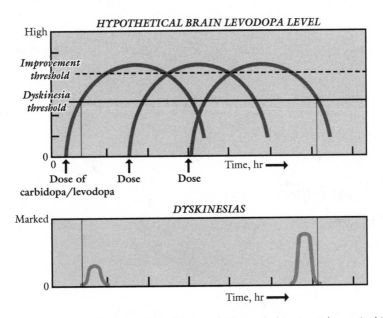

17.7 A strategy for working around troublesome biphasic dyskinesias. Inherent in this scheme is the assumption that only three to four doses of carbidopa/levodopa will be tolerated. Doses taken about 2 hours apart defer the end-of-dose dyskinetic phase, allowing several hours of good time, plus accumulation of the long-duration levodopa benefit.

With the scheme illustrated in Figure 17.7, a dyskinetic episode is expected 2–4 hours after the last carbidopa/levodopa dose. If not too many doses of carbidopa/levodopa are overlapped, this should last about 30–60 minutes. In my experience, if more than three to four doses are overlapped, the end-of-dose dyskinetic period becomes more severe and prolonged.

During the time of the overlapped doses, people typically do very well, perhaps near normal. After the last dyskinetic episode at the end of the cycle has resolved, the anti-parkinsonian benefit is not as good as during the overlapped levodopa doses, but it is usually acceptable. This benefit usually lasts overnight and well into the following morning. The benefit typically starts to tail off around mid-day, which is when most people choose to restart the carbidopa/levodopa. The time when the three or so carbidopa/levodopa doses are overlapped can be arranged to fit with the day's activities. Similarly, the end-of-dose dyskinetic episode is best timed so that people are home and can experience this in the quiet of their own room.

18

◆ ◆ ◆

Supplemental Drugs for Motor Fluctuations and Dyskinesias

In the first edition of this book, much text was devoted to the use of ancillary drugs added to carbidopa/levodopa for unstable levodopa responses. This especially involved the use of supplementary dopamine agonist medications. In the intervening decade, I have increasingly favored optimizing carbidopa/levodopa as the primary strategy (described in Chapter 17), rather than adding supplementary drugs. In part, this changing approach has related to side effects from the adjunctive medications. The dopamine agonists used 10 years ago included bromocriptine and pergolide, which were subsequently shown to frequently cause inflammatory fibrotic scarring in the heart, lungs, or near the kidneys. Pergolide is off the market and bromocriptine is no longer used for PD treatment. The currently available dopamine agonists, especially pramipexole and ropinirole, have now been recognized to frequently cause pathological behaviors, such as gambling or sexual indiscretions (discussed in Chapter 10). These behavioral problems were documented in a quarter of our patients taking therapeutic doses of pramipexole or ropinirole. These agonists also may induce sleepiness and are more likely to provoke hallucinations. Hence my prescriptions for dopamine agonists have declined. Finally, tolcapone, which blocks an enzyme that degrades levodopa, and which appeared very promising, was shown to rarely cause potentially fatal liver failure; I no longer prescribe this drug. I also discussed anticholinergic drugs, such as trihexyphenidyl and benztropine, in the last edition of this book, primarily to maintain a broad focus. Now, I believe it is unwise to even consider those anticholinergic drugs because the side effects usually offset the modest benefits. Hence the content of this chapter has markedly shortened, which reflects my current practice.

Levodopa Fluctuations

Carbidopa/levodopa doses initially have a long-duration effect, but after several years of PD, short-duration levodopa responses (wearing off) become apparent. Chapter 17 emphasized strategies for treating this with carbidopa/levodopa adjustments. However, adjunctive drugs are also used for that purpose. In the order of efficacy, dopamine agonists, entacapone, and the MAO-B inhibitors selegiline and rasagiline are used to help stabilize and prolong levodopa responses. We will discuss these in the order of likely benefit.

DOPAMINE AGONISTS ADDED TO CARBIDOPA/LEVODOPA

Ideally, one should first optimize the carbidopa/levodopa dosing scheme as discussed in Chapter 17. If short-duration responses remain problematic, then pramipexole, ropinirole, or the rotigotine patch may be added, with the dosing schemes outlined in Chapter 13. These agonists are not nearly as efficacious as carbidopa/levodopa, but they have a longer-lasting effect, potentially improving parkinsonism control during levodopa off-states. This might allow longer carbidopa/levodopa dosing intervals.

Note that dopamine agonist drugs are always started with a low dose and slowly raised. Improvement of parkinsonism will be minimal with the initial doses; it will probably take several weeks of dosage escalation to appreciate any benefit. The agonist doses can be raised until the off-states are better controlled. This may require escalation to the so-called target doses shown in Chapter 13.

Once the dose of the agonist is sufficiently high to provide benefit, you may then try increasing the interval between the carbidopa/levodopa doses, perhaps by 30–60 minutes. The intent is to arrive at the longest duration between carbidopa/levodopa doses that allows continued control of parkinsonism.

Do not reduce the carbidopa/levodopa doses when starting the agonist unless occurrence of dyskinesias requires this. The initial agonist doses shown in Chapter 13 are too low to have a substantial effect. The carbidopa/levodopa dose may not need to be reduced later when the agonist dose is therapeutic, unless levodopa dyskinesias surface. If dyskinesias develop, the carbidopa/levodopa doses can be reduced by a small amount, such as half of a 25/100 tablet each dose.

Perhaps the most common reason for dopamine agonists to fail relates to an insufficient dose. The starting doses are too low to benefit. Hence, if committing to a dopamine agonist, follow through with the dose escalation scheme, assuming it is tolerated.

If you are prone to orthostatic hypotension (low blood pressure when standing), check the standing blood pressure as the agonist dose is escalated. Dopamine agonists are additive with carbidopa/levodopa in lowering the standing blood pressure in susceptible people.

There is no purpose in starting a second dopamine agonist drug when the first is insufficient. The three available dopamine agonists (pramipexole, ropinirole, rotigotine) have very similar properties and are somewhat interchangeable. If one of these is insufficient, despite adequate dosing, adding another agonist will be unlikely to provide further benefit and may provoke side effects. By the same token, if one of these three dopamine agonists has been given an adequate trial with the dosage escalated, it is unlikely that another of the three will prove more efficacious.

SWITCHING DOPAMINE AGONIST MEDICATIONS DUE TO SIDE EFFECTS

The three available dopamine agonists have a similar spectrum of side effects, thus a switch from one to another may not be advantageous. If one of the agonists provokes pathological behaviors (e.g., gambling, sexual proclivities, etc.), massive leg edema (swelling), hallucinations, or sleepiness, trying another is unlikely to prove successful. Whether nausea would be reduced by switching from agonist pills to the rotigotine patch is unclear, since this nausea is mediated at the brainstem level rather than in the stomach; nonetheless, it may be tried. Expense may be a factor forcing a switch; see the cost of these drugs shown in Table 11. 3, in Chapter 11.

A switch of one agonist to another using comparable doses may be done overnight. In other words, it is not necessary to taper off one and slowly escalate the other; this may be done by stopping one agonist after the last dose of the day and starting the other in a comparable dose the following morning. The comparable doses are relatively easy to calculate. As a crude approximation, one may assume that ropinirole and rotigotine are approximately equivalent in their milligram (mg) potency (i.e., 6 mg of ropinirole is equally efficacious as 6 mg of rotigotine). To be equivalent to pramipexole, either of these two drugs must be about three times the dose (i.e., 2 mg of pramipexole = 6 mg ropinirole = 6 mg rotigotine). For example, if switching from 3 mg of pramipexole per day (either 1 mg three times daily or the 3 mg extended-release), a comparable dose of ropinirole would be 9 mg (3 mg three times daily). If switching to the sustained-release ropinirole formulation, note that there is no 9 mg Requip tablet; choose the closest size, which would be 8 mg of ropinirole extended-release.

INHIBITING COMT WITH ENTACAPONE TO PROLONG THE LEVODOPA EFFECT

Entacapone (Comtan) inhibits an enzyme that degrades levodopa, catechol-O-methyltransferase (COMT). Entacapone does not enter the brain but protects levodopa from being broken down in the circulation. It prolongs the levodopa effect by 30–60 minutes and also mildly enhances the levodopa response. Entacapone has no effect on PD when used alone; it requires levodopa for benefit.

Entacapone comes in only one pill size, 200 mg. This captures the full benefit, and there is no purpose in taking more or less per dose. With each dose of entacapone, the effect on levodopa lasts about 4 hours. Typically it is administered with each dose of carbidopa/levodopa. If the carbidopa/ levodopa dosing interval is very short, such as every 2 hours, it may be taken with every other dose (the 4-hour effect makes dosing every 2 hours unnecessary). There is no harm and no benefit in taking more than 200 mg at a time, but doubling the dose increases the expense (see Table 11.3 in Chapter 11 for cost).

Since entacapone makes each dose of carbidopa/levodopa slightly more potent, it may increase dyskinesias. This can be controlled by reducing the carbidopa/levodopa doses by a small amount (e.g., one-half of a 25/100 tablet each dose). If dyskinesias are already bothersome, then the addition of entacapone may not be desirable, at least not until they are brought under control. Other entacapone side effects are rarely problematic. Uncommonly, it causes nausea or loose stools. It may turn the urine slightly orange but this is not of concern.

Entacapone is easy to use. A 200 mg tablet may be taken with each carbidopa/levodopa dose (or with every other dose if the carbidopa/levodopa interval is 2 hours). The effect occurs with the first dose. If effective, the carbidopa/levodopa dosing interval can be increased by 30–60 minutes, but not substantially longer than that. Entacapone is also formulated with carbidopa/ levodopa in a single pill, with the brand name Stalevo. I would not recommend starting dose adjustments with Stalevo because the amount of carbidopa/ levodopa in each Stalevo tablet is a fixed amount. The flexibility of being able to lower or raise the amount of levodopa is then lost. However, if the dosage of carbidopa/levodopa is stabilized, a switch to Stalevo may be considered. Stalevo comes in multiple sizes, each with 200 mg of entacapone but with different amounts of carbidopa/levodopa in each pill. The pills are named for the amount of levodopa (e.g., Stalevo-100 contains 100 mg levodopa, plus 25 mg carbidopa and 200 mg entacapone). The available sizes are Stalevo-50, Stalevo-75, Stalevo-100, Stalevo-125, Stalevo-150, and Stalevo-200.

Entacapone may be abruptly started and stopped. No tapering is necessary. However, if taking carbidopa/levodopa in the form of Stalevo, the carbidopa/levodopa component should not be stopped.

MAO-B INHIBITION WITH SELEGILINE OR RASAGILINE FOR LEVODOPA FLUCTUATIONS

MAO-B is a brain enzyme that degrades dopamine. Selegiline and rasagiline inhibit MAO-B and are mildly beneficial for treating parkinsonism. Although they theoretically should smooth fluctuating levodopa responses, they are only modestly beneficial in that regard. The primary advantage of these two drugs is the ease of use, requiring only 1 tablet each morning, either 1 mg of rasagiline or 5 mg of selegiline. Parenthetically, selegiline (5 mg) is often recommended to be taken twice daily; however, once daily should provide the same effect. The effect of these two drugs on brain dopamine is long-lasting (half-life of 40 days) and they may be stopped abruptly. As discussed in Chapter 10, combining these MAO-B inhibitors with certain classes of drugs is discouraged, including nearly all the antidepressants, as well as many prescription pain medications.

Side effects are infrequent when selegiline or rasagiline are used by themselves. However, they may cause or enhance side effects when added to other PD drugs. For example, if added to carbidopa/levodopa, they infrequently may provoke hallucinations. Selegiline and rasagiline should not be raised above the recommended doses, as a higher dose may inhibit both MAO-A and MAO-B, with potentially serious consequences.

APOMORPHINE RESCUE THERAPY

Rescue therapy implies the use of a medication for a quick anti-parkinsonian response. In the previous chapter we discussed liquifying carbidopa/levodopa, which induces the response in about 20 minutes. Much quicker is the unique dopamine agonist apomorphine. This drug is administered by subcutaneous (under the skin) injection. A full response, equivalent to levodopa, develops in 10 minutes or slightly less. The effect lasts 60–90 minutes.

Although a dopamine agonist, apomorphine is quite different from the other dopamine agonists—pramipexole, ropinirole, and rotigotine. These three agonists have limited potential to activate brain dopamine receptors, primarily binding to only the D3 receptors (with limited affinity for D1, D2, D4, or D5 receptors). Apomorphine has broad affinity for dopamine receptors and produces a response similar to that of full doses of carbidopa/levodopa.

Apomorphine is not a new PD drug. In early PD treatment trials 40 years ago, apomorphine was administered in pill form with demonstrable efficacy;

however, it damaged kidneys, precluding use of this drug as oral therapy. It was subsequently recognized that administration by other routes, such as injection, carries no risk of kidney injury. Apomorphine by injection has been used for PD treatment outside the United States for decades.

Apomorphine side effects include potential for nausea, dyskinesias, and occasionally hallucinations or psychosis. It has substantial potential for inducing orthostatic hypotension (low standing blood pressure); if this is a preexisting problem, apomorphine is best avoided. Sudden sleepiness may occur with apomorphine administration; avoid driving when using apomorphine until you have taken it often enough to be sure sedation will not occur. Irritation around the injection site can occur, but is usually is not severe. The apomorphine solution contains sodium metabisulfite and should not be used by people with known sulfite sensitivity.

INITIATING APOMORPHINE

For apomorphine to reverse a levodopa off-state, it must be administered in an appropriate dose, which varies from person to person. Determination of the correct dose is initially done in the clinic where a clinician can observe the responses. This includes not only monitoring the parkinsonism response but also assessing the standing blood pressure.

Apomorphine is packaged in a 3.0 milliliter (mL) cartridge that fits into an injector pen, which is relatively easy to self-administer. Each milliliter contains 10 milligrams (mg) of apomorphine; hence the cartridge contains a total of 30 mg of apomorphine. Be aware that the dose is conventionally given in milliliters (mL), not milligrams (mg); there is a 10-fold difference in these numbering schemes, so do not mix this up. The injector pen has a dial that allows you to determine the dose.

Dose determinations in the physician's office start in a levodopa off-state. The clinician will start with a 0.2 mL (2 mg) apomorphine dose, then observe the response. If the initial 0.2 mL (2 mg) dose fails to produce a satisfactory on-state, a higher dose is tried, typically 0.3 mL or 0.4 mL (3 to 4 mg). The clinician will allow a minimum of 2 hours to elapse between each injection trial. The typical dosing range for apomorphine is 0.2 to 0.6 mL (2 to 6 mg). During each of the dosing assessments, the standing blood pressures are checked.

Apomorphine may induce nausea, and an anti-nausea drug is conventionally started 3 days before the first apomorphine injection. Trimethobenzamide (Tigan) in a dose of 300 mg three times daily is recommended (outside the United States, the more potent anti-nausea drug domperidone is available). As discussed in Chapter 6, certain of the other anti-nausea drugs worsen parkinsonism and should not be used, specifically metoclopramide (Reglan) and prochlorperazine (Compazine). It is recommended that the trimethobenzamide (or other nausea medication) be continued for at least the first

6 weeks of apomorphine use. If you have tolerated apomorphine on numerous occasions without nausea, you might try omitting trimethobenzamide to see if you can get by without it. Do not use ondansetron as the anti-nausea drug, as this combination may cause a severe drop in blood pressure. It is also advisable to avoid other drugs in the ondansetron class: dolasetron, granisetron, palonosetron, and alosetron.

Once the ideal dose is determined in the doctor's office, you can then administer this on your own. Use carbidopa/levodopa to maintain an on-state throughout the day as best you can. However, if stuck in an off-state, anticipate that within 10 minutes after the injection you should be mobile again. Plan ahead, recognizing that the effect will wear off in 60–90 minutes. However, this gives you time for your carbidopa/levodopa pills to start working.

How often can you safely administer apomorphine injections? There are no recognized limits; however, there are some practical constraints. The brief response, skin irritation from too many injections, hassle factor, and the cost will limit how often you choose to use this.

WHERE SHOULD APOMORPHINE BE INJECTED?

Apomorphine is injected subcutaneously, which means under the skin. You can pick up a fold of skin and insert the needle into that fold. Usually, it is injected into the thigh, upper arm, or stomach area. You should shift the injection site each time; if you inject into the same region, it may become irritated. You must wipe clean the injection site with an alcohol swab before each injection. You must use a new, sterile needle each time. Don't inject through your clothes as they are not sterile. Also, do not inject it by some other route, such as into a vein.

What if you are out in public wearing a suit or dress and don't want to be conspicuous with the injection? The easiest strategy is to unbutton a couple of the lower buttons on your shirt or blouse, exposing a limited area of your abdomen for the injection. (Don't wear an undershirt.) If the weather is warm and you are wearing shorts, then injection into the thigh is an easy strategy.

Supplemental Drugs for Dyskinesias

AMANTADINE

Dyskinesias are the involuntary movements that reflect an excessive response to levodopa, discussed in prior chapters. The easiest strategy to eliminate dyskinesias is a reduction of the levodopa dose, addressed in detail in Chapter 17. Unfortunately, a small minority of people are unable to eliminate their dyskinesias with levodopa dose reduction without causing increased parkinsonism. In this circumstance amantadine may prove helpful. It is the only drug that reduces levodopa dyskinesias without reducing the levodopa benefit.

Before considering amantadine, review the description of dyskinesias in Chapter 17. Commonly, tremor, inner restlessness (akathisia), or dystonia are misinterpreted as levodopa-induced dyskinesias. Since the treatment is exactly the opposite, be certain you are correct in assuming levodopa dyskinesias are the problem.

Amantadine has been around for several decades, first introduced around the time that levodopa initially became available. It was recognized to have a mildly beneficial effect on parkinsonian symptoms. Interestingly, it took about 20 years for physicians to recognize that it also tends to reduce levodopa dyskinesias. Currently, that is its primary role in PD treatment.

Amantadine does many things in terms of brain chemistry, none very prominently. The primary substrate for attenuating dyskinesias is thought to be inhibition of one class of receptors for the brain neurotransmitter glutamate: NMDA receptors. Restated, drugs blocking glutamate NMDA receptors tend to reduce levodopa dyskinesias. Unfortunately, the most potent drugs in this category have too many side effects to allow them to be used. Amantadine has a mild glutamate-blocking effect, which is enough to reduce dyskinesias, but not so potent as to provoke troublesome side effects.

Memantine (Namenda) is used in the treatment of dementia and shares the same pharmacological properties as amantadine (i.e., glutamate NMDA antagonist). It should not be used concurrently with amantadine.

AMANTADINE DOSING

Amantadine comes in only one size, 100 mg tablets. It may taken with food or on an empty stomach. If levodopa adjustments are insufficient to control dyskinesias, settle on the carbidopa/levodopa that results in the best balance between parkinsonism control and dyskinesias. Amantadine can then be added to reduce the dyskinesias. Start with 1 amantadine tablet each morning or 1 tablet twice daily. The doses should be taken earlier in the day when dyskinesias are problematic; dyskinesias are absent during sleep, so the amantadine is usually not taken near bedtime. Twice-daily amantadine is often insufficient, and after a week or so the dose may be raised to 1 tablet three times daily. Over the next few weeks, if tolerated, amantadine can be raised further to 1 tablet four times daily. Doses are not raised beyond 5 tablets per day.

AMANTADINE SIDE EFFECTS

In low doses, amantadine is typically well tolerated. A common side effect is redness or red-purple discoloration of the legs (sometimes arms) in a fishnet pattern. This is not worrisome and if it doesn't bother you, the dose does not need to be lowered.

Among those who are disposed, amantadine may provoke hallucinations, paranoia, or confusion. This is more likely to occur with the higher doses, beyond 3 tablets daily. This happens in only a small minority of people, but when it occurs, it usually signals the need to taper off the amantadine altogether.

PART NINE

◆ ◆ ◆

Other Treatment Problems: Not Just a Movement Disorder

19

♦ ♦ ♦

Subjective Parkinson's Disease Symptoms Due to Dopamine Deficiency

Parkinson's disease (PD) notoriously impairs movement, with variable degrees of slowness, tremor, or gait difficulties. These movement problems primarily reflect brain dopamine deficiency, and they respond to medications that restore the effect of dopamine. However, the problems of PD are not confined to these *objective* movement manifestations. Many *subjective* symptoms are also a part of the PD experience, which are only apparent to the person with PD. Because these symptoms cannot be seen, they often are unrecognized as components of PD. If attributed to other conditions, treatment may be sidetracked. Like tremor, slowness, or walking problems, certain of these subjective symptoms respond to levodopa, such as anxiety and shortness of breath. Subjective symptoms that often prove responsive to carbidopa/levodopa are listed in Table 19.1 (not an exhaustive list). This chapter focuses on such levodopa-responsive subjective symptoms, while recognizing that they may also be caused by other conditions and hence not respond to carbidopa/levodopa.

Table 19.1. Subjective PD Symptoms That May Respond to Carbidopa/Levodopa*

• Anxiety	• Cramps
• Panic attacks	• Sciatica and other pain
• Restlessness (akathisia)	• Tingling (paresthesia)
• Inner tremor	• Increased urinary urgency
• Fatigue	• Hot flashes, sweating (diaphoresis)
• Shortness of breath (dyspnea)	• Poor concentration; slowed thinking (bradyphrenia)

*These symptoms may have causes other than PD and, if so, carbidopa/levodopa will not prove very helpful. Sleep disorders, restless legs syndrome, and depression may also benefit from these PD drugs and are discussed in subsequent chapters.

How to Tell If Subjective Symptoms Are Due to Parkinson's Disease

We should not simply jump to the conclusion that each and every symptom listed in Table 19.1 is always due to PD. For example, if the person is short of breath, then heart and lung problems should be excluded before considering PD as the cause. Similarly, sciatica is common and may have nothing to do with PD. Clinical acumen is often necessary to sort this out. When PD is the cause, the response to carbidopa/levodopa may be a clue, such as the following:

1. PD symptoms resolve with carbidopa/levodopa if the dose is sufficient. Many of these symptoms respond "all-or-none"—completely or not at all—and adequate dose escalation is often necessary to determine responsiveness.

2. With longer-standing PD and short-duration carbidopa/levodopa responses, the subjective symptoms may be time-locked to the levodopa cycles:

  • The symptoms resolve at the time of the peak levodopa effect, starting about 1 hour after a dose of immediate-release carbidopa/levodopa.
  • The symptoms recur 2–6 hours after a dose of levodopa, when the levodopa effect has worn off.

Carbidopa/levodopa is typically necessary to determine responsiveness; the other PD drugs (e.g., dopamine agonists) are often insufficient.

The symptoms listed in Table 19.1 are common among people in general. Causes other than PD are suggested if:

1. The symptoms fail to respond to aggressive carbidopa/levodopa therapy (as outlined in Chapter 12).

2. The symptoms have been lifelong, or predating parkinsonism by years.

3. There is another obvious cause, such as low thyroid or anemia in the case of fatigue.

Anxiety, Panic Attacks, and Akathisia

ANXIETY IS A COMMON SYMPTOM OF PARKINSON'S DISEASE

Anxiety implies nervousness, apprehension, or worry. In the mildest form, it may simply represent an uneasy feeling that something will go wrong. In the most severe form, it is experienced as a panic state, often without insight or objectivity. Sometimes anxiety is appropriate, such as the nervousness that precedes a college examination or starting work in a new job. However, it becomes problematic when it is out of proportion to life's events or develops in the absence of any inciting factors.

Anxiety may be one of the first symptoms of PD, preceding the tremor, gait, and movement problems by many years. Among people of Olmsted County, Minnesota, those with PD were significantly more likely to have experienced anxiety states early in life, compared to the general population. These anxiety problems were documented well before the onset of parkinsonism, suggesting that these may have been among the earliest PD symptoms. On the other hand, anxiousness is common in general, and most people who are anxious worriers will not ultimately develop PD.

AKATHISIA

Akathisia implies an inner restlessness or an inability to sit still or be comfortable. It is experienced as an antsy feeling, and for no apparent reason. Occasionally, it is confused with anxiety and sometimes they occur together. Akathisia is among the more common subjective symptoms of PD and responds to levodopa and sometimes dopamine agonist therapy.

Some people with PD also experience an inner tremor, which cannot be seen. It is debatable whether this is a variant of akathisia or actually a low-grade, imperceptible tremor.

PANIC

Panic is anxiety taken to its highest level. Panic states are uncommon among those with PD, but in rare cases may be the most troublesome symptom. When it occurs, this typically is experienced in discreet episodes. Most often, panic will occur as a manifestation of a levodopa off-state. In other words, it represents loss of the levodopa effect, when the levodopa response has worn off. Often, the relationship to levodopa goes unrecognized.

Panic attacks also occur in those who do not have PD. In that setting, the drugs for PD are ineffective. Thus not all panic attacks are due to PD.

RECOGNITION AND TREATMENT
OF ANXIETY AND PANIC ATTACKS

If troublesome anxiety newly develops in the context of PD, appropriately aggressive use of carbidopa/levodopa should be considered. Rarely, anxiety may overshadow the other symptoms of PD. Carbidopa/levodopa is usually necessary (Chapter 12) and the other PD drugs will often fail to help; the response is often all-or-none.

In later PD, anxiety or panic may surface at the end of carbidopa/levodopa dose cycles. Clues to this scenario include the following.

- The anxiety states come and go. (Consider whether they have a relationship to the times of the levodopa doses.)

- A dose of carbidopa/levodopa is followed by resolution of the anxiety state (unless that dose was taken with a meal).

- Anxiety is minimal when the levodopa effect is most prominent (i.e., during the on-state).

- The anxiety state tends to occur during times of the day when no levodopa doses have been administered, such as in the middle of the night.

- Anxiety tends to occur around the time that the next dose of carbidopa/levodopa is due (i.e., at the time of wearing off).

This fluctuating pattern suggests that the anxiety is occurring when the levodopa effect has worn off. Just as tremor and stiffness may recur several hours after a dose of carbidopa/levodopa, so may anxiety. Fluctuating anxiety can be treated the same way as fluctuating movement problems. This typically responds to shortening of the carbidopa/levodopa dosing interval and adding extra doses as necessary, as discussed in Chapter 17.

Optimization of carbidopa/levodopa dosage as outlined in Chapter 12 is usually appropriate for initial treatment of anxiety in the context of PD. If insufficient, dopamine deficiency is apparently not the primary problem and other strategies may be necessary.

A non-dopamine substrate is likely if anxiety has been lifelong and unchanged after PD. In that case, it may be wise to consult a psychiatrist if the anxiety is substantial. The general medication strategies for treating non-PD anxiety are beyond the scope of this book, but a cursory overview and discussion of side effects may be helpful.

LIMITED COMMENTS ABOUT ANXIETY TREATMENT WHEN NOT DUE TO PARKINSON'S DISEASE

People who ruminate and worry endlessly about the same issues may be helped by drugs from the selective serotonin reuptake inhibitor (SSRI) class. This is the group of medications that includes Prozac (fluoxetine), plus an assortment of drugs with similar properties; they tend to enhance brain serotonin neurotransmission. This class of drugs is primarily used as treatment for depression, but it is also helpful for rumination and anxiety; they are discussed in detail in Chapter 22. They tend to be well tolerated by those with PD and are easy to use.

The primary anti-anxiety drugs are from the Valium (diazepam) class; this includes the medications listed in Table 19.2. They are effective in attenuating anxiety in the short term, including anxiety linked to PD. However, they have several side effects that can be concerning, especially for long-term use:

- Sedation

- Imbalance

- Cognitive impairment

- Habit-forming

These drugs tend to be less well tolerated in seniors, especially regarding the first three of these side effects. Limited use of these drugs when the anxiety

Table 19.2. **Commonly Prescribed Anti-Anxiety Medications**

Generic	Brand Name
Diazepam	Valium
Clonazepam	Klonopin
Alprazolam	Xanax
Lorazepam	Ativan
Chlordiazepoxide	Librium
Clorazepate	Tranxene

escalates may be reasonable, but unrestricted, as-needed self-administration can easily lead to habitual use. They are less effective after weeks or months of regular use. If prescribed, limits on use should be set, with follow-up to ensure that excessive drowsiness, unsteadiness, or memory impairment is not provoked. It is wise to defer these anxiety medications if the symptoms are treatable with carbidopa/levodopa.

Occasionally, antipsychotic medications are prescribed for augmenting the effects of antidepressants, most notably aripiprazole (Abilify). Aripiprazole and related drugs block dopamine receptors and should not be used in PD. The exceptions are quetiapine and clozapine, which very rarely are used for anxiety disorders.

One last caveat is not to mistake levodopa-dyskinesias as a sign of anxiety. Dyskinesias are the dancing, fidgety movements that occur when the levodopa effect is too prominent. These may convey the appearance of nervousness, but just the opposite is subjectively experienced. Anxious people with PD will be least nervous when their PD medications are working, even if working excessively to cause dyskinesias.

Shortness of Breath

The medical term for shortness of breath is *dyspnea*. Dyspnea is occasionally experienced as a symptom of PD and responds to carbidopa/levodopa therapy. Obviously, lung conditions (e.g., pneumonia, asthma) or heart failure may cause dyspnea, as may a variety of serious medical conditions, such as fluid retention from kidney failure. When physicians hear the complaint of dyspnea, they appropriately think first about lung, heart, or other serious medical conditions. However, if these have been excluded, then PD may be considered.

MEDICAL ASSESSMENT OF DYSPNEA

The dyspnea evaluation typically starts with a general medical history and examination, including listening to the heart and lungs. Tests may include a chest x-ray, electrocardiogram, pulmonary functions tests (breathing tests), as well as routine blood tests. An echocardiogram may be performed, which evaluates the function of the heart muscle and valves. If all tests are negative, the focus may then shift to parkinsonism.

WHY SHOULD PARKINSON'S DISEASE CAUSE DYSPNEA?

Note that PD does not cause heart or lung malfunction. Rather, PD-related dyspnea is due to reversible impairment of breathing muscle function.

The muscles that move air in and out of the lungs include the diaphragms and the muscles of the rib cage. The diaphragms are the large muscles underneath the lungs (i.e., between the chest and abdomen). The muscles of the rib cage are located between the ribs. These two sets of breathing muscles are responsible for the bellows function of the lungs. The muscles of the rib cage and diaphragms repetitively contract to expel air, and relax to expand the lung cavity. These repetitive movements of our breathing muscles unconsciously move air in and out of the lungs. Recall that PD typically attenuates the amplitude of movements, for example, reducing arm swing, or the repetitive movement of handwriting. Among those with PD-related dyspnea, the chest excursions are unconsciously reduced.

The good news is that the amplitude of breathing movements tends to respond to carbidopa/levodopa treatment, similar to other motor aspects of PD. Notably, the response is typically all-or-none; an adequate levodopa dose is required. If the levodopa effect wear offs in the context of short-duration responses, dyspnea may develop in parallel.

RECOGNITION AND TREATMENT OF DYSPNEA FROM PARKINSON'S DISEASE

If no evidence implicates heart or lung disease to account for dyspnea, PD may be considered. Note that the dyspnea linked to PD is typically experienced fairly continuously, even when not exerting effort or exercising. This contrasts with all but the most serious heart and lung conditions, where the shortness of breath tends to be provoked by exertion. PD-related dyspnea may come and go, but not in association with exercise; rather, fluctuating PD dyspnea correlates with levodopa responses, surfacing when the carbidopa/levodopa effect has worn off. Restated, if dyspnea is time-locked to recurring signs of parkinsonism, consider wearing-off of the carbidopa/levodopa effect.

Dyspnea developing when the carbidopa/levodopa effect wears off is treated like other off-symptoms, as discussed in Chapter 17. Typically, this would involve shortening the carbidopa/levodopa dosing interval to match the levodopa response duration. If dyspnea is continuously present, carbidopa/levodopa dosage may be insufficient; that is, the doses are too low, or they are not being taken correctly, such as being administered with meals (see Chapter 12). Be reminded that dyspnea, like certain other PD symptoms, usually responds all-or-none to carbidopa/levodopa.

Fatigue

A sense of fatigue is common among those with PD. It should be distinguished from sleepiness, although sleep-deprived people feel fatigued as well as drowsy. Fatigue in the context of PD has a variety of substrates, some treatable and some not. Sometimes it is a direct consequence of PD and improves with levodopa. However, it often is not that simple. Causes to consider include the following:

1. *Other medical problems.* This might warrant a general medical examination and routine blood tests to exclude some other disorder; appropriate blood tests might include a complete blood count, thyroid and chemistry panel, plus whatever seems warranted by the medical history.

2. *Medications.* These may include the following:

   - Sleep aids, especially those that are long-acting like clonazepam
   - Anxiety medications, such as alprazolam (Xanax) or lorazepam (Ativan)
   - Certain older allergy medications, most notably diphenhydramine (Benadryl)
   - Seizure medications
   - Muscle relaxants, or drugs for spasms (such as cyclobenzaprine, baclofen, or tizanidine)
   - Prescription pain relievers, such as narcotics, fentanyl or tramadol

3. *Low blood pressure, orthostatic hypotension.* People with PD are predisposed to orthostatic hypotension (low blood pressure when upright), and this is exacerbated by the medications used to treat PD. Although lightheadedness and feeling faint are typical symptoms of orthostatic hypotension, general fatigue may also be a consequence. This can be diagnosed by measuring standing blood pressures during times of fatigue. If the systolic blood pressure is less than 90, this could be the problem. See Chapter 21 for more details.

4. *Poor sleep at night.* Poor energy during the day may be a consequence of inadequate sleep at night. There are various reasons why those with PD may experience poor nighttime sleep. Contributing factors include inadequately controlled parkinsonism (impairing sleep) or sleep apnea (disordered breathing during sleep). These conditions and their treatment are discussed in Chapters 20.

5. *Depression.* Lack of energy and interest are common depressive symptoms. Depression is common in PD and often requires medical treatment, which is addressed in Chapter 22.

6. *Deconditioning.* Lack of exercise may also contribute to fatigue, although is unlikely to be the primary cause. This can become a self-perpetuating problem where fatigue reduces activity and reduced activity potentiates the fatigue state.

When these causes have been treated or excluded, we are then left with PD as the probable cause of fatigue. PD-related fatigue typically improves, but rarely resolves with PD medications. Those who were extremely energetic prior to PD may find that their high energy levels never return, despite otherwise optimum treatment. They may no longer be able to burn the candle at both ends. However, this is not to say that they cannot continue to be productive in their careers and hobbies; they simply must pace themselves appropriately.

Apathy occasionally surfaces in PD and is sometimes misinterpreted as a fatigue state or due to depression. Apathy implies disinterest, indifference, or disinclination to engage in usual activities. When this occurs, it usually is after many years of PD, perhaps in the early stages of dementia and especially in advanced age. Prototypically, apathetic people behave as if they no longer care about things that previously were of interest. Thus, they may stop reading the newspaper or prefer spending the day in their easy chair rather than going out with family. Unfortunately, apathy does not respond to carbidopa/levodopa or any other medications.

Cramps, Tense Muscles, Sciatica, Pain, or Tingling

Pain and a variety of abnormal sensations may be due to PD. These especially are experienced in the limb or side of the body most affected by PD. These sensations tend to be at least partially responsive to carbidopa/levodopa.

CRAMPS, TENSE MUSCLES

Almost everyone has experienced cramps, such as after vigorous exercise. Cramps are especially common in PD, and in that context are caused by the brain dopamine deficiency state. They respond to adequate carbidopa/levodopa treatment. PD cramps may affect the calves, but especially the toes, manifesting as toe-curling or upward toe deviation. PD cramps presumably represent a form of dystonia and may develop during levodopa off-states. Some people recognize cramps as a signal to take their next dose of levodopa.

Nighttime cramps often occur because of the relatively long interval since the last dose of carbidopa/levodopa. These nocturnal cramps respond to carbidopa/levodopa coverage, which is discussed in more detail in Chapter 20, on sleep.

Tense muscles are also common in PD and occur especially in the limb(s) first affected by PD. The tension typically improves with carbidopa/levodopa therapy, but the response may be incomplete.

SCIATICA

Sciatica, experienced as pain radiating down a leg, is commonly due to a protruded lumbar disc irritating a nerve root. However, a similar pain may also be caused by the brain dopamine deficiency state of PD. If this is the cause, it should resolve with adequate carbidopa/levodopa, and this treatment may establish the diagnosis. If a dose of carbidopa/levodopa completely takes away the sciatica pain, even for just a few hours, dopamine deficiency, rather than a disc, is the likely culprit. Note, however, that leg pain from an irritated lumbar nerve root may improve but not resolve with adequate carbidopa/levodopa (see next section).

NON-PD PAIN IS WORSE WHEN PARKINSON'S DISEASE IS UNDERTREATED

Frequently unrecognized by those with PD is that pain from other causes is exacerbated during levodopa off-states or with levodopa underdosage. Pain thresholds are reduced during levodopa off-states, documented in clinical studies. For example, if someone with PD fractures their leg, the resulting pain will be magnified if carbidopa/levodopa is withheld. For those with PD who also have painful injuries or arthritis, maintaining satisfactory parkinsonism control with carbidopa/levodopa is crucial to pain control.

Surgeries are typically associated with pain from the incisions. This is not the time to stop carbidopa/levodopa. Maintaining a levodopa on-state will help control the surgical pain. Carbidopa/levodopa by itself will not be sufficient, but will reduce the need for even higher doses of potent pain medications.

TINGLING (PARESTHESIA)

A pins-and-needles sensation, numbness, or tingling is sometimes a symptom of PD. Most often, it is most prominent in the first affected arm or leg. This could also be a symptom of one of a variety of other neurological conditions. However, if it began around the time that parkinsonism first developed, or if this fluctuates with the levodopa response, it may well be a parkinsonian symptom.

Other Symptoms That May Relate to Parkinson's Disease

EXACERBATION OF URINARY URGENCY

Urinary symptoms are common among those with PD, and often this relates to autonomic nervous system dysfunction (so-called neurogenic bladder).

However, age-related causes may also translate into bladder symptoms, such as prostate enlargement in men. While bladder symptoms do not directly respond to carbidopa/levodopa, they may partially benefit from adequate levodopa coverage. For example, urinary urgency or frequent urination during the night may be reduced with optimized carbidopa/levodopa treatment. Conversely, those with urinary urgency often experience an exacerbation of this problem during levodopa off-states. This is discussed in more detail in Chapter 27.

HOT FLASHES, SWEATING (DIAPHORESIS)

"Hot flashes" or "hot flushes" are common among menopausal women, which typically respond to estrogen therapy. Men and women with PD may experience a similar phenomenon, although not due to estrogen loss. In that setting, this typically signals wearing-off of the levodopa response several hours after the last dose. Occasionally, this is associated with profuse sweating, especially at night when the last carbidopa/levodopa dose was taken many hours before. The nighttime sweating episodes occurring during the transition to the off-state may be enough to soak the bed clothes.

Minimizing levodopa off-states most effectively treats episodes of profuse sweating. Nighttime perspiration episodes are often most troublesome; strategies for improving nighttime levodopa coverage are discussed in Chapter 20, on sleep.

SLUGGISH THINKING

Impaired concentration and slowed thinking are common experiences in PD. The physicians' term for this is *bradyphrenia*. The slowed or inefficient thinking of PD tends to improve with carbidopa/levodopa treatment of PD. This condition should not be considered a forerunner of dementia. Unfortunately, carbidopa/levodopa does not directly improve memory or treat dementia, topics covered in Chapter 23.

OTHER SYMPTOMS THAT MAY RESPOND TO CARBIDOPA/LEVODOPA

Occasionally other subjective symptoms occur as a consequence of the PD dopamine deficiency state. The relationship to dopamine and PD may not be immediately apparent. However, if the symptoms abate when the levodopa effect kicks in, or when the carbidopa/levodopa dosing scheme is optimized, dopamine deficiency is the likely substrate.

20

◆ ◆ ◆

Sleep Problems: Insomnia, Daytime Sleepiness, and Nighttime Disruptions

For people with PD, sleep is frequently disrupted, and this may impact the waking day. Daytime drowsiness, poor energy, reduced attention and concentration, as well as cognitive impairment can all be consequences of a poor night's sleep. Causes of disordered sleep are treatable.

Insomnia

Insomnia is a common problem, in general, and increases with aging. Young people typically have no trouble getting adequate sleep. Witness teenagers left undisturbed on a Saturday morning, who sleep till noon. With age, getting to sleep or staying asleep often becomes more difficult. Depression and stress are common reasons for insomnia, whereas for some people insomnia is part of their constitutional makeup.

Insomnia is especially frequent and troublesome among people with PD. They have trouble getting to sleep and, once they do, may awaken after a few hours and experience another cycle of sleeplessness. Consequently, many with PD are chronically sleep-deprived and thus sleepy during the daytime.

Table 20.1.   Common Causes of Insomnia in Parkinson's Disease

Cause	Comments
Primary insomnia	Predates onset of parkinsonism and is an unrelated problem
Insomnia due to PD	Typically relates to insufficient treatment of parkinsonian symptoms at bedtime and during the night (i.e., dopamine deficiency problem)
Urge to urinate	Common among seniors, who awaken to urinate and have trouble returning to sleep
Restless legs syndrome	Responds to medications
Depression	Improves with treatment of the depression
Medications	Certain medications may cause insomnia if taken in the evening, e.g., duloxetine, selegiline

A variety of factors may contribute to insomnia among those with PD; these are summarized in Table 20.1. By far the most common reason for their insomnia is the discomfort of parkinsonism itself. This is highly treatable with carbidopa/levodopa, and this cause should not be overlooked.

INSOMNIA DUE TO PARKINSON'S DISEASE

The dopamine-deficient state of PD makes it difficult to become comfortable, which is the necessary prelude to sleep. The stiffness and muscle tension (rigidity) of parkinsonism are not compatible with a relaxed state, nor is tremor. The inability to easily turn over in bed may leave one stuck in the bedcovers. Perhaps most important factor, however, is the akathisia of PD. *Akathisia* is defined as an inner restlessness; an inability to feel relaxed or a sense of nondescript discomfort when sitting or lying still. Very few with PD volunteer such a complaint to their physician, but recognize akathisia if asked. This is a very common symptom of PD.

Akathisia, rigidity, tremor, and immobility are all symptoms that are treatable with carbidopa/levodopa. Carbidopa/levodopa is key to treating the insomnia caused by PD. Liked other aspects of PD, an adequate carbidopa/levodopa dose is necessary, and with longer-standing PD, the timing of the doses is crucial.

INSOMNIA IN EARLY PARKINSON'S DISEASE

In nearly all those who have had PD for only a few years, the levodopa response has the long-duration pattern, discussed in Chapters 15 and 17.

In other words, the levodopa benefit stabilizes after a week on a consistent dose, with an effect that lasts around-the-clock. As you might infer, adequate doses (sufficient to capture a good long-duration effect) should treat nighttime symptoms. Thus optimized daytime doses should treat bedtime akathisia and stiffness, allowing normal sleep. For those people with PD, a carbidopa/levodopa dose at bedtime is not necessary; the dosage during the daytime must simply be sufficient to capture an adequate long-duration response. As discussed in earlier chapters, this often requires 6–8 of the 25/100 immediate-release carbidopa/levodopa tablets per 24 hours.

INSOMNIA LATER IN PD

Commonly, those with PD experience new-onset insomnia after several years while on stable doses of daytime carbidopa/levodopa. This signals the development of short-duration levodopa benefit (described in Chapter 17). Thus the last carbidopa/levodopa dose of the day, taken before supper, fails to provide persistent coverage lasting until bedtime; that is, the anti-akathisia effect has worn off. The strategy for this is obvious: take another *full dose* of carbidopa/levodopa an hour before bedtime (it takes about an hour to kick in). Note that a *full dose* is stipulated here. This is very important, as the benefit for sleep responds all-or-none. In other words, a half dose fails, as does a three-quarter dose; it requires the full dose to become comfortable, allowing natural sleep to occur. Intuitively, many people assume that since the carbidopa/levodopa bedtime dose is simply for sleep, less is needed, but it does not work that way.

Unfortunately, some who are able to sleep following the bedtime dose of carbidopa/levodopa do not sleep through the night but rather awaken in a few hours. Often this is due once again to the short-duration levodopa effect, or wearing-off. What should one do? Again, the obvious solution is to take another full dose of carbidopa/levodopa upon awakening. I advise people to have the pills and a glass of water on their nightstand to take upon awakening. As long as at least 3–4 hours elapse between doses, there should not be an excessive effect. This nighttime dose will not work immediately, but it will kick in and allow natural sleep in about an hour. I generally discourage people from setting an alarm during the night to awaken them for another dose, because sometimes they are able to sleep longer than anticipated. Rather, I advise people to sleep as long as they can and to take the carbidopa/levodopa upon awakening. It is acceptable to do this more than once during the night. For example, if retiring around 10 p.m. but awakening at 2 a.m., a dose at that time may not last until it is time to get out of bed in the morning. Hence a second carbidopa/levodopa dose may be taken at 5–6 a.m. As discussed in Chapter 17, there are no limits on the number of doses per 24 hours, except as limited by common sense.

SUSTAINED-RELEASE CARBIDOPA/LEVODOPA TO SUSTAIN SLEEP

Regular carbidopa/levodopa (immediate-release) should be the formulation used at bedtime to facilitate natural sleep. This formulation kicks in within an hour, thus the advice to take it about an hour before bedtime. Sustained-release carbidopa/levodopa (also called Sinemet CR; controlled-release carbidopa/levodopa) may have a role in allowing a longer sleep duration when taken precisely at bedtime.

For sustained-release carbidopa/levodopa to be used, the dynamics need to be appreciated. This formulation is slow to kick in; thus regular carbidopa/levodopa should be used to initiate sleep, taken an hour before bedtime. Sustained-release carbidopa/levodopa takes up to 2 hours to kick in (twice as long as regular carbidopa/levodopa). At night, it persists about 120 minutes longer than regular carbidopa/levodopa. With that knowledge, you can infer how to use the sustained-release tablets. It should be taken immediately before falling asleep (i.e., an hour after the late-evening dose of regular carbidopa/levodopa taken to facilitate sleep onset). The sustained-release dose taken at the very last minute before falling asleep has a 2-hour onset delay, which kicks in while one is asleep. This allows sleep to persist longer at night, provided the dose is correct.

The situation is not quite that simple, however, as we have yet to address the appropriate dose of sustained-release carbidopa/levodopa. As discussed in Chapter 17, there is no mg-to-mg correspondence of regular (immediate-release) carbidopa/levodopa to the sustained-release formulation. For this sleep benefit, the bedtime sustained-release levodopa content needs to be comparable to the optimized dose of daytime regular carbidopa/levodopa (detailed in Chapter 17); in other words, it needs to be about 50% greater than the daytime levodopa doses (assuming the daytime doses have been adjusted to the optimum level). Because sleep responds all-or-none, too small a levodopa dose will not allow sleep.

To illustrate the conversion, if the daytime optimized dose of regular carbidopa/levodopa is 2 of the 25/100 tablets (200 mg levodopa), the appropriate dose of sustained-release carbidopa/levodopa is 3 tablets (300 mg levodopa; 50% more). Rarely, the absorption of sustained-release carbidopa/levodopa is poor and even a slightly higher dose may prove necessary. In our illustration, if 3 of the 25/100 sustained-release tablets fails to sustain sleep, it would be appropriate to try 4 sustained-release tablets (400 mg levodopa).

Taking regular (immediate-release) carbidopa/levodopa an hour before bedtime ensures that the levodopa effect is present when trying to fall asleep (assuming it takes an hour to work); the interval before bedtime could be longer than that. If that doses is taken an hour before going to sleep, the sustained-release drug taken just before falling asleep will kick in about 3 hours after the dose of regular carbidopa/levodopa, which typically is sufficient so that the doses of these two formulations do not overlap, with a doubling of their effects.

The sustained-release dose at bedtime should be helpful, but some people still awaken before their ideal rising time because of loss of the levodopa effect. In other words, the prolonged response from sustained-release carbidopa/levodopa may still only extend the effect to 4–5 a.m. What to do then? The answer is to take another full dose of regular (immediate-release) carbidopa/levodopa to allow a return to sleep. Have that on the nightstand with a glass of water, ready to take. Note that regular, not sustained-release, is stipulated for this middle-of-the-night dose, because of the slow kick-in time of the sustained-release formulation.

BEDTIME SNACKS

Often forgotten in the focus on carbidopa/levodopa for sleep is the inhibitory effect of food on the levodopa response. Evening snacks will block the levodopa effects. Recall the rule that for carbidopa/levodopa to work, it must be taken at least an hour before and at least 2 hours after the end of meals. Typical evening snacks containing protein will all be problematic, for example, milk, yogurt, nuts, and ice cream. Fruit or toast with only jelly (minimal protein) should be tolerated.

OTHER TREATABLE CONTRIBUTORS TO INSOMNIA

Although inadequate levodopa coverage during the night is the most common cause of insomnia in PD, other factors or conditions may also play a role. These include restless legs syndrome, urinary symptoms, depression, and other medications.

RESTLESS LEGS SYNDROME

Restless legs syndrome is a common disorder, estimated to occur in at least 2–3% of adults. Although there are some similarities to the nocturnal symptoms experienced in PD, these are fundamentally different disorders. Under the microscope, Lewy bodies are the brain hallmark of PD; these are not present in restless legs syndrome. Those with restless legs syndrome do not have evidence of brain dopamine deficiency (although they do respond to dopamine-based treatment; see later discussion in this chapter). Because both PD and restless legs syndrome are fairly common, they may occur together by chance.

Those with restless legs syndrome describe an uncomfortable sensation in their legs when trying to sleep at night or when relaxing and reading in the evening. These leg sensations are described in a variety of ways: crawling, itching, or pulling. In bed, people with this disorder cannot lie still and need to move their legs or get up and walk to relieve the discomfort. Obviously, this can severely interfere with sleep.

Most people with restless legs syndrome also have periodic limb movements of sleep. These are jerks of the legs occurring during sleep. They are periodic in that they typically recur about every 20–40 seconds throughout the night. People with these periodic movements will be unaware of them while they are asleep; however, the sleep partner may be keenly aware! This periodic kicking of the legs may force a spouse into another bed.

Iron deficiency occasionally causes restless legs syndrome, and blood iron studies (e.g., serum ferritin level) are an appropriate part of the evaluation. Iron supplementation may reverse the symptoms if low iron or ferritin is discovered (including low-normal). While most people with restless legs are not iron deficient, if they are, this is a simple to assess and treat.

The subjective symptoms of restless legs syndrome resemble akathisia, described in Chapter 19. It may be difficult to distinguish these two conditions among those with PD. However, those with restless legs syndrome focus primarily on their legs, whereas akathisia is typically not confined to the legs or lower body.

The medications that effectively treat restless legs syndrome in the general population are the same drugs used to treat PD. Low doses of carbidopa/levodopa or the dopamine agonist medications are often dramatically beneficial. The dopamine agonist drugs (pramipexole, ropinirole, rotigotine) have been the conventional therapy for routine restless legs syndrome for a number of years. These are also effective in treating periodic limb movements of sleep.

Dopamine therapy for restless legs with either carbidopa/levodopa or a dopamine agonist works well in the short term, but longer-term treatment may cause augmentation or rebound. This implies that the medication effect is transient, lasting hours, but with later recurrence of the symptoms. Thus an evening dose of medication may allow good sleep overnight, but with recurrence of the restlessness the following morning or later in the day. Rarely, dosing every few hours becomes necessary. For those without PD, such dosing can be very problematic when the initial problem was only in the evening and required only a dose or two near bedtime. This augmentation seems to be driven by the potency of the dopamine drug. Carbidopa/levodopa is most likely to cause this; higher doses of dopamine agonists may do the same. For some people with restless legs, low doses of these medications work well for years, whereas others require higher and higher doses to treat the restlessness, and then augmentation and rebound become problematic.

For those with both PD and restless legs, augmentation is often not an issue, since conventional daytime administration of carbidopa/levodopa for parkinsonism also treats the daytime restlessness. In other words, carbidopa/levodopa may be sufficient. Thus, if restless legs symptoms become apparent after PD is diagnosed, I typically try treating that with an evening or bedtime coverage of carbidopa/levodopa. If that proves insufficient, then other medications may be added.

Treatment of Restless Legs Syndrome with Dopamine Agonists

Dopamine agonists have been a standard treatment for restless legs syndrome for a number of years. They are administered as a single dose 2–3 hours before bedtime. If the restlessness starts much earlier in the evening, the agonist may be started just before the anticipated onset. The sustained-release forms of pramipexole and ropinirole as well as the rotigotine patch require just one dose daily. The regular formulations of pramipexole or ropinirole may require two doses, one in the late afternoon or early evening and a second before bedtime.

The agonist drugs usually do not need to be raised to very high doses to treat restless legs. If they work in low doses this is ideal, since the higher doses are more likely to cause augmentation. Note that even with low doses, there is still the potential for pathological compulsive behaviors, described in Chapter 10, and one should be vigilant in watching for these.

These agonists are started at the lowest doses possible and raised every few days until a satisfactory response is achieved. This should be done under a clinician's guidance. The starting doses of the three available agonists reflect the smallest pill or patch sizes available and are as follows:

Pramipexole (Mirapex)

    Regular 0.125 mg

    Sustained-release 0.375 mg

Ropinirole (Requip)

    Regular 0.25 mg

    Sustained-release 2 mg

Rotigotine patch (Neupro) 1 mg

Be aware that the sustained-release formulations are much more expensive than the regular pills, and the rotigotine patch is very expensive; review Table 11.3 in Chapter 11 if cost is an issue.

Non-dopamine Medications for Restless Legs

Gabapentin (Neurontin) and pregabalin (Lyrica) each effectively treat restless legs and do not interact with brain dopamine systems. A typical evening starting dose of gabapentin is 300 mg. It can be raised by 100 to 300 mg increments up to 1200 mg as a single evening dose. If restless legs symptoms are prominent around the clock, it may be taken up to three times per 24 hours. A prolonged effect with once-daily dosing occurs with gabapentin enacarbil extended-release tablets, although this formulation is more expensive. Pregabalin also effectively treats restless legs symptoms with efficacy in higher doses (300 mg daily).

Narcotics have been prescribed for restless legs for many years. In my experience, the doses and potency necessary to control symptoms have been substantial; I do not use this class of drugs for restless legs.

The anti-anxiety medication clonazepam is also occasionally used to treat restless legs. It probably works via a sedating effect. It may cause imbalance or sedation and tends to have a long-lasting effect that occasionally persists the following morning. This is not a preferred drug for restless legs syndrome. However, clonazepam is the most efficacious medication for treating dream enactment behavior, described later in this chapter. When that condition plus restless legs are both present, clonazepam may be the preferred drug.

THE NEED TO URINATE AT NIGHT (NOCTURIA)

Seniors, especially senior men, often need to urinate during the night, often more than once. Light sleepers are more prone to this problem. Improving sleep with adequate levodopa dosing, as described earlier, may help override some of the nighttime urinary urges.

Simple contributors should also be considered. Fluid intake late in the evening should be reduced. Review the medications taken in the evening to determine if this list includes diuretics (water pills), which induce urination; common diuretics are listed in the Chapter 21. Also, don't drink caffeinated or alcoholic beverages before bedtime as these have a mild diuretic effect.

If nighttime urination is very frequent, and especially if it is associated with daytime urinary difficulties, urinalysis is advisable. Ultimately, evaluation by a urologist may be appropriate.

Certain medications may be taken at bedtime to dampen the urge to urinate. Most share a common mechanism: they block the neurotransmitter acetylcholine; that is, they are anticholinergic drugs. This class of anticholinergic medications has several side effects, but sometimes the benefits justify their use. If nocturia is the primary urinary problem, a single bedtime dose of trospium, 20 mg, may prove helpful. A new medication without anticholinergic side effects, mirabegron (Myrbetriq), was recently introduced for reducing bladder urgency. Presumably this drug may also reduce the need to urinate at night, although I have no current experience prescribing this drug. Drugs for urinary symptoms are addressed in more detail in Chapter 27.

DEPRESSION AND SLEEP

Psychological depression is frequent in PD, and insomnia is a common manifestation of depression. The person who feels blue, has lost appetite and interest in life, and can't sleep may have an underlying depression that requires specific treatment. This is addressed in more detail in Chapter 22.

Antidepressant medications tend to reverse insomnia due to depression, but some may inhibit sleep if taken at bedtime. This includes SSRI drugs (selective serotonin reuptake inhibitors), such as fluoxetine (Prozac), sertraline (Zoloft), and paroxetine (Paxil). Insomnia is even more likely with the antidepressants that additionally block the neurotransmitter norepinephrine, such as venlafaxine (Effexor) and duloxetine (Cymbalta). These are best administered in the morning and not beyond mid-day if insomnia is a problem. If insomnia persists, another antidepressant that induces sleep is often added at bedtime: trazodone in low doses of 50 to 100 mg before bedtime. Trazodone is not a very potent antidepressant in this dose, but tends to make people sleepy.

DRUGS CAUSING INSOMNIA

A variety of medications may cause insomnia. This includes the PD drug selegiline and, perhaps, rasagiline, if taken late in the day. Certain asthma drugs, such as dyphylline (Lufyllin) or theophylline (Theo-Dur), may cause arousal and are best avoided in the evening if asthma allows. Medications for attention deficit, such as methylphenidate (Ritalin) or amphetamines, notoriously inhibit sleep and should be avoided late in the day. Note that the sustained-release release forms of these stimulants may carry over to evening. Finally, do not forget that caffeinated beverages (e.g., colas, tea, coffee) also tend to cause insomnia and are best avoided in the evening.

PRIMARY INSOMNIA

Insomnia may develop independent from PD, urinary symptoms, or depression. In other words, it may have separate origins; we will refer to this as primary insomnia ("primary" implying that it is not secondary to some other obvious cause).

Primary insomnia is common among adults, and entire books and careers have been devoted to treatment. While a detailed and comprehensive discussion of treatment is beyond the scope of this book, certain simple measures deserve discussion here. Two basic strategies for treating primary insomnia include modification of behavior and use of sleep-inducing medications.

Modifying sleep behavior

Insomnia may improve with measures directed at lifestyle, stressors, and behavior. Experts in sleep disorders typically counsel their insomniac patients about sleep hygiene. Sleep hygiene tips include the following:

- Avoid caffeine beyond the early afternoon.

- Avoid alcoholic beverages; these may induce sleep, but increase the likelihood of awakening in the middle of the night.

- Avoid evening activities that increase stress. This includes good stress, such as late-night sporting events.

- Sleep in a quiet, dark room. Light stimulates brain mechanisms associated with wakefulness, whereas darkness does the opposite.

- Clock-watchers should move their alarm clocks out of sight.

- Slightly cooler room temperatures are often more conducive for sleep (but with adequate bed covers).

- Avoid engaging in other activities in bed, such as television watching or balancing the checkbook. Reserving the bed for sleep allows the bedroom environment to trigger sleep-related thoughts.

- Avoid daytime naps. A single, relatively brief nap after lunch is usually not a problem. However, a long afternoon nap (e.g., 2–3 hours) or naps after supper will sabotage nighttime sleep. If tempted to nap after supper, leave the easy chair and engage in some activity, such as walking, or working on a hobby.

- Establish fairly regimented sleep patterns. Avoid having to reset your biological clock repeatedly.

- Get adequate exercise. Avoid exercise right before bedtime, when it can produce a stimulating effect.

- Develop strategies for managing your stress. Do not be a ruminator; avoid carrying unpleasant thoughts.

One common reason for nighttime insomnia among seniors with PD is *reversal of the day–night cycle*. Retirees have the luxury of being able to sleep during the day if they don't get a good night's sleep; sometimes this habit evolves, and most sleep occurs during the daytime. If this is becoming a problem, specific measures to revert to a more normal sleep pattern are necessary.

If your day–night cycle is reversed, transition to a more conventional sleep pattern will be aided by the following measures:

- Avoid naps beyond the early afternoon.

- Limit the afternoon nap to 60 minutes.

- Avoid sedentary activities after supper (don't sit in the easy chair to read the paper or watch TV, where sleep is inevitable).

- Stay active during the daytime. If you are feeling sleepy when engaged in a sedentary activity, force yourself to get up and go for a walk, or do something active.

It may also be necessary to use a sleep medication at bedtime to help the body re-time the sleep cycle. In other words, if forcing yourself to stay up during the daytime does not result in sleepiness at bedtime, you can use one of the medications from the next section to elicit sleep, and entrain the sleep cycle. It may not be necessary to use this for long, once the normal sleep cycles are restored and the body gets used to this new schedule.

Medications to Aid Sleep

When simpler strategies fail, a medication for sleep taken at bedtime may be appropriate. Clinicians are very familiar with insomnia treatment, and every doctor typically has a favored medication for that purpose. A detailed discussion of drugs used to induce sleep could fill a separate text, but a few general comments are appropriate here.

The antihistamine *diphenhydramine* has been used as a mild sleep aid for decades. It is available as an over-the-counter drug, which goes under a variety of names, such as Benadryl. It is an ingredient in combination sleep-aids, such as Tylenol PM (Tylenol is the brand name for acetaminophen) and Excedrin PM. A conventional adult dose of diphenhydramine for sleep is 50 mg, the amount contained in two Tylenol PM caplets. Diphenhydramine administration is compatible with PD. Some who take this medication feel drugged, but it usually is tolerated. Diphenhydramine has mild anticholinergic properties, which potentially translate into mild memory impairment, dry mouth, and constipation; however, these are typically not problematic if solely used at bedtime. Note that the newer antihistamines now commonly prescribed for allergies are not sedating and have no role as sleep aids, including such drugs as fexofenadine (Allegra), cetirizine (Zyrtec), and loratadine (Claritin).

Melatonin is a natural hormone, produced by the pineal gland in the center of the brain. It plays a role in the normal sleep–wake cycle, with increased levels present during the evening, which persist overnight. It is not particularly sedating but may help trigger sleep initiation, especially if other behavioral factors have been addressed (described in the previous section). It is available over the counter as a sleep aid. The starting dose for sleep is 1 mg, which can be raised up to as high as 3 mg before bedtime. It has minimal side effects. Note that it is used in higher doses for REM sleep behavior (dream enactment), discussed later in this chapter.

Ramelteon (Rozerem) is a prescription sleep aid that was designed to stimulate brain melatonin receptors. It appears to have very similar properties to natural melatonin and limited side effects. It is unclear whether it has advantages over melatonin but certainly is much more expensive.

Certain antidepressant medications are also used to treat insomnia. Already mentioned is trazodone, which is a fairly potent sleep aid. The antidepressant mirtazapine (Remeron) is often used when depression and insomnia are combined; the starting dose is typically 15 mg before bedtime.

A variety of medications have been specifically designed as sleep aids. Some of the older medications in this category, such as flurazepam (Dalmane), have longer durations of action and may cause daytime grogginess or clumsiness persisting to the following morning. These are no longer recommended. Several shorter-acting drugs are commonly prescribed for sleep initiation. Because they have brief half-lives (on the order of 1–3 hours), they have been assumed to not cause sedation or imbalance after nighttime. However, recent publicity has been given to such short-acting drugs as zolpidem (Ambien), which in higher doses have been blamed for automobile accidents the following morning, although this is a rare occurrence. Hence clinicians have been advised to prescribe conservative doses. Medications in this category include Eszopiclone (Lunesta), Zaleplon (Sonata), as well as zolpidem. It is generally recommended that these medications not be used for long-term treatment of insomnia, as they might cause dependency.

Daytime Sleepiness

An adequate night's sleep should translate into alertness throughout the daytime. If one is very drowsy during the day, this could be due to too brief or disturbed sleep, as well as to sedating medications. Such problems are suggested if any of the following are frequent occurrences:

- Falling asleep after breakfast
- The need for long daytime naps (more than 2 hours)
- Falling asleep while reading or watching TV
- Nodding off during conversations or while eating

A brief nap after lunch or following exercise is acceptable; frequent long naps or the inability to stay awake during sedentary activities suggests a problem. Causes to consider include the following:

1. Insomnia—problems either getting to sleep or staying asleep
2. Impaired sleep quality: sleep apnea
3. Abbreviated sleep (going to bed too late; rising too early)

4. Sedating medications

5. A primary sleep disorder: excessive sleepiness from Lewy disease (or narcolepsy)

Daytime sleepiness is a common problem among those with PD and detracts from quality of life. Not only does it reduce initiative and curtail activities, it may also contribute to cognitive impairment. The cause or causes need to be addressed and treated as best possible.

Driving safety is an important issue for those with daytime drowsiness. Do not drive if sleepy. This is a very common cause of car accidents.

Specific Causes and Treatment of Daytime Sleepiness

INSOMNIA

If you are unable to get to sleep or stay asleep, the need for sleep carries over to the waking day. In my PD practice, the most likely cause of insomnia is insufficient carbidopa/levodopa coverage. The akathisia, stiffness, and impaired turning in bed prevent normal sleep. Treatment of insomnia with carbidopa/levodopa was discussed in detail earlier in this chapter. A sleep medication may be considered if the simpler strategies outlined earlier are insufficient.

SLEEP APNEA

Disrupted breathing during sleep prevents deep sleep and impairs sleep quality. The term for this is *sleep apnea; apnea* implies cessation of breathing. This is a very frequent cause of daytime sleepiness but is unrecognized by the sleeper, who only appreciates the lack of restful sleep after morning awakening. The spouse or bed partner may hear the loud snoring associated with this condition, which is often a red flag for sleep apnea. Restated, daytime drowsiness plus nighttime snoring suggests sleep apnea.

By far the most common cause of sleep apnea is obstructed breathing; hence the term *obstructive sleep apnea*. Normally, we cycle through successive stages of sleep during the night, starting with light sleep, then deeper sleep stages, and vice versa. People with obstructive sleep apnea typically breathe normally during the lighter stages of sleep but breathing becomes impaired with deeper sleep. In most cases, this is due to the throat closing off and obstructing the flow of air. Specifically, deep sleep causes the muscles of the body to relax and become flaccid; when muscles in the back of the throat become too relaxed and collapse, breathing is impeded. With this obstruction to air flow, the blood oxygen declines and is sensed by the brain. The brain then reflexively arouses the sleeper just enough to return to a lighter sleep stage and restored air flow.

As a consequence of this process, deep sleep is never achieved. Sleeping only in lighter stages of sleep does not fully meet the body's needs and nonrestorative sleep is the consequence. This nonrestorative sleep may translate into not only drowsiness but also other symptoms such as poor energy, headaches, achiness, fatigue, hypertension, and even heart rhythm disorders (e.g., atrial fibrillation). Obstructive sleep apnea is more likely to occur in overweight people but also may develop in people with a normal body habitus.

The other primary cause of sleep apnea is dysfunction in the brainstem center that programs breathing. This is termed *central sleep apnea* and manifests as pauses in breathing during deep sleep that are not due to airway problems. This is much less common than obstructive sleep apnea and may not be associated with loud snoring.

If sleep apnea is suspected, this can be assessed with polysomnography at a sleep center. Polysomnography involves an overnight recording of brain waves (EEG), breathing, and blood oxygen during sleep. Sometimes physicians do a screening test for sleep apnea, termed *overnight oximetry*. A simple device is used at home to measure blood oxygen while one is asleep (oximeter). The circulating oxygen is detected by a component that slips over a fingertip and is connected to a digital recorder. This generates an ongoing record of blood oxygen saturation. If the blood oxygen periodically plummets during sleep, sleep apnea is suspected.

If sleep apnea is documented during polysomnography, treatment is usually initiated the night of this study. This typically consists of a trial of continuous positive airway pressure (CPAP). CPAP is administered via a mask that fits over the mouth and nose. It is connected via a tube to a bedside compressor that generates higher air pressure, which keeps the airway open. This is effective in most people with sleep apnea. People generally feel so much better after their sleep apnea has been treated that they gladly put up with the minor aggravation of the CPAP device.

ABBREVIATED SLEEP

Fully restorative sleep typically usually requires 7–8 hours of sound sleep each night (and sometimes 9 hours). Occasional people do well with less sleep, but they are a minority. If you are sleepy during the day and sleeping less than 7 hours each night, too little time in bed may be causing this. There may be obvious related factors, such as setting an alarm clock; going to bed too late; a dog that awakens the family; or too many commitments. These are all fixable issues if recognized.

MEDICATIONS CAUSING SLEEPINESS

A wide variety of drugs may induce drowsiness. It may be helpful to recall when the sleepiness began and consider whether a new medication was initiated around that time. Drugs that cause sleepiness typically provoke the drowsiness time-locked to doses. If each time you take a given medication you become sleepy an hour later, that is a crucial clue.

Certain general categories of drugs are notorious for causing daytime drowsiness, which are listed in Table 20.2. If daytime drowsiness is a problem, drugs from these classes should be minimized, if possible. This is not an exhaustive list, and other drugs may also be offenders. The physician prescribing the medication should be a party to the decision to discontinue

Table 20.2. General Classes of Medications That May Cause Daytime Sleepiness

Medication Classes	Examples of Drugs from Each Class
Dopamine agonists for PD	Pramipexole (Mirapex), ropinirole (Requip), rotigotine (Neupro patch)
Anti-anxiety drugs	Alprazolam (Xanax), diazepam (Valium), lorazepam (Ativan), clorazepate (Tranxene)
Muscle relaxants, drugs for spasticity	Cyclobenzaprine (Flexeril), orphenadrine (Norflex), tizanidine (Zanaflex), baclofen (Lioresal)
Narcotics	Codeine (in Tylenol #3), hydrocodone (in Vicodin), oxycodone (in Percodan, Oxycontin), fentanyl (Duragesic)
Non-narcotic prescription pain relievers	Tramadol (Ultram)
Seizure drugs	Phenytoin (Dilantin), carbamazepine (Tegretol), phenobarbital
Non-prescription anti-histamines	Diphenhydramine (Benadryl)*
Longer-acting drugs for insomnia (may carry over to next day)	Clonazepam (Klonopin)**, flurazepam (Dalmane)**
Drugs for hallucinations/psychosis	Quetiapine (Seroquel)**, clozapine (Clozaril)**, olanzapine (Zyprexa)**
Certain drugs for depression	Amitriptyline, nortriptyline, mirtazapine (Remeron)**

*Newer non-prescription antihistamines, such as cetirizine, fexofenadine, loratadine, do not cause drowsiness because they do not enter the brain.

**These may or may not have effects carrying over to the next day after a single bedtime dose.

the drug. Often drugs need to be slowly reduced before stopping them, and your physician can advise you how best to do that.

It is also helpful to know which medications are unlikely to cause daytime drowsiness. General classes of drugs unlikely to induce sleepiness are shown in Table 20.3. If you are taking one of these, there should be no reason to worry that it is making you sleepy.

The dopamine agonist drugs, pramipexole (Mirapex), ropinirole (Requip), and rotigotine (Neupro patch), induce sleepiness in a minority of people with PD. With use of the regular (immediate-release) formulations of pramipexole or ropinirole, the sleepiness tends to follow each dose. By contrast, the sustained-release forms of these two drugs and the long-acting rotigotine patch have no such timed relationships. In that case, a clue would be whether the sleepiness started after one of these drugs was initiated. If you are uncertain, withhold using the drug for 36–48 hours to see whether this is indeed the case; that is, if this period of abstinence reverses the drowsiness, then the agonist may be responsible. The agonist can then be restarted and slowly tapered off.

CARBIDOPA/LEVODOPA SLEEPINESS

Carbidopa/levodopa infrequently causes drowsiness. When it does, this usually occurs in someone who sleeps poorly at night because of inadequate levodopa coverage. As discussed earlier in this chapter, levodopa underdosage in the evening or at nighttime may be associated with akathisia and stiffness preventing sleep. With the first carbidopa/levodopa dose in the morning, the akathisia and stiffness that prevented sleep resolves and sleepiness ensues. This is appropriately treated with bedtime (and, if necessary, nighttime) carbidopa/levodopa in full doses. After a week or two of good sleep, the morning carbidopa/levodopa usually no longer induces sleepiness.

Rarely, carbidopa/levodopa induces drowsiness in someone who is not sleep-deprived. In other words, this cannot be blamed on poor nighttime sleep, but rather is a direct side effect of levodopa. This does not preclude use of carbidopa/levodopa but simply a change in strategy. This treatment strategy capitalizes on the long-duration benefit from carbidopa/levodopa, with carbidopa/levodopa exclusively administered at bedtime and during the night. Recall that the long-duration benefit from carbidopa/levodopa requires a certain minimum amount of levodopa to be taken every 24 hours. Typically, 6–8 of the 25/100 carbidopa/levodopa tablets (immediate-release) daily are necessary to capture the benefit. The response slowly develops over about a week and is then stable, regardless of when during the 24-hour cycle the carbidopa/levodopa is taken. If the sleep is interrupted by the need to urinate during the night, that provides an opportunity for taking a dose. In this scenario, carbidopa/levodopa (25/100) could be started with a single tablet an hour before bedtime and then two additional doses when awakening

Table 20.3. **Commonly Prescribed Medications Unlikely to Cause Daytime Sleepiness**

Medication Classes	Examples of Drugs from Each Class
Drugs for lowering cholesterol	Atorvastatin (Lipitor), pravastatin (Pravachol), simvastatin (Zocor)
Most drugs for lowering blood pressure	Amlodipine (Norvasc), enalapril (Vasotec), losartan (Cozaar)
Diabetic agents	Insulin, metformin (Glucophage), glipizide (Glucotrol)
Antibiotics	Penicillins (Amoxacillin), sulfa/trimethoprim (Bactrim, Septra)
Diuretics (water pills)	Furosemide (Lasix), hydrochlorothiazide
Prescription anti-inflammatory drugs	Celecoxib (Celebrex), diclofenac (Cataflam), etodolac (Lodine), fenoprofen (Nalfon), ketoprofen (Orudis), ketorolac (Toradol), nabumetone (Relafen), oxaprozin (Daypro), rofecoxib (Vioxx), sulindac (Clinoril), tolmetin (Tolectin)
Non-prescription anti-inflammatory drugs	Aspirin, ibuprofen (Motrin, Advil), naproxen (Aleve)
Non-prescription pain relievers	Acetaminophen (Tylenol)
Estrogen, progesterone, or thyroid hormones	Premarin, oral contraceptives, levothyroxine (Synthroid)
Bronchodilators for asthma (but may cause insomnia)	Dyphylline (Lufyllin), Theophylline (Theo-Dur)
Steroids (but may cause insomnia)	Prednisone
Anticoagulants	Warfarin (Coumadin), dabigatran (Pradaxa), clopidogrel (Plavix)
Drugs for gastritis, ulcers, acid reflux	Cimetidine (Tagamet), esomeprazole (Nexium), famotidine (Pepcid), nizatidine (Axid), omeprazole (Prilosec), pantoprazole (Protonix), ranitidine (Zantac), sucralfate (Carafate)
Drugs for osteoporosis	Alendronate (Fosamax), calcitonin (Miacalcin)
Newer generation of antihistamines	Fexofenadine (Allegra), loratadine (Claritin, Alavert)

during the night. As long as at least 3 hours elapse between doses, there should be no important overlap. After a week, the doses could be raised to 1 ½ tablets three times, then 2 tablets, then 2 ½ tablets three times, at bedtime and during the night. That should capture the long-duration benefit. It is unclear whether 3 tablets three times at night would be more effective than 2 ½ or 2 tablets three times nightly; one may systematically experiment to determine which dose works best.

For people prone to orthostatic hypotension, a caveat is in order. Note that carbidopa/levodopa tends to provoke the drop in blood pressure when the body is upright. Carbidopa/levodopa doses during the night are not problematic when lying in bed, but could cause low blood pressure when walking to the bathroom. If lightheadedness is experienced, then measurement of the standing blood pressure at that time would be important. If the standing systolic blood pressure is less than 90 mmHg, this should be addressed to avoid fainting. This is treatable and is discussed in Chapter 21.

Other strategies for drowsiness induced by daytime doses of carbidopa/levodopa include a brief (e.g., 20-minute) nap after each dose, as well as a cup of strong coffee at appropriate times. Avoidance of driving when sleepy cannot be overemphasized.

DRUGS TO COMBAT SLEEPINESS

Stimulants to counter drowsiness are sometimes considered after other causes have been addressed. A cup of strong coffee might be used at times when sleepiness is anticipated. Prescription stimulant drugs in this setting often lose their effectiveness with continued use. Common prescription stimulants include modafinil (Provigil), armodafinil (Nuvigil), and methylphenidate (Ritalin; sustained-release formulation, Concerta). Except for the regular formulation of methylphenidate (Ritalin), these drugs are long-acting and might impair sleep.

PSEUDO-SLEEPINESS: LOW BLOOD PRESSURE

If your blood pressure drops too low, you may faint. Sometimes, fainting from low blood pressure can be confused with sleep, as illustrated in the following case.

> Mrs. Jones reported that her husband falls asleep after breakfast most mornings. "He just slumps over and sleeps with his head on the table." His blood pressure during that afternoon clinic appointment was normal in the lying position (130/70), a little low when sitting (85/60), but very low when standing (70/50).

With such obvious hypotension, an astute clinician would need to consider the possibility that these "sleep attacks" after breakfast might be faints. Measuring the blood pressure at that time would provide the answer. In this gentleman's case, several other factors suggested this possibility, which was later confirmed. Specifically, a dose of carbidopa/levodopa was regularly taken an hour before breakfast, which can lower the blood pressure, as can a meal (so-called postprandial hypotension). Moreover, a night's sleep will also translate into lower blood pressure levels in the morning. This is an uncommon scenario but one that is important to recognize. This type of problem is the primary topic in the next chapter.

Disruptions During the Night

A variety of happenings may occur while asleep. Some of these may be disruptive and prevent you or your sleep partner from getting a good night's sleep. At the very least, it is useful to understand what these represent.

VIVID DREAMS AND NIGHTMARES

All of us have occasional nightmares or vivid dreams, and the medications used to treat PD occasionally increase this tendency. This is not a serious problem, unless you find it disturbing. However, the development of vivid dreams needs to be distinguished from acting out your dreams, which we discuss in the next section. Acting out your dreams is due to PD, and rarely due to your medications.

Bear in mind that any medication that passes into the brain could trigger nightmares. This includes PD drugs, as well as medications for psychiatric conditions (e.g., anxiety), insomnia, or nighttime urinary symptoms (e.g., oxybutynin); prescription pain medications; and muscle relaxants. These same medications may also contribute to nighttime confusion in susceptible individuals.

ACTING OUT DREAMS: REM SLEEP BEHAVIOR DISORDER

When humans dream, they typically are quiet and unmoving in bed. This is because the normal brain turns off the connection between the dreaming circuits and the movement control centers. Often in PD, the connection is not turned off, and people act out their dreams while asleep. The dream behavior may be dramatic, with thrashing, hitting, or yelling during sleep. Some people may jump out of bed to chase some character in their dream.

This phenomenon of acting out dreams is termed *rapid eye movement sleep behavior disorder*, or REM sleep behavior disorder. The term *rapid eye movement sleep* relates to a specific sleep state. We normally cycle through various stages of sleep over the course of the night, going from lighter to deeper stages, and then back. Most dreaming occurs during the rapid eye movement (REM) stage of deep sleep. In this stage, our bodies are paralyzed except for eye movements. Thus, in normal individuals, dreams are acted out only with eye movements (hence the term *rapid eye movement*), but not with our bodies. This obviously has practical consequences, preventing us from injuring ourselves or our bed partners while fighting bad guys in our dreams.

PD predisposes to this dream enactment behavior. Although PD drugs may get blamed for this behavior, they are not responsible. REM sleep behavior disorder may be an early sign of PD and related conditions, predating any other PD manifestations by many years.

Those with REM sleep behavior disorder do not necessarily have a serious problem. It only becomes significant if the dream enactment behavior endangers the sleeper or sleep-mate. Falling out of bed while mentally running from a dream-state pursuer may result in injury. Hitting your sleep partner while dreaming is equally serious.

Treatment is considered if there is potential for injury. Otherwise, it requires no specific therapy. Practical strategies for the bedroom may be appropriate. This may include a separate bed for your sleep partner. For those who are at risk of falling out of bed, surround the bed with padding and remove furniture with sharp corners (such as a nightstand). Bedrails may also be fabricated to prevent falls to the floor.

If acting-out dreams are troublesome, and especially if potentially dangerous, medications are appropriate. The definitive treatment is with clonazepam (Klonopin). This drug is from the benzodiazepine class of medications, which includes diazepam (Valium). Clonazepam is typically administered as a single dose, a little before bedtime. It induces sleep, so it may be additionally helpful for that reason. However, it does have side effects, which include potential for morning sleepiness, clumsiness, as well as nighttime confusion. In my experience, most people tolerate this drug when taken at bedtime. Clonazepam is prescribed in low doses to avoid side effects, starting with ½ to one 0.5 mg tablet before sleep. It may be raised up to 1 mg if necessary and tolerated.

Melatonin has also been used for REM sleep behavior. This is available over the counter and started with a dose of 3 mg for this condition. It may be increased every few days up to 3–12 mg at bedtime, guided by the response. Note that the doses for REM sleep behavior (3–12 mg) are higher than conventionally used for insomnia (1–3 mg). These higher melatonin doses, however, are not increasingly sedating.

DON'T CONFUSE REM SLEEP BEHAVIOR WITH HALLUCINATIONS

REM sleep behavior may sometimes be mistaken for hallucinations. Hallucinations are visual illusions experienced during wakefulness, that is, seeing things that are not there. Hallucinations occur in a minority of people with

PD, and there are ways to control these (see Chapter 24). They are, however, fundamentally different from dream enactment behavior and the treatment distinctly differs. The primary distinction is based on whether the person is asleep or awake. Hallucinations occur when one is awake, whereas REM sleep behavior occurs during sleep. The following are clues to help you sort this out.

- You can have a conversation with someone who is hallucinating. They respond to questions. Those acting out their dreams are engaged in the dream and do not answer questions or obey commands.

- Those acting out their dreams will do this for only the length of the dream, which may be a few minutes or less. Those hallucinating tend to persist in this state for longer periods of time.

- Those acting out their dreams can be awakened. However, if the dream has been very vivid, they may be mentally caught up in this for a few minutes after awakening.

- Those acting out their dreams may remember the dream the next day, but not events in the bedroom that took place during the dream. For example, they will not recall what the bed partner said to them during the dream. Those hallucinating may not have a clear memory of the events, but typically remember components of this experience.

If the distinction between nighttime hallucinations and REM sleep behavior disorder is unclear, monitoring overnight in a sleep laboratory (polysomnography) will usually sort this out.

NIGHTTIME CONFUSION

Dementia may occur in advanced PD. For people with impaired thinking, the most troublesome time is often during the night. During the waking day, they may be fairly well compensated and the cognitive impairment may not be too troublesome. However, these same people may become very confused in the middle of the night, and their antics may disrupt the sleep of everyone in the household. Why do these problems seem to surface during the night? There are multiple reasons:

- External stimulation is less during the night; the lights are out and the room is quiet.

- Awakening from a deep sleep may have a disorienting effect.

- Medications taken at bedtime may contribute.

- Mental fatigue from a long day may accrue and culminate in the late evening.

Treatment depends on the extent of the problem. If hallucinations (seeing things that are not there) or delusions (imagining bizarre things) are commonly present at night, specific medications may be necessary; this is addressed in Chapter 24. For treatment of simple nighttime confusion, consider the following:

1. A nightlight and familiar surroundings help people stay oriented. Dark rooms and unfamiliar bedrooms (e.g., hotel rooms) can be disorienting after awakening from sleep. Sleeping in the same bedroom with unchanged furniture arrangements helps orientation.

2. Sedating medications taken in the evening may need to be reduced or discontinued. A sleep medication may initially induce sleep, but the persistent sedation may contribute to confusion during the night when awakened. Melatonin is not problematic in this regard.

3. Focus on strategies that reduce the likelihood of awakening during the night, including the following:

   • A quiet bedroom and comfortable bed and bedclothes may facilitate sleeping through the night.
   • Adequate levodopa coverage during the night will reduce the likelihood that parkinsonism will cause awakening, as discussed earlier.
   • Alcohol should be avoided, since it may initially induce sleepiness, but increase the likelihood of awakening in the middle of the night.

4. A medication that prolongs sleep may be helpful, although it may also contribute to nighttime confusion. A drug such as low-dose trazodone (50 mg) could be tried; if it worsens the problem, then obviously it would need to be stopped.

5. For those with a reversed sleep–wake cycle, institute measures to prevent sleeping during the day. A single nap after lunch (an hour or less) is acceptable, but avoid napping beyond this, especially after supper.

PERIODIC LIMB MOVEMENTS OF SLEEP

Periodic limb movements of sleep are jerks that occur during sleep, mainly of the legs, but sometimes in the arms or trunk. The typical movement is a sudden drawing up of one leg, which then quickly relaxes after no more than a few seconds. This is termed *periodic* because this recurs periodically throughout the night at fairly reproducible intervals, often 20 to 40 seconds apart. Most people with restless legs syndrome also have periodic leg movements of sleep, although these also occur in people without restless legs syndrome.

Several years ago, the prevailing opinion among sleep experts was that these periodic leg movements disrupt deep sleep. The current conventional opinion is that this usually is not disruptive. Hence, they are not specifically treated unless the sleeper or sleep partner is unable to sleep through these. Obviously, if restless legs syndrome is associated with periodic leg movements, the restless legs component is appropriately treated. Treatment of periodic leg movements involves the same medications and strategies used to treat the restless legs syndrome, discussed earlier in this chapter.

NIGHTTIME SWEATING (NOCTURNAL DIAPHORESIS)

Occasionally during sleep, the transition from a levodopa on-state to an off-state is accompanied by profound perspiration, soaking the bedclothes. This is typically due to the long interval since the last (daytime) dose of carbidopa/levodopa. Why this should be especially likely during sleep is unclear, but one reason probably reflects the many hours since the last dose of carbidopa/levodopa. The most effective treatment strategy is to improve levodopa coverage during the night, as outlined earlier in this chapter.

21

◆ ◆ ◆

Orthostatic Hypotension and Other Causes of Dizziness: Different Types and Different Treatments

Dizziness is a common word in our vocabulary and is often used by those with Parkinson's disease (PD) to describe one of their symptoms. However, the term *dizziness* has more than one meaning. In fact, there are three basic types of dizziness, and each may be experienced by those with PD. It is critical to distinguish these, since the causes and treatments are quite different. The three categories of dizziness are

- Imbalance

- Vertigo

- Faintness due to low blood pressure (hypotension)

The concepts behind these dizziness subtypes are summarized in Table 21.1. To correctly treat dizziness, avoid confusing these terms. Parenthetically, there is one other category of dizziness, which is a nondescript feeling in the head provoked by certain medications; it is not due to low blood pressure. This is uncommon and experienced as time-locked to the administration of a drug. We will not discuss this type further in this section.

Table 21.1.   The Word *Dizziness* Is Used for Three Different Conditions

Type of Dizziness	Description	Cause
Imbalance	Unsteadiness; head is clear	Parkinsonism or other process affecting brain balance centers
Vertigo	Sense of spinning in the head; if mild, it is experienced as head wooziness; often provoked by certain head positions or quick head movements	Most often due to non-worrisome problems affecting the inner ears (vestibular system); not caused by PD or medications, but common with aging
Orthostatic hypotension	Low blood pressure when standing or walking (Orthostatic = standing; hypotension = low blood pressure). Symptoms are lightheadedness, faintness	Due to problems within the autonomic nervous system plus medications

One Form of Dizziness: Imbalance

The word *dizziness* may be used to describe feeling unsteady, that is, a tendency to lose balance. This imbalance is not associated with lightheadedness, faintness, spinning sensations, head wooziness, or other head sensations; the head is clear. To distinguish this from the other two major forms of dizziness, your physician may ask if the dizziness is experienced in the head or the body. If the head is clear but there is a sense of unsteadiness, then imbalance is being experienced.

Imbalance is a symptom of parkinsonism. Typically, it is not prominent during the initial years of PD, although it may become troublesome after many years. Medications that cause sedation, such as sleep aids or anti-anxiety drugs, may also induce imbalance. However, the usual drugs for PD do not cause unsteadiness. Those with parkinsonism-plus syndromes, such as progressive supranuclear palsy or multiple system atrophy, may experience marked imbalance and falls early in the disease course (see Chapter 6).

Treatment of imbalance with carbidopa/levodopa may help to compensate for unsteadiness by facilitating leg and trunk movements to avoid falls. However, we have no medications that improve balance.

Another Form of Dizziness: Vertigo

Many seniors occasionally experience vertigo, another type of dizziness. This is not a symptom of PD. However, since many with PD are senior citizens, they are susceptible to problems of vertigo because of age. Occasionally, younger people also develop vertigo.

Vertigo implies a sense of spinning or movement in the head (or the room is spinning). When mild, it is experienced as a sense of head "wooziness" (swimming in the head). Those with vertigo typically complain that certain head positions or quick head movements will transiently provoke these symptoms. If the vertigo is severe, then a sense of imbalance is also experienced. Obviously, this is different from the experience of simply being unsteady but with a clear head, as just described.

Most of the time, vertigo originates from problems within the inner ear. The inner ears contain sensors that inform the brain about our head position. These sensors monitor the speed and direction of head movements and also sense the direction of gravity. Each ear has such a sensing apparatus, with the right and left sensors perfectly in sync. If signals from the right ear mirror those from the left, the brain is able to easily interpret this. However, symptoms develop if one ear malfunctions and the signals from the two ears do not match. When the brain receives two different signals, vertigo is the result (or at least wooziness).

These inner ear sensors may malfunction for a variety of reasons, but most are not worrisome. As mentioned, it is common with aging. Often it develops for no identifiable reason, developing out of the blue. It becomes apparent when making quick head movements or assuming certain head positions. Such vertigo due to inner ear malfunction is termed *benign positional vertigo* or *benign paroxysmal positional vertigo*. Ear infections may also provoke vertigo. Only rarely is vertigo a sign of a brain disorder.

A much less common cause of vertigo is Meniere's syndrome. This is associated with severe attacks of vertigo plus hearing loss and ringing in the ears.

The medications used to treat PD do not induce vertigo. Vertigo neither improves nor worsens with treatment of Parkinson's disease.

Vertigo usually does not require much testing. If the neurological and ear examinations are normal, it may then be appropriate to simply observe, without any testing. If there are concerns, vestibular system testing can be performed, and a brain scan may be done to exclude other causes.

For very troublesome vertigo, a vestibular-ear specialist should be consulted. For many with typical position-related vertigo, specific maneuvers may effectively treat this, termed *canalith repositioning*.

From our perspective, it is important that the common symptom of vertigo not be confused with dizziness due to low blood pressure, which we will discuss next. The dizziness of low blood pressure is not vertigo.

The Third Type of Dizziness: Faintness Due to Hypotension

The physician's term for low blood pressure is *hypotension*. A common manifestation of hypotension is the sense that one might pass out. Other symptoms often accompany this faint feeling, including lethargy, general weakness, and blurring or graying of vision. The lower the blood pressure, the more severe the symptoms; if the blood pressure drops very low, then an actual faint does occur. Spinning in the head (vertigo) is not a symptom of hypotension. Similarly, simple imbalance or fear of falling is not reflective of hypotension.

Among all seniors, the two most common causes of hypotension are medications and abnormal heart rhythms. Medications prescribed to treat hypertension (high blood pressure) occasionally reduce the blood pressure too much, resulting in faintness. Certain drugs used to treat other problems may likewise do this. Abnormal heart rhythms may cause faintness (hypotension) if the heart rate is very slow or rapid. This results in inefficient pumping of blood and a corresponding drop in blood pressure.

People with PD, however, are especially likely to experience hypotensive symptoms for two quite different reasons:

1. Dysfunction of the autonomic nervous system

2. Medications used to treat parkinsonism

These two factors make people with PD especially prone to low blood pressure, and specifically when standing or walking. This syndrome of low blood pressure in the upright (standing/walking) position is termed *orthostatic hypotension*, already briefly mentioned in previous chapters. We will now focus on this problem, including accurate detection and appropriate treatment.

Orthostatic Hypotension

Orthostatic hypotension implies a low blood pressure when on your feet (*orthostatic* = upright), but typically with a normal blood pressure when sitting or lying down. Rarely, the sitting (but not lying) blood pressure values are also low. Restated, the symptoms of orthostatic hypotension are primarily or exclusively experienced when one is upright. Orthostatic hypotensive symptoms will be relieved by sitting and certainly by lying down. Symptoms include lightheadedness/faintness, generalized weakness, and sometimes graying of vision, but not spinning or vertigo. Orthostatic hypotension may also result in a chronic fatigue state.

If the blood pressure drops very low, loss of consciousness occurs. Typically, such loss of consciousness is brief if the person collapses to the ground, because the blood pressure and blood flow to the brain are reestablished in the collapsed (lying) position.

Orthostatic hypotension may be missed with routine blood pressure testing. Blood pressure recordings are conventionally checked in the seated position. While seated, the blood pressure among those with orthostatic hypotension is typically normal. Thus, the blood pressure should be checked in both the seated and standing positions if you have PD.

PREDISPOSITION TO ORTHOSTATIC HYPOTENSION RELATES TO THE AUTONOMIC NERVOUS SYSTEM

Dysfunction within the autonomic nervous system predisposes to orthostatic hypotension, as discussed in previous chapters. The autonomic nervous system is the internal network of nerves that control function of many of our internal organs. It modulates blood vessel diameter, heart rate and pumping function, as well as sweating and bladder and bowel activity. In PD, Lewy body neurodegenerative changes occur in the autonomic nervous system, similar to what happens in the substantia nigra in the brain.

Normally, our blood pressure is stabilized by the autonomic nervous system, which appropriately modulates blood vessel diameter (resistance) and heart function. In normal humans, the blood pressure is regulated so that it is maintained at approximately the same value, whether lying, sitting, or standing. If not for the autonomic nervous system, blood would tend to pool in the blood vessels of our feet and legs whenever we stood up, pulled there by gravity. Normally, when we stand, blood vessels in the lower half of the body constrict, under the direction of the autonomic nervous system. In effect, this squeezes the blood up to our heads and maintains a constant blood pressure throughout the body, regardless of position.

When the autonomic nervous system malfunctions in PD, the internal reflexes that stabilize the blood pressure do not work properly. A failing autonomic nervous system will result in pooling of blood in the vessels of our feet and legs when standing. In this upright position, the brain does not receive enough blood. A mild reduction in blood flow to the brain will result in lightheadedness and, if severe, a faint occurs.

PD MEDICATIONS PROVOKE ORTHOSTATIC HYPOTENSION IN SUSCEPTIBLE PEOPLE

Typically in PD, autonomic nervous system malfunction is not severe, and in the absence of medications, orthostatic hypotension does not surface. Medications, however, provoke this problem; importantly, these include the medications used to treat PD. For the majority of people with PD this is not a problem, but this should always be considered when starting PD drugs.

The tendency of these drugs to reduce the blood pressure is roughly in proportion to their potency in treating PD symptoms. Lower doses are less likely to provoke orthostatic hypotension than higher doses. Less efficacious dopamine-replenishing drugs are less likely to lower the blood pressure than the more potent medications. Drugs used as supplements to levodopa therapy may not cause orthostatic hypotension when prescribed alone, but they will exacerbate this tendency from levodopa if they are added. The combination of orthostatic hypotension and PD complicates treatment and confuses medical management.

It is important to check the standing blood pressure before starting or increasing PD medications. If the pressure is low, measures to raise it should be implemented before commencing more aggressive treatment of PD, addressed later in this chapter. Although carbidopa/levodopa exacerbates orthostatic hypotension, this situation is treatable.

Orthostatic Hypotension: Detection and Treatment

There is a logical order of addressing this issue. First, a reliable strategy for detecting orthostatic hypotension is necessary. Second, other causes of low blood pressure must be addressed, such as non-PD drugs, anemia, or other medical problems. Third, effective strategies for treatment of orthostatic hypotension need to be implemented.

THE BASICS OF BLOOD PRESSURE: SYSTOLIC AND DIASTOLIC READINGS

Blood pressure measurements are recorded using two values, which relate to the two cycles of the heart. The first value is termed the *systolic* blood pressure and is the peak pressure generated by the pumping action of the heart. The second value, the *diastolic* blood pressure, relates to the low pressure point of the heart pumping cycle. Thus blood pressure readings are expressed as the systolic over the diastolic, for example, 120/80. The units of measurement are given in millimeters of mercury (mmHg). This relates to the pressure required to raise a column of mercury in a tube. Although we now rarely use columns of mercury to measure blood pressure, this system has survived as the unit of measurement. Throughout this book, when addressing blood pressure, we will abandon the units, mmHg, to keep this simple.

HOW MUCH CAN THE BLOOD PRESSURE DROP WITHOUT CAUSING PROBLEMS?

Faintness and other symptoms of low blood pressure do not occur unless the reading drops below a certain level; in other words, there is a threshold. By definition, readings above this threshold do not cause faintness or other symptoms and vice versa. This threshold varies from person to person, but some general guidelines have pragmatic utility. Note that the drop in blood pressure from sitting to standing can be profound, but if the standing blood pressure does not drop below a certain threshold level, symptoms will not occur. Thus, the change in blood pressure going from sitting to standing is not what translates into symptoms or faints; rather, the absolute blood pressure when upright determines whether symptoms develop, or the symptom threshold.

There is no specific threshold value that is true for everyone, given the variability between people. However, we can provide general practical guidelines. To simplify this exercise, we will focus on the systolic (upper) blood pressure value (e.g., the number 120, from a blood pressure reading of 120/80). Since the systolic and diastolic values tend to run in parallel in any given person, using one number instead of two makes this manageable. Throughout this book, we will maintain focus on the upper number, the systolic, and use that to help guide detection and treatment of low blood pressure. With that in mind, a general rule of thumb has practical utility:

> A systolic blood pressure that is always above 90 is adequate and will not result in low blood pressure symptoms.

Extrapolating from that rule of thumb, consider the following examples that illustrate this rule.

- Mrs. Stone has a sitting blood pressure of 200/110, which drops to 110/70 when standing. Since the systolic value of 110 is still well above 90, no symptoms result. This is despite a drop in the systolic blood pressure of 90.

- Mr. James has a sitting blood pressure of 110/70 that drops to 70/40, which results in faintness. Here, the systolic drop in blood pressure is only 40, but is sufficient to reduce the pressure below threshold and cause symptoms.

In general, a systolic blood pressure of 90 or higher provides adequate blood flow to the brain. Values below this may result in faintness, more likely if much below 90. This is not to say that if your blood pressure drops below 90 you will feel faint. If it is slightly below 90 and your body is used to this, you may feel fine. However, the risk of faintness starts at about that level. As a corollary to this rule:

> *Dizziness experienced at a time that the systolic blood pressure is above 90 is not due to low blood pressure.*

In that case, consider other explanation for your dizziness. It is important to emphasize, however, that this is valid if the blood pressure reading was taken *when* you are dizzy. This rule is not appropriate if the blood pressure reading was taken *after* feeling dizzy. Here is a scenario illustrating this oversight:

- Mr. Thomas walked across the living room and felt dizzy. He sat down and his wife measured his blood pressure. It was perfect, at 120/80. They concluded that his dizziness was not due to a low blood pressure. What was wrong in reaching this conclusion?

  Answer: If he truly has orthostatic hypotension, his blood pressure likely reverted to normal when he sat. His wife should have checked it in the standing position (assuming he tolerated standing without fainting).

Thus, if you feel dizzy, check the blood pressure when you are dizzy and in the position in which you feel dizzy (assuming you are not so dizzy that you will faint).

BLOOD PRESSURE VALUES MAY VARY DRAMATICALLY: IMPORTANCE OF TIMING

The tendency toward orthostatic hypotension typically fluctuates throughout the course of the day. This variation is especially related to the times of the carbidopa/levodopa doses. Thus, low pressure tends to occur when the levodopa effect is most prominent, 1–4 hours after the last dose. When the levodopa effect has worn off, the blood pressure typically reverts to normal or even high.

Other factors may also contribute to orthostatic hypotension and play a role in its variability (see Table 21.2). Meals tend to exacerbate orthostatic hypotension because of diversion of blood to the gut, plus circulating factors released in the digestive process. Hence, those with orthostatic hypotension tend to experience symptoms after meals, termed *postprandial hypotension*.

The tendency toward orthostatic hypotension is also increased by a night's sleep. It tends to be more of a problem in the morning than later in the day.

A very hot environment, such as soaking in a hot tub, will also tend to lower the blood pressure, because heat causes our blood vessels to dilate (expand). Vigorous exercise, increasing body heat, also tends to lower the blood pressure.

Table 21.2. Factors Predisposing to a Low Standing Blood Pressure

Factor	Effect on Standing Blood Pressure (BP)
Carbidopa/levodopa	Will tend to substantially lower BP beginning about 1 hour after each dose and lasting up to 4 hours
Dopamine agonist medications (pramipexole, ropinirole, rotigotine)	Will tend to lower BP in proportion to dose
Supplemental drugs: selegiline, rasagiline, entacapone	Will increase the tendency of levodopa to lower BP
Meals	Will tend to lower BP for about 2 hours after eating
Night's sleep	Will tend to lower morning BP
Hot environments, such as hot tub, summer heat; vigorous exercise	Heat tends to dilate blood vessels and lower BP
Fluid losses from diarrhea, vomiting, or blood loss	Reductions in the blood volume tend to lower the BP

Finally, any loss of the body's fluid volume, such as occurs with vomiting, diarrhea, or profuse sweating, tends to lower the blood pressure. Conversely, intake of fluids helps counter this. Blood loss notoriously lowers blood pressure.

Given these factors, the blood pressure of someone with PD may be normal at one point in the day and low at some other time. Hence a single blood pressure reading is insufficient to draw any conclusions.

When will blood pressure be lowest? *Answer:* Usually right after breakfast. The combined effects of a night's sleep, a meal, and a dose of carbidopa/levodopa (taken before breakfast) will converge and may provoke orthostatic hypotension. Thus after breakfast is a good time to routinely check the standing blood pressure if there is concern about orthostatic hypotension. Record these values so that they may be reviewed by your clinician.

OTHER CAUSES OF LOW BLOOD PRESSURE

If a low blood pressure is detected, there may be other factors that are contributing, especially non-PD drugs as well as other medical problems, such as anemia. These should be addressed before using any specific measures to raise the blood pressure.

NON-PD DRUGS LOWERING BLOOD PRESSURE

A myriad of medications lower blood pressure, such as antihypertensive drugs and water pills (diuretics). Thus a review of the medication list is appropriate at the first sign of orthostatic hypotension. Unnecessary medications can then be discontinued. The most common offenders are in the following categories:

- *Antihypertensive medications (blood pressure–lowering drugs).* Sometimes high blood pressure treatment started years ago is no longer necessary. This category includes many drugs from a variety of classes that are too numerous to individually list and includes some of the drugs listed next.

- *Diuretics (water pills).* These includes furosemide (Lasix), hydrochloro-thiazide (Hydrodiuril), triamterene (Dyrenium), hydrochlorothiazide plus triamterene (Dyazide, Maxzide), metolazone (Zaroxolyn), inda-pamide (Lozol), spironolactone (Aldactone), amiloride (Midamor), torsemide (Demadex), bumetanide (Bumex), and ethacrynic acid (Edecrin). These are used for a variety of problems, including swelling of the legs, blood pressure reduction, and heart failure.

- *Certain heart medications.* Not all heart drugs aggravate orthostatic hypotension but a few may do this, such as the nitrate drugs used to treat angina or carvedilol (Coreg) for congestive heart failure. Reduction in these drugs often requires the approval of the cardiologist.

- *Beta-blockers.* These are used for a variety of problems, including heart conditions, hypertension, tremor control, and migraine. They include atenolol (Tenormin), metoprolol (Lopressor, Toprol), propranolol (Inderal), nadolol (Corgard), timolol (Blocadren), and Pindolol (Visken).

- *Calcium channel blockers.* These are used for various conditions, including hypertension, cardiac problems, and migraine. These include verapamil (Calan, Isoptin, Verelan), diltiazem (Cardizem, Tiazac, Dilacor), nifedipine (Adalat, Procardia), amlodipine (Norvasc), felo-dipine (Plendil), isradipine (DynaCirc), and nicardipine (Cardene).

- *Certain prostate drugs.* The so-called alpha-blockers used to treat an enlarged prostate causing urinary hesitancy are commonly problematic in men with orthostatic hypotension. Drugs from this class include alfuzosin (Uroxatral), doxazosin (Cardura), silodosin (Rapaflo), tam-sulosin (Flomax), and terazosin (Hytrin).

- *Certain antidepressant drugs, especially those from tricyclic class.* These drugs are taken at bedtime and usually are not major offenders. They include amitriptyline (Elavil), nortriptyline (Pamelor), protriptyline (Vivactil), imipramine (Tofranil), and desipramine (Norpramin). Three other antidepressants may also mildly aggravate orthostatic hypotension: doxepin (Sinequan), mirtazepine (Remeron), and trazodone (Desyrel).

- *Male impotence medications.* These drugs include sildenafil (Viagra), vardenafil (Levitra, Staxyn), tadalafil (Cialis), and avanafil (Stendra).

Some of the medications on this list are for serious medical conditions. Your physician needs to advise whether any of these medications may be safely discontinued in the setting of orthostatic hypotension.

MEDICAL PROBLEMS CONTRIBUTING TO HYPOTENSION

A low blood pressure may be a clue to another medical disorder, such as anemia. Ongoing fluid losses from vomiting or diarrhea may cause hypotension. Thus, general medical disorders should be considered by the clinician if hypotension surfaces. Routine blood work, to include a complete blood count and blood chemistries, may be considered if not recently checked.

GENERAL PRINCIPLES IN TREATING ORTHOSTATIC HYPOTENSION

First, medications that may be contributing to hypotension should be eliminated if possible. Second, other medical conditions should be excluded, such as anemia. As this is being done, regular and reliable standing blood pressure measurements should be recorded. At that point, specific treatment of orthostatic hypotension may proceed.

In orthostatic hypotension, the blood tends to pool in blood vessels of the legs when standing. There are two general strategies for increasing the standing-up blood pressure.

- Increase the volume of blood in your blood vessels.

- Constrict the blood vessels with medications or compressive stockings.

Each strategy may be used to treat orthostatic hypotension. We will begin our discussion with the simplest natural strategies first, and will initially address this in general terms before providing very specific guidelines later in this chapter.

INCREASING BLOOD VOLUME

Increasing fluid intake (e.g., water, juice) tends to raise the volume of blood in the circulation. However, this alone is insufficient. The kidneys regulate water balance, and extra ingested water (or other fluids) is rapidly excreted into the urine. A crucial element that effectively holds the water in the circulation is sodium, or salt (sodium chloride). Salt is the primary source of sodium. In general, the more water held in the bloodstream by sodium, the higher the blood pressure. This drawing of water into the bloodstream with sodium occurs by osmosis, the process we studied in high school biology. Thus, adding salt and fluids to one's diet are simple initial steps in treating orthostatic hypotension.

Ingesting salt may fail to adequately raise the blood pressure. Again, this is because of the kidneys. The kidneys also tend to excrete extra salt into the urine. Sometimes this tendency can be overcome by administering large amounts of salt, in the form of salt tablets. Also, the tendency for the kidneys to remove salt from the bloodstream can be countered with a medication, fludrocortisone (Florinef). Fludrocortisone administration specifically causes the kidneys to retain sodium (salt). Hence, this medication is often used to treat orthostatic hypotension.

The over-the-counter anti-inflammatory medications used for pain relief also tend to cause sodium retention. These are the nonsteroidal anti-inflammatory drugs (NSAIDs), such as ibuprofen (Advil) and naproxen (Aleve); there are also a variety of prescription drugs from this class. However, their effect on blood pressure is slight, and these have not been very effective in treating the orthostatic hypotension of PD.

COMPRESSIVE STOCKINGS

The tendency for blood to pool in the vessels of the legs can be offset by wearing compressive stockings. Tight-fitting compressive stockings that go up to thigh or waist level are often effective treatments. These must be specifically fitted to match the size of your legs. Unfortunately, there is a major hassle factor with these compressive stockings; they are hard to put on, and some people find these uncomfortable and hot in the summertime. They must be washed carefully with gentle detergents in cold water to avoid damaging the compressive elastic. Also, they are expensive, as they must be custom-fit to the leg size. Despite the efficacy of compressive stockings, many people discontinue using these because of the expense, discomfort, and inconvenience. In my practice, it is rare for someone to tolerate these beyond a few weeks.

OTHER MEASURES

As mentioned earlier, those with orthostatic hypotension will tend to have lower blood pressure levels in the morning. Elevation of the head of the bed by about 6 inches may tend to partially offset this. You can put boards or some other 6-inch platform under the bedposts at the head of the bed.

Large meals contribute to orthostatic hypotension. If you frequently experience low blood pressure symptoms after eating a big meal, do the obvious: eat smaller meals. High-carbohydrate foods seem to be especially problematic at aggravating orthostatic hypotension, and reducing carbs may additionally be helpful. Alcohol dilates blood vessels. Those with significant orthostatic hypotension should avoid alcoholic beverages.

MEDICATIONS TO CONSTRICT BLOOD VESSELS

Certain adrenaline-like medications raise the blood pressure. Some of these are available as over-the-counter drugs, such as ephedrine or phenylpropanolamine. However, the over-the-counter drugs also stimulate the heart and may cause too rapid a heart rate. Hence, these are not recommended. The prescription drug midodrine (ProAmatine) raises the blood pressure by a similar adrenalin-like effect, but sparing the heart rate; it raises the blood pressure primarily by constricting blood vessels. This has proven very effective in countering the blood pressure–lowering effect of carbidopa/ levodopa; these two drugs have similar durations of action but with opposite effects on the blood pressure. Thus, if taken together, the blood pressure effects tend to be offset.

An old medication used for decades to treat a different disorder, myasthenia gravis, is also used to treat orthostatic hypotension: pyridostigmine (Mestinon). This drug modestly elevates the standing blood pressure but does not substantially elevate sitting or lying blood pressure values. It may be added to midodrine to complement that effect. It has a similar duration of action as midodrine.

NEW BLOOD PRESSURE ELEVATING DRUG, DROXIDOPA

In early 2014, the U.S. Food and Drug Administration approved droxidopa (Northera) for treatment of orthostatic hypotension. At the writing of this book, it had just become available, thus I do not have experience with using this drug.

Because of its pharmacology, it is unclear if droxidopa will benefit people with PD taking carbidopa/levodopa. Droxidopa is the precursor to norepinephrine (noradrenalin); norepinephrine is a hormone neurotransmitter that elevates blood pressure. Droxidopa has no direct influence on blood pressure and the effect is exclusively after it is converted to norepinephrine. Circulating norepinephrine appears to be the primary source of blood pressure elevation. Although norepinephrine stimulation in the brain may also raise blood pressure, it is unclear if this has a meaningful effect. Norepinephrine generated in the bloodstream does not cross the blood-brain barrier.

The conversion of droxidopa to the active agent norepinephrine is via the enzyme dopa decarboxylase (aromatic amino acid decarboxylase). As you may recall from Chapter 10, carbidopa blocks dopa decarboxylase, and therefore blocks the conversion of droxidopa to norepinephrine in the circulation. Thus, if you are taking carbidopa/levodopa, the primary mechanism of blood pressure elevation from droxidopa will be inhibited. We will not address droxidopa further in this chapter.

WHAT TO DO IF FEELING FAINT

In orthostatic hypotension, the blood pressure is low when standing and should normalize when sitting. With that knowledge, it is obvious what to do if feeling faint: sit down. If you are still feeling faint when sitting, lie down. The intent is to allow gravity to pull blood to your brain, not to your feet. Inform your family to not prop you up to standing. Instead, they should assist you to sit and, if necessary, lie down.

If the lightheadedness is mild while standing and you are not able to easily sit, cross your legs and squeeze your thigh muscles together. This muscle contraction state helps squeeze the blood upstream. Squatting may also be effective. Remember, however, that if you feel very faint, you need to sit or lie down. Sit on the ground if necessary.

If orthostatic symptoms develop, how long will they persist? Typically they are time-locked to the effect of your last carbidopa/levodopa dose. The blood pressure will rise when the levodopa effect wears off, typically 3–4 hours after the last carbidopa/levodopa dose.

PRELUDE TO TREATMENT: NEED FOR FREQUENT BLOOD PRESSURE CHECKS

Blood pressure monitoring is imperative to adequately treat orthostatic hypotension. If you have orthostatic hypotension, purchase a home blood pressure measurement device. When buying a blood pressure testing instrument, don't choose the cheapest; some of the less expensive instruments may not be calibrated for accurate readings in low ranges. If no one in the household has experience in taking blood pressure, have the nurse in your doctor's office instruct you.

Once you start checking your blood pressure, remember to check both the sitting and standing values. A common mistake is to record only the sitting pressure, which obviously misses the crucial readings when you have orthostatic hypotension.

When is the best time to check the blood pressure? As we discussed, the lowest readings will typically be in the morning after breakfast. This is a good time for one of your measurements. A second reading in the afternoon, after lunch, may also be helpful to determine if low readings persist. Once measures are taken to elevate the blood pressure, a third reading while lying in bed at the time you retire is appropriate. This is to make certain the readings don't go too high with treatment.

Be certain that blood pressure readings are taken between 1 and 2 hours after a levodopa dose. Blood pressure values may vary greatly between the levodopa on-state (when levodopa is working) and the levodopa off-state; it will typically be much lower when there is a good levodopa effect. In fact, it is often only low during levodopa on-states or within a few hours of a dose.

TREATMENT TARGETS: WHAT RANGE OF BLOOD PRESSURE?

When treating orthostatic hypotension, it is difficult if not impossible to consistently achieve perfectly normal blood pressure values. Hence, we will need to accept that. An occasional aberrant reading should not be cause for alarm unless it is some very extreme value.

As discussed, the aim is to maintain the standing systolic blood pressure at 90 or higher. This will provide adequate blood flow to the brain. If the systolic blood pressure is occasionally in the 80s, that is acceptable if you don't feel faint and if most of the readings are higher than that.

What is the optimal blood pressure? In a perfect world, we would shoot for a systolic blood pressure of between 100 and 120. Similarly, the diastolic readings would be between 60 and 80. However, those with autonomic dysfunction cannot control the pressure precisely, so you should anticipate substantial deviations, even with the best of treatment. Again, we will not aim for perfection, but rather target a broader range of blood pressure values that are acceptable.

HOW HIGH IS TOO HIGH A BLOOD PRESSURE?

Recognizing the practical impossibility of achieving perfect blood pressure control in this setting, I am satisfied with systolic values up to 160; if most of the readings are in this range but infrequent readings run a little higher to 180, I generally accept that as well. Most diastolic blood pressure values should be below 95, allowing for occasional diastolic readings up to 100. Since the highest blood pressure values are recorded lying down, this is a good position to monitor for excessive values (see Table 21.3).

Is it dangerous to have too high a blood pressure? It is not dangerous unless it is dramatically elevated, far beyond the values in Table 21.3, or if this level is sustained over months to years. The primary problem with chronic high blood pressure is that this contributes to hardening of the arteries, termed *atherosclerosis*. Atherosclerosis leads to heart attacks and strokes. Atherosclerosis represents a buildup of plaque inside artery walls and, if severe, cuts off the flow of blood. Aging contributes prominently

Table 21.3. Treating Orthostatic Hypotension: Blood Pressure Targets

Blood Pressure	Value*	Position to Detect These Readings**
Too low?	Less than 90 systolic	Standing
Perfect	Systolic = 100–120; diastolic = 60–80	
Too high?	Systolic over 160, but accept occasional systolic pressure values up to 180	Lying down
	Diastolic over 100; accept occasional diastolic values of 95–100	

* *Systolic* represents the upper number in blood pressure readings and *diastolic*, the lower number.

** The lowest readings will be when standing and the highest when lying down. Hence, these are the positions to assess the extremes.

to this, as do other risk factors such as smoking, high cholesterol, and diabetes mellitus. The atherosclerotic plaque in the artery eventually narrows the lumen, restricting blood circulation. If blood flow to the heart muscle is restricted, a heart attack occurs. If blood flow to an area of the brain is restricted, this results in a stroke. This buildup of plaque inside artery walls is a slow, insidious process, occurring over many years. Hence occasional, brief blood pressure elevations are not dangerous unless extremely high.

What is an extremely high blood pressure that requires immediate attention? This varies, depending on your usual blood pressure. However, systolic readings over 220 or diastolic readings over 120 that persist for more than a few hours should be brought to your physician's immediate attention. If substantially higher than those values, a trip to the emergency room is appropriate.

For elevated blood pressure values when in bed at night, elevation of the head of the bed by 6 inches will reduce these values. This was the same strategy discussed earlier to attenuate low blood pressure when getting up in the morning. Also, if the lying-down blood pressure values are very high, supplementary salt and fludrocortisone therapy to raise the blood pressure may have to be stopped. These elevate the blood pressure around the clock.

When orthostatic hypotension is a problem during the day, but the blood pressure is very high in bed at night, a short-acting blood pressure–lowering drug such as hydralazine may be added at bedtime. If this strategy is employed, however, caution is advised to avoid low blood pressure during the night that might lead to faints when going to the bathroom. This strategy is almost never necessary.

REMINDER: HEART RHYTHM PROBLEMS
MAY ALSO CAUSE FAINTNESS

Faintness developing in someone with PD is most often due to orthostatic hypotension. However, do not forget that heart rhythm irregularities are also a cause of faintness. If the heart beats too fast, too slow, or pauses, the blood pressure may plummet. In contrast to the symptoms of orthostatic hypotension, faintness due to heart irregularities occurs in any body position and is not linked to standing. Heart rhythm spells tend to be infrequent and occur haphazardly. If faints or near-faints develop in the seated or lying positions, heart irregularities should be considered.

If you think a heart rhythm problem might be the cause of your spells, learn to feel your pulse or have family members learn to do this. Then if symptoms develop, assess whether the heartbeat is very irregular, very slow, or very fast. This information could be very helpful to your physician.

Specific Guidelines for Treating Orthostatic Hypotension

The strategies for elevating low blood pressure outlined here need to be organized into a pragmatic scheme. Experience indicates that certain of these measures work better than others. The approach we will take to treat orthostatic hypotension is based on several premises. First, it makes sense to do the simplest things first. Second, strategies that are theoretically effective but modestly helpful in practice will not be emphasized. Third, tolerability will be considered; strategies that are helpful but unworkable will likewise not be emphasized here. Throughout this section, continued monitoring of blood pressure values will be encouraged, since ongoing readings are necessary to make the correct treatment decisions. The goal is a standing systolic blood pressure that is consistently at least 90.

The general strategy can be organized into a series of steps, listed below. For some people, blood pressure control will be accomplished early in this sequence and nothing further is necessary. Recall that the blood pressure–lowering effect of carbidopa/levodopa is related to the size of the individual doses (i.e., higher doses tend to further reduce the pressure). Thus, if the carbidopa/levodopa doses are raised, implementation of additional steps in this sequence may be necessary.

1. Review your medications with the clinician to determine if any drugs are contributing to a low blood pressure and can be eliminated. The list of possible offending drugs earlier in this chapter may help identify which drugs to consider. Discuss with your clinician whether there might be another medical condition contributing to the low pressure

(e.g., anemia); blood work might then be appropriate if not done recently.

2. Increase the salt in your diet. Often, senior citizens are instructed to maintain a low-salt diet, since high blood pressure is common in the general population.

3. For salt supplementation to be effective, adequate intake of fluids is necessary. The salt (sodium) in the bloodstream draws in water, and adequate fluid intake is necessary. Water, per se, isn't mandatory; juice and soda pop work as well. About 6 to 10 tall (10 ounce) glasses daily should satisfy this fluid requirement. Don't go overboard on drinking fluids. You don't need more than about 10 glasses daily. If you drink milk, recall that this is a protein drink and that protein may block levodopa passage to the brain (restrict milk to mealtimes).

4. Elevate the head of the bed by about 6 inches using blocks under the bed posts. This may help counter the very low blood pressure that sometimes occurs in the morning after arising. It may also help prevent high blood pressure during sleep.

5. If increasing the salt (sodium chloride) in the diet is insufficient, then the use of salt tablets is appropriate. These are available over the counter; one common brand is Thermotabs, but any brand is acceptable. Start with one-half salt tablet twice daily and increase to a whole tablet twice daily, if necessary. It is often tolerated best if taken with meals, but this isn't mandatory.

Salt caveats:

- Those with heart, liver, or kidney failure are cautioned to limit salt. If a serious heart, liver, or kidney problem is present, a physician review is required.
- Increasing dietary salt may cause mild swelling in your legs. If this becomes very pronounced, talk with your physician. Elevating the legs to about chest level when seated is often an effective treatment. This helps gravity draw off the fluid, returning it to the circulation where the kidneys can excrete it. Remember that water pills (diuretics) are not an advisable treatment for leg swelling in this situation; they lower blood pressure.
- High salt intake may be associated with increased calcium excretion in the urine. If this continues for years, this may lead to bone weakening (osteopenia/osteoporosis) from calcium loss. If a high salt intake is maintained, make certain that you are consuming

adequate calcium and vitamin D. Note that vitamin D facilitates calcium absorption in the gut. The daily elemental calcium intake from diet or supplements should be about 1200 mg, plus 800–1000 units of vitamin D per day. This is discussed further in Chapter 30.

At this juncture, if these measures have proven insufficient to maintain the blood pressure in the setting of carbidopa/levodopa administration, I often go directly to midodrine, which is step #8.

6. If the simpler measures are inadequate, physicians sometimes prescribe fludrocortisone (Florinef). Fludrocortisone causes the kidneys to retain sodium, rather than being excreted into the urine. This is mildly helpful to elevate blood pressure. The starting fludrocortisone dose is one 0.1 mg tablet daily. It takes about a week to appreciate the response. It can be raised to one 0.1 mg tablet twice daily and over the next 2 weeks raised as high as two 0.1 mg tablets twice daily. Remember that fludrocortisone requires salt to work, so salt supplementation and adequate fluid intake remain necessary. Fludrocortisone may cause loss of potassium into the urine, and the blood (serum) potassium level should be checked after the fludrocortisone dose is stabilized and occasionally thereafter. Fludrocortisone is more effective when the potassium concentration in the blood is normal. Hence, a potassium supplement may be necessary. The downside of fludrocortisone is the around-the-clock effect, tending to raise the blood pressure when one is in bed at night.

7. Compressive hose are very effective for countering orthostatic hypotension, provided that they are of the proper type and combined with an abdominal binder. The reason for the benefit is that they externally constrict the blood vessels in the lower half of the body. Recall that a normal autonomic nervous system triggers the internal constriction of these vessels when going from sitting to upright; in orthostatic hypotension, this fails. Squeezing from the outside with constrictive garments therefore makes good sense. For these to be effective, however, the stockings and binder must constrict most or all of the lower half of the body. Hence the compressive stockings must be waist-high or at least thigh-high and combined with a girdle-like garment known as an abdominal binder. Few people in my practice are willing to try this strategy and those that have, abandon it after a few weeks. The garments are hard to put on, hot, and expensive, and they require special washing (to avoid damaging the elastic). If you think you might tolerate these, see the section on compressive hose later in this chapter. Note that calf-length support hose have no utility in this setting.

8. Midodrine (ProAmatine) has properties that make it a very useful agent to counter the blood pressure–lowering effect that occurs with each dose of carbidopa/levodopa. It often is used in conjunction with some of the measures listed here, not necessarily in place of them. Midodrine will *elevate* the blood pressure for about 3–4 hours following each dose, similar in duration to the blood pressure–*lowering* effect of levodopa. Thus, if midodrine and carbidopa/levodopa are taken together, the blood pressure effects should offset and cancel each other (if the midodrine dose is sufficiently high).

Midodrine is usually started in a low dose and then raised, guided by the blood pressure readings. Because this drug works for only 3–4 hours, doses typically need to be repeated throughout the waking day, usually with each daytime dose of carbidopa/levodopa. Effective midodrine doses are between 5 mg and 15 mg. It is conventionally started with a dose of 2.5 mg, but in my experience, that is too low to be effective. I start with 5 mg doses.

Some people experience low blood pressure symptoms only during the first half of the day. For these people, midodrine may only be required with the initial daily doses of carbidopa/levodopa.

Occasionally, I see people who are prescribed midodrine in a dose of t.i.d., which translates into three times daily. This sets up the possibility of gaps in coverage, since such a dosing schedule is often, by convention, at intervals of 6 hours (e.g., 6 a.m., noon, and 6 p.m.). When prescribed, it should either be administered at 3- to 4-hour intervals or with each dose of carbidopa/levodopa. For those whose hypotension is only problematic in the morning, a single morning midodrine dose, perhaps followed by second dose 3–4 hours later, may be sufficient.

Midodrine is taken only when one is up and about, and is not to be taken within 3–4 hours before bedtime. By definition, those with orthostatic hypotension do not have low blood pressure when lying down. Hence, taking midodrine before bedtime could cause the blood pressure to go from normal to high. Midodrine in usually well tolerated without side effects, although occasional people experience tingling or similar sensory effects.

9. An optional treatment is the addition of pyridostigmine to midodrine. Pyridostigmine (Mestinon) elevates only the standing blood pressure and for 3–4 hours after each dose, paralleling the durations of midodrine and carbidopa/levodopa. The advantage of this drug is that it has a different mechanism of action from that of midodrine and is less likely to elevate the sitting or lying blood pressure. However, it is not as potent as midodrine. Some clinicians add pyridostigmine if the lower doses of midodrine are insufficient. Pyridostigmine can be administered with each carbidopa/levodopa (and midodrine) dose,

starting with 30 mg (one-half of a 60 mg pyridostigmine tablet). It can be raised to a full 60 mg tablet, if indicated. Side effects are primarily gastrointestinal, including loose stools or nausea. The primary downside of pyridostigmine in this setting is the addition of yet another drug to an already complicated medication regimen.

SPECIFIC INSTRUCTIONS FOR MIDODRINE

Midodrine can be very effective and the administration is straight-forward. It has a 3- to 4-hour effect, and the response is directly in proportion to the dose; that is, the higher the dose, the greater the blood pressure elevation. Midodrine doses between 5 mg and 15 mg are nearly always adequate in PD.

In PD, orthostatic hypotension in the absence of carbidopa/levodopa is typically manageable without midodrine. It is the exacerbating influence of carbidopa/levodopa that requires midodrine in PD. If orthostatic hypotension is highly problematic even without carbidopa/levodopa, review the discussion in Chapter 6 relating to multiple system atrophy.

In this context of PD, we will assume that people requiring midodrine will be taking carbidopa/levodopa. Hence, each midodrine dose will be administered with carbidopa/levodopa doses to offset the levodopa orthostatic hypotensive effect. The basic principles are as follows:

- Before starting midodrine, record the sitting and standing blood pressure values in the morning after breakfast, and again in the afternoon, after lunch. If only the morning standing systolic blood pressure values are frequently below 90, then afternoon doses of midodrine will not be necessary. Otherwise, take midodrine with each daytime dose of carbidopa/levodopa.

- Do not take midodrine within 3 hours of going to bed at night. Also, avoid taking this before any long daytime naps.

- The effect from midodrine lasts 3 to 4 hours; do not take it at intervals less than this. If taken at too brief intervals, the effects will overlap and summate.

- If carbidopa/levodopa is taken at 2-hour intervals, take midodrine with every other dose of carbidopa/levodopa, recognizing that the midodrine effect lasts up to about 4 hours.

- The conventional recommendation is for midodrine to be started with one-half of a 5 mg tablet each dose. This is too low to provide adequate benefit in most people and will likely need to be raised to at least 5 mg doses.

- After starting midodrine, check the standing blood pressure 1 to 2 hours after each dose. After just a few readings, it will become apparent if the dose of midodrine is sufficient. If the standing systolic blood pressure is still frequently below 90, then the doses can be raised. Typically, the same amount of midodrine is used for each dose.

- If one-half of a 5 mg tablet is insufficient (as expected), based on the blood pressure readings, raise all doses to a whole 5 mg tablet. With ongoing blood pressure recordings it will be apparent after just 2–3 days if this dose is adequate. If not, raise to 1 ½ tablets each dose (7.5 mg). Ultimately, 2 whole tablets (10 mg) each dose may be used. Rarely is it necessary to go higher, the ceiling dose being 15 mg (3 tablets).

- If the carbidopa/levodopa dose is subsequently raised, recheck the blood pressure, since a higher dose of midodrine might then be required.

- The treatment goal is to maintain the standing systolic blood pressure over 90.

- Note that excessively high blood pressure values more than 4 hours after the last dose of midodrine are not due to this drug (e.g., systolic values over 160). By that time, the effect will have worn off.

Midodrine comes in three tablet sizes, 2.5 mg, 5 mg, and 10 mg. Dose initiation and adjustments are easiest with the 5 mg tablet size. How many doses are required each day depends on how many hours per day you are up and whether you need coverage beyond the morning.

SPECIAL INSTRUCTIONS FOR USE OF COMPRESSIVE HOSE

Compression of leg veins with tight-fitting hose can be very helpful in treating orthostatic hypotension. They prevent the pooling of blood in the lower extremities, essentially squeezing blood out of the lower half of the body toward the brain. As mentioned, there are drawbacks, including difficulty putting these on, expense, and discomfort on hot days. In their defense, they work continuously throughout the waking day and should not substantially elevate the blood pressure when lying down. They are removed at night, so they do not impair sleep.

If you are able to tolerate compressive hose, try these as a first option, rather than as a last resort. Here are a few things you should know about compressive hose for orthostatic hypotension.

- They must be thigh-high or waist-high for treating orthostatic hypotension. Knee-high hose do not work for this purpose. Knee-high stockings reduce leg swelling but do not counter low blood pressure. The waist-high hose work a little better than thigh-high hose. Problems of urinary urgency may preclude use of waist-high hose.

- The hose must be fitted to your leg size. There are specific sites on your legs to take the measurements. You will need to refer to instructions from the stocking company or the medical supply store advising exactly how to do this. This is best done by the person waiting on you in the medical supply store or by a physical therapist (physical therapists are knowledgeable about these stockings).

- There are two standard pressure values, 20 to 30 mmHg (millimeters of mercury, a measurement of pressure) and 30 to 40 mmHg. The 30 to 40 mmHg stockings are a little more effective (squeeze a little tighter) but are also a little harder to get on. You might start with the 20 to 30 mmHg stockings and see if they are adequate. Physiatrists and physical therapists are in a position to assist and advise about these garments.

- Pay close attention to the washing instructions, since very hot water and certain harsh detergents may damage the elastic and make these baggy and useless.

- An abdominal binder complements these hose, and these are available from medical supply companies. They fit around the waist, similar to women's girdles worn in the last century. Compression from the binder helps reduce the pooling of blood in the abdominal blood vessels. This can be very helpful for those individuals susceptible to postprandial hypotension (low blood pressure after meals).

- Put the hose on first thing in the morning before you get out of bed. Often, blood pressure is lowest early in the morning and faintness may be a risk on your way to the bathroom.

- Purchase two pairs of hose to start, recognizing that you will need to wear one while the other is being washed.

- Measure the standing blood pressure just before putting these garments on and again afterward to confirm their utility.

- There are tricks to putting these on and the manufacturer typically provides advice. They may go on more easily using rubber dishwashing gloves for a better grip. Often this is a two-person job.

Avoid any tight bands around your legs, such as rubber bands or stockings with a very tight elastic band that cuts into your leg. Compressive hose facilitate the flow of blood out of your legs because of the widespread pressure gradient. However, narrow bands around your legs may do the opposite;

Table 21.4.   Strategies for Maintaining an Adequate Blood Pressure (BP)

Target = Consistent Systolic Readings of at Least 90 (Standing)

Strategy (Simplest Things First)	Comment
1. Review medication list	Physician to eliminate unnecessary drugs that lower BP
2. Exclude other causes of low BP	Clinician evaluation, which may include complete blood count and blood chemistry profile
3. Increase salt and fluids*	Fluid intake: about 6–10 tall glasses of water, juice, soda pop daily
4. Elevate head of bed	Raise head of bed 6 inches
5. Salt tablets *	One-half to 1 tablet two times daily
6. Optional: fludrocortisone (Florinef)*	Dose of 1 tablet daily, up to 2 tablets twice daily. Induces the kidneys to retain sodium rather than excreting it into the urine
7. Optional: compressive hose and abdominal binder	Waist- or thigh-high compressive stockings specially fitted to the leg size can be a very effective treatment, if tolerated.
8. Midodrine (ProAmatine)	BP is raised for about 3–4 hours after each dose. Same duration of action as carbidopa/levodopa to offset that effect
9. Optional: pyridostigmine (Mestinon)	This drug may be added to carbidopa/levodopa and midodrine; it also has about a 3- to 4-hour effect.

*If there is severe heart, kidney, or liver failure, salt is typically restricted; this must be discussed with your physician.

they may block the flow of blood and may even lead to a blood clot in your leg (thrombophlebitis).

SUMMARY

People with PD and orthostatic hypotension will probably not require most of the strategies outlined in this chapter. It is not imperative that the scheme cited here be followed precisely in this order, but it does go from simpler to more complex. For people with primarily carbidopa/levodopa-induced orthostatic hypotension, midodrine may be used earlier, since it has properties that allow offsetting the levodopa hypotensive effect. Table 21.4 summarizes this scheme.

RECORD BLOOD PRESSURE READINGS

Remember that it is very important to record your blood pressure values. You and your physician need these data to make therapeutic decisions. At the end of this chapter is a blood pressure record that you may reproduce for this purpose (Supplement 21.1).

Supplement 21.1.   Blood Pressure Chart
Record your blood pressure (BP) values to guide you and your physician.

Date and Time	Symptoms (If Present)	Sitting BP	Standing BP	Lying BP

22

◆ ◆ ◆

Depression

What Is depression?

Depression is a mental state, synonymous with feeling blue, unhappy, sad, gloomy, hopeless, or melancholy It is a perceptual state; the glass is always half-empty rather than half-full. One sees only the dark side of things. It is tied to daily activities; it sabotages motivation and saps energy. It affects the most basic elements of lives, causing insomnia, loss of appetite, and sexual dysfunction. Sometimes it's linked to obsessive worry and rumination, always anticipating and expecting the worst to happen.

Why Do People Become Depressed?

Certainly, we all encounter things in our life that eat at our souls; who would not be depressed when a loved one dies or illness strikes the family? If you have Parkinson's disease (PD), the prospect of a chronic disease is discouraging in and of itself. If you have had to restrict your lifestyle because of PD, that is all the more reason to become discouraged. Hence depression is a part of the normal human existence and is appropriate during times when things are going very badly. Depression, however, becomes pathological when it is prolonged, severe, and out of proportion to events in our lives. Although depression may be triggered by major life trauma, it often comes out of nowhere.

When depression becomes pathological and disabling, it presumably is associated with changes in brain chemistry. Deficient activity of certain brain neurotransmitters such as serotonin, norepinephrine, and dopamine are believed to underlie depressive states. PD predisposes to depression by virtue of the neurodegenerative process also affecting these systems. In PD, the same process that causes degeneration of the dopamine-containing neurons in the substantia nigra leads to degeneration of brain neurons containing serotonin, norepinephrine, and other dopamine systems. Hence it is not surprising that people with PD are predisposed to depression. This recognition of the biochemical substrates of depression, however, has opened the door to medical treatment.

How Do I Know If I Am Depressed?

It may be difficult to be objective about one's emotional state. Reading your own psyche in an unbiased manner is not something most of us are good at doing. It is helpful to discuss this with a loved one, your physician, clergy, or a professional psychologist or psychiatrist. The typical symptoms are summarized in Table 22.1.

You will note from this table that PD causes symptoms that may resemble depression. Family members may notice that you don't smile anymore, but this may reflect the facial masking of PD. Activities and initiative may be diminished, but perhaps that has to do with the reduced energy that is part of PD. Similarly, some of the signs that psychiatrists use as indicators of depression, such as reduced appetite, insomnia, and reduced libido, may be due to PD, PD medications, or both.

The decision to treat depression may be made by the family physician, internist, neurologist, or a psychiatrist. If the problem is straightforward, the primary physician may feel comfortable initiating treatment.

"I'm Not Depressed!"

Typically there is a tendency to resist and deny a diagnosis of depression. Some people view this as a sign of weakness; "I should be able to deal with this on my own!" Being stubborn about this, however, may deprive you of experiencing life's pleasures once again; this capability might be right around the corner with appropriate treatment. In most cases, the treatments are effective and well tolerated; they should be welcomed. Years

Table 22.1. Symptoms of Depression*

Symptom	Comment
Sadness, tearfulness, feeling blue	
Loss of interest	Apathy may be a component of advancing PD
Reduced activities and energy (but sometimes agitation)	But PD also reduces energy levels
Rumination and worry	
Everything seems bleak and hopeless	
Focus on the negative; failing to see the positive	
Poor self-esteem, guilt, worthlessness	
No longer smiling	But hard to tell, since PD causes masking
Loss of appetite (sometimes increased appetite)	Poor appetite could be due to medications
Insomnia	Insomnia may be due to PD (and responds to PD drugs, as discussed in Chapter 20)
Sleeps excessively	But this may be related to medications, or the effects of PD on sleep patterns (see Chapter 20)
Reduced libido	But may have other causes such as age, medications, as well as PD (see Chapter 28 on sexual functioning)
Thoughts of death, suicide	Suggests urgent attention necessary

* Considered significant when depressed mood and other symptoms interfere with daily functioning and persist beyond 2 weeks.

ago there was stigma tied to a diagnosis of depression. Now, with celebrity lives made public by the media, we have grown accustomed to seeing our favorite and most respected public figures treated for depression and related disorders. Like stomach ulcers and asthma, depression is now recognized for what it is—a bonafide medical illness. This is even more apparent in the case of PD; depression is typically caused or exacerbated by changes in brain chemistry as part of the underlying neurodegenerative process.

Suicide

Depression may make a life look so bleak that it may seem that life is not worth living, with thoughts like "I would rather be dead." If depression reaches these proportions, objective thought is often no longer possible. It may produce thoughts so twisted and dark that perceptions of the world are turned inside out. One may think that everything is evil and worthless, especially oneself. Why live in this world?

If the depression is sinking to these depths and suicide is being contemplated, it is absolutely critical to ask for help. You will not be able to work through this type of a depressive illness when suicidal thoughts are becoming prominent; thinking is no longer objective and help is necessary. Meet with your doctor, and when you meet in the office, be open about the depths of the depression. If you have contemplated suicide, this must be put on the table. Your doctor will know what to do.

Origins of Depression in Parkinson's Disease

PD predisposes to depression for a variety of reasons:

- It may be a reaction to the disability of PD. Such depression should improve with carbidopa/levodopa treatment of parkinsonism.

- It may directly relate to the dopamine deficiency state. For example, some individuals with fluctuating motor responses note that depression coincides with their levodopa off-states; it lifts when the levodopa response kicks in. Appropriate treatment is the same as for the motor symptoms of PD.

- It may relate to a deficiency of the brain neurotransmitter serotonin, caused by the PD neurodegenerative process. This can be adequately treated with drugs that enhance serotonin activity within the brain. Drugs from the medication class called *selective serotonin reuptake inhibitors* (SSRIs) are often effective.

- Other brain chemistry problems linked to PD may also play a role in depression. For example, the PD neurodegenerative process also affects brain systems containing the neurotransmitter norepinephrine. Deficient activity of this neurotransmitter is known to cause depression, and antidepressant drugs are available that target norepinephrine.

Pseudodementia

People who are depressed may seem dull and uninterested. This may become so pronounced that they actually seem demented. In other words, depression can affect your ability to think and remember. Physicians call this *pseudodementia*, and recognize that this possibility must be considered when evaluating people with impaired thinking. The good news is that this is treatable; once depression is controlled, memories and thoughts flow once again.

Treatment of Depression

As you might surmise, the treatment needs to fit the problem. The therapeutic strategies differ depending on the severity, the cause(s), the family, and other support systems. The basic elements of the treatment approach start with the following:

- *Treat the symptoms of PD with carbidopa/levodopa.* Unless the depression is severe, I typically do this first. Often the improvement in gait, tremor, and mobility are sufficient to improve one's outlook and reverse depression. Moreover, the replenishment of brain dopamine with levodopa may have a direct antidepressant effect.

- *Treat insomnia.* Although insomnia may be a symptom of depression, it may also be a contributor to depression if sleep deprivation is marked. Many people with PD require levodopa therapy at bedtime or during the night to attain a good night's sleep (refer back to Chapter 20).

- *Make a conscious effort to be active.* It's easy to sit back on the couch in front of the TV if not feeling 100%. However, this feeds into the depressive process. If physically able to be up and about, force yourself, little by little, to engage in social and recreational activities.

When to start an antidepressant drug is based on the severity of symptoms and circumstances. The medications for treating depression are usually effective, easy to use, and well tolerated. Doctors typically have a low threshold for starting one of these drugs.

Note that drugs used to treat depression are slow to work. They do not produce a high, but exert the beneficial effects slowly and gradually over weeks. They change brain chemistry to allow a more positive outlook on life. It is often several weeks later that you realize that you are feeling much better. Those who worried about every small incident begin to focus on the good things in life and appreciate that these ruminations are fading away. Given the insidious and slow responses with these medications, patience is necessary. Anticipate that it may take 6 weeks or so for the benefits to become apparent.

Table 22.2 lists the medications commonly used to treat depression. The first two categories in the table list the SSRI and SNRI drugs. These are the antidepressants most commonly prescribed in the current era.

SSRI stands for selective serotonin reuptake inhibitor.

SNRI stands for serotonin-norepinephrine reuptake inhibitor.

Table 22.2. Medications Commonly Used to Treat Depression

Class of Drug	Medication	Typical Starting Dose	Usual Dose Range
SSRI			
	Fluoxetine (Prozac)	10 mg each morning	10–50 mg each morning
	Sertraline (Zoloft)	25 mg each morning	50–150 mg each morning
	Paroxetine (Paxil)	10 mg each morning	10–40 mg each morning
	Paroxetine sustained release (Paxil CR)	12.5 mg each morning	25–50 mg each morning
	Fluvoxamine (Luvox)	50 mg at bedtime	100 mg once at bedtime to 300 mg daily in two divided doses
	Citalopram (Celexa)	10 mg once daily	20–40 mg once daily
	Escitalopram (Lexapro)	10 mg once daily	10–20 mg once daily
SNRI			
	Venlafaxine (Effexor)	25 mg twice to three times daily	25 mg to 75 mg three times daily
	Venlafaxine sustained-release (Effexor XR)	37.5 mg to 75 mg once daily	75 mg to 225 mg once daily
	Duloxetine (Cymbalta)	20 mg once to twice daily	20–30 mg twice daily (or 60 mg once daily)
	Desvenlafaxine (Pristiq; extended-release)	50 mg once daily	50 mg once daily
Tricyclics			
	Amitriptyline (Elavil)	10–25 mg at bedtime	75–150 mg at bedtime
	Desipramine (Norpramin)	10–25 mg at bedtime	75–150 mg at bedtime or divided into two daily doses

(continued)

Table 22.2.   Continued

Class of Drug	Medication	Typical Starting Dose	Usual Dose Range
	Doxepin (Sinequan)	10–25 mg at bedtime	75–150 mg at bedtime
	Imipramine (Tofranil)	10–25 mg at bedtime	50–150 mg at bedtime
	Nortriptyline (Pamelor, Aventyl)	10–25 mg at bedtime	50–150 mg at bedtime
	Protriptyline (Vivactil)	5 mg once to twice daily	5 mg three to four times daily
	Trimipramine (Surmontil)	25 mg at bedtime	50–150 mg daily as either a bedtime dose or divided into two daily doses
	Clomipramine (Anafranil)	10–25 mg at bedtime	75–150 mg at bedtime
Others	Bupropion (Wellbutrin)	75–100 mg each morning	100 mg two to three times daily
	Bupropion sustained-release (Wellbutrin SR)	150 mg each morning	150 mg once to twice daily
	Maprotiline (Ludiomil)	25 mg to 75 mg once daily	50 mg to 150 mg as a single dose or divided doses
	Mirtazapine (Remeron)	15 mg at bedtime	15 mg to 45 mg at bedtime
	Nefazodone (Serzone)	100 mg at bedtime	100 mg to 200 mg twice daily
	Trazodone (Desyrel)	50 mg at bedtime	50 mg to 200 mg twice daily

SSRI = selective serotonin reuptake inhibitor; SNRI = serotonin-norepinephrine reuptake inhibitor.

The middle column in the table lists the typical starting dose for each drug. In many cases, this is too low to be consistently effective. However, the medication is started conservatively to make certain that it is tolerated before escalating to doses more likely to be effective. If the starting dose is tolerated for 1 to 2 weeks, it is then raised. The medications listed in Table 22.2 tend to have similar efficacy in treating depression, in general. However, some are sedating and others energizing; side effects differ. These properties influence the choice of antidepressant.

SSRI Medications Target Serotonin

Serotonin is a neurotransmitter found in brain circuits associated with affective states, that is, states spanning elation to depression. The SSRI drugs increase the activity of brain serotonin systems by blocking the "reuptake" of serotonin.

What is reuptake? In general, the concentration of neurotransmitters in the synapse is modulated by the nerve terminal (refer back to Figure 2.2 in Chapter 2). Nerve terminals releasing the neurotransmitter subsequently remove it from the synapse by reuptake; that is, they effective suck it back up. If reuptake is blocked by a drug, this allows more neurotransmitter at the receptor, enhancing the effect. SSRI drugs target only serotonin terminals and block the reuptake of serotonin. This mildly enhances serotonergic neurotransmission.

Brain serotonin activity is reduced in some people with depression, and enhancing serotonin neurotransmission effectively treats this depression. Note that brain serotonin levels tend to be reduced among people with PD due to the underlying neurodegenerative process affecting brain serotonin neurons. Thus SSRI drugs that enhance serotonin effects treat depression in general, as well as depression among those with PD.

Among the SSRI drugs listed in Table 22.2, none stand out as superior. If one fails, this does not mean that another may not work. These drugs typically do not make people sleepy (with the exception of fluvoxamine) and are usually taken in the morning. They require only one dose daily, although fluvoxamine (Luvox) is often administered twice a day.

Years ago, there were several published reports of SSRI medications inducing or worsening parkinsonism. I personally cannot recall encountering this problem in caring for hundreds, if not thousands of people with PD on one of these drugs. I regard this as a safe class of medications for people with PD.

My usual medication choice for treating depression in someone with PD is a drug from this SSRI class. They are usually effective, are easy to use, and have few side effects.

SNRI Medications Target Serotonin and Norepinephrine

A newer class of antidepressants, the SNRI drugs, enhances neurotransmission in not only brain serotonin but also norepinephrine systems. Norepinephrine neurons are also involved in affective states. Enhancing norepinephrine neurotransmission reduces depression and tends to be mildly energizing. Blocking reuptake in both serotonin and norepinephrine neurons should be especially effective for treating depression, although in practice, the antidepressant effect does not appear to be dramatically superior to the SSRI drugs. The SNRI class tends to enhance motivation and activity and is often selected for that purpose. These drugs may cause insomnia if taken later in the day or evening. They are also used in the treatment of chronic pain problems. The three medications in this class are venlafaxine (Effexor), duloxetine (Cymbalta), and desvenlafaxine (Pristiq).

Insomnia and SSRI, SNRI Drugs

The SSRI and SNRI medications may induce insomnia if taken later in the day; hence they are usually administered in the morning. If insomnia is a problem, it may be appropriate to add a low dose of one of the sedating antidepressants at bedtime. Typically, the drug chosen for that purpose is trazodone. Trazodone in a dose of 50 mg, taken a little before bedtime, is usually adequate to induce sleep. If ineffective, the trazodone dose may be raised to 100 mg at bedtime.

Tricyclic Medications

The tricyclic antidepressants are named for their chemical structure: three chemical rings. They are the oldest class of antidepressants and were the primary medications used to treat depression before the advent of the SSRI drugs. They are approximately equally efficacious for treating depression as the SSRI and SNRI drugs. They have more side effects than the newer drugs and for that reason are prescribed less often. Except for protriptyline, they tend to be sedating; however, this is often not a problem since they are usually administered as a single bedtime dose. They also tend to have anticholinergic side effects, which include constipation, dry mouth, visual blurring, and, rarely, mild memory impairment. They tend to dampen the urinary flow, which may be advantageous if you are experiencing urinary urgency, but problematic if you have trouble starting your stream.

Tricyclic medications block reuptake of serotonin, norepinephrine, or both, depending on the drug. Those with sedating effects are used as sleep aids, and certain of these medications are used in the treatment of chronic pain as well as headaches.

Other Medications for Depression

The last group of drugs shown in Table 22.2 ("Others") is a heterogeneous group of medications that cannot easily be classified and have more than one mechanism of pharmacological activity. Mirtazapine and nefazodone tend to be sedating and sometimes are prescribed for people who are agitated or can't sleep in addition to being depressed. Trazodone is rarely prescribed as an antidepressant but commonly used to treat insomnia (as discussed earlier), often as a bedtime supplement to an SSRI or SNRI.

Talk Therapy

For some people, mental baggage may prevent turning the corner on depression. Without doubt, people who are depressed benefit from talking to someone. In some circumstances, a non-psychiatrist, non-psychologist may be appropriate, such as clergy. Family or friends may also serve that purpose, provided they are good listeners, nonjudgmental, are patient and have common sense. Usually personal physicians with busy practices are not in a position to be a good listener, as much as they would like, because of time constraints. However, they could refer you to a counselor, psychologist, or psychiatrist.

Vigorous Exercise to Treat Depression

Throughout this book, the benefits of aerobic exercise have been emphasized; they may even slow the progression of PD (see Chapter 9). Not to be overlooked is the role that regular exercise plays in the treatment of depression. Whereas less demanding exercise routines may be beneficial (e.g., stretching and toning), vigorous exercise that makes you hot, sweaty, and tired helps clear the mind and reduce rumination. Exercise with friends or family has the added benefit of the company of others, which is helpful when depression is present. Moreover, exercise costs little and has few side effects (assuming no orthopedic injuries).

Severe, Refractory Depression: Electroconvulsive Therapy (ECT)

Electroconvulsive therapy, or ECT, has been used for many years to treat severe depression that proves resistant to simpler forms of therapy. Rarely is it required to treat depression in the context of PD, but when necessary, it often works well. In fact, for a brief time following ECT treatment (days to weeks), parkinsonian movement symptoms are improved. This is most apparent on the day of the ECT and often requires a reduction of carbidopa/levodopa on that treatment day.

ECT involves administering an electrical shock to the brain. It briefly convulses the brain, and in doing this appears to wipe clean many bad thoughts and memories. For several days memory may be impaired, but when it comes back, it tends to return without the baggage of the dark thoughts and ruminations.

Usually, ECT is initially performed in the hospital. However, once benefit is achieved and the problems stabilized, it can be done in an outpatient clinic. For people with the most severe and disabling depression that has failed all other forms of treatment, this treatment can be life-saving.

23

♦ ♦ ♦

Thinking, Memory, and Dementia

Although Parkinson's disease (PD) notoriously affects movement, cognition may later become impaired. Cognition is the clinical term for thinking, judgment, and memory. By definition, if such thinking and memory problems do not interfere with life, this is termed *mild cognitive impairment*. *Dementia* implies cognitive impairment that is sufficient to interfere with activities of daily living.

Dementia that develops in PD primarily represents progression of the Lewy body disease process. The risks are especially related to two factors:

1. How long you have had PD

2. Age

When the prevalence of dementia is assessed in PD clinics, it is found in a minority of patients and usually late in the course of PD. Just because you have PD does not necessarily mean that you are destined to become demented. Moreover, not everyone with PD who complains of memory impairment is demented. There are other reasons why thinking and memory may be affected, some very treatable. Let's consider this in more detail.

Forgetting as We Get Older

Our brain ages, just like the rest of our body. Consequently, memory declines with age. Those over the age 70 typically have occasional difficulties recalling names and phone numbers. If you fall into this age class and this is your problem, you may consider this part of the normal aging process.

Slowed Thinking: Bradyphrenia

People with PD experience slowed movements, termed *bradykinesia* (*brady* = "slow"). Similarly, they also may experience slowness of thinking, termed *bradyphrenia*. Those with bradyphrenia arrive at the right answer; it just takes longer. The checkbook still balances but the answers come more slowly and deliberately. Bradyphrenia is not necessarily an early sign of dementia.

Treatment of bradyphrenia is the same as for bradykinesia. Just as levodopa therapy improves movements, it also tends to speed the thought process. This requires optimization of the carbidopa/levodopa dose, as outlined in Chapter 12.

Pseudodementia: Depression

People with prominent depression often become apathetic and uninterested. Such people may seem dull, indecisive, and unable to engage in life's activities. They may say nonsensical things, not because they are confused, but because they don't care. As such, severe depression may occasionally be mistaken for dementia. This is an important distinction, since depression is a very treatable disorder.

Diagnosing depression and gauging the severity can be difficult in PD; many of the clues pointing to depression are also signs of parkinsonism, as discussed in Chapter 22. The facial masking of PD makes people appear depressed. People with PD may restrict their social and recreational activities, not because of depression but because it simply is harder to do these things. Appetite loss may not be a sign of depression but due to PD medications or PD-related problems of the digestive system (Chapter 26). PD-related loss of the sense of smell (olfaction) may reduce interest in eating. Insomnia, another sign of depression, is also a product of PD.

To determine whether depression is masquerading as dementia sometimes requires consultation with a psychiatrist. This is usually supplemented with formal testing of intellectual function (psychometric testing).

Poor Sleep and Cognition

If one is sleep deprived, it is difficult to think straight. Those chronically deprived of good sleep may behave like someone in the early stages of dementia. Sleep deprivation should be obvious; after all, we know if we are not sleeping. However, it could also be occurring in a subtle fashion, due to the disordered breathing of sleep apnea. With sleep apnea, people are deprived of *deep* sleep, as discussed in Chapter 20. If deep sleep is deficient, thinking will be affected.

Medication Effects on Thinking and Memory

Certain medications may compromise memory and occasionally lead to confusion. This is more likely among seniors with major medical problems or if age-related mild memory impairment is already present.

In the setting of newly developing cognitive impairment, the medication list should be reviewed. Medication classes that may affect cognition are listed in Table 23.1. These drugs are not necessarily the cause of cognitive problems but have the potential to contribute to them, at least in some people. This is not an all-inclusive list; for example, cancer drugs and medications used to suppress the immune system of organ transplant patients are not listed.

This potential for a medication to impair cognition must be balanced against the benefit. For example, the heart drug amiodarone occasionally causes one of a variety of neurological problems, including cognitive impairment. However, it is perhaps the most effective drug for controlling life-threatening cardiac rhythm problems. Hence, even though there might be concern that it is causing side effects, it may be necessary to continue it. These are issues that the physician should address.

One clue that a medication may be responsible for cognitive impairment relates to the time the cognitive problem first developed. If confusion developed on the heels of a newly prescribed medication, this raises suspicions. This is especially likely if the onset was rather sudden and otherwise unexplained,

Other Medical and Neurological Problems May Impair Cognition

It's easy to blame everything on PD. However, other conditions may be superimposed, contributing to cognitive problems. These are likely if the cognitive problems developed over minutes, days, or a few weeks. The dementia of PD is more insidious and evolves over months to years.

Table 23.1. Medications That May Contribute to Memory Impairment or Confusion

Medication Classes	Commonly Prescribed Medications in These Classes
Anticholinergic drugs for controlling the bladder	Hyoscyamine (Levsin, Levsinex, Cystospaz), oxybutynin (Ditropan), solifenacin (VESIcare), tolterodine (Detrol)
Anticholinergic drugs for PD	Benztropine (Cogentin), biperiden (Akineton), procyclidine (Kemadrin), trihexyphenidyl (Artane)
Anticholinergic drugs for loose stools, irritable bowel	Atropine, hyoscyamine, clidinium (ingredient in Librax), dicyclomine (Bentyl), propantheline (Pro-Banthine), scopolamine (ingredients in a variety of antidiarrheals)
Anti-anxiety drugs	Alprazolam (Xanax), clonazepam (Klonopin), clorazepate (Tranxene), diazepam (Valium), hydroxyzine (Atarax, Vistaril), lorazepam (Ativan)
Muscle relaxants, anti-spasticity drugs	Cyclobenzaprine (Flexeril), baclofen (Lioresal), carisoprodol (Soma), chlorzoxazone (Parafon Forte), orphenadrine (Norgesic, Norflex), tizanidine (Zanaflex)
Narcotics	Codeine (in Tylenol #3), hydrocodone (in Vicodin, Lortab), fentanyl (Duragesic patch), oxycodone (in Percodan, Oxycontin, Roxicet)
Certain non-narcotic prescription pain relievers	Butalbital (used in headache preparations), tramadol (Ultram)
Seizure drugs	Carbamazepine (Tegretol), phenytoin (Dilantin), phenobarbital, gabapentin (Neurontin), lamotrigine (Lamictal), levetiracetam (Keppra), oxcarbazepine (Trileptal), primidone (Mysoline), topiramate (Topamax), zonisamide (Zonegran)
Non-prescription antihistamines	Diphenhydramine (Benadryl); contained in many over-the-counter sleep aids
Longer-acting sleep medication	Flurazepam (Dalmane), clonazepam (Klonopin)
Heart rhythm medication	Amiodarone (Cordarone, Pacerone)
Tricyclic drugs for depression	Amitriptyline (Elavil), desipramine (Norpramin), doxepin (Sinequan), imipramine (Tofranil), nortriptyline (Pamelor), trimipramine (Surmontil)

A variety of medical conditions potentially affect cognition, such thyroid disease, severe anemia, and major liver or kidney problems. Thus the evaluation of cognitive problems in those with PD should include a review of the general medical status plus the blood tests that internists and family physicians typically order for routine medical screening (see the next section).

Other disorders affecting the brain may also occur in people with PD. If cognitive impairment develops suddenly, then strokes, brain hemorrhage, or seizures need to be considered. Less commonly, more diffuse conditions may affect the brain, such as infections (e.g., Lyme disease, HIV) or inflammatory disorders (e.g., Lupus, or other autoimmune disease). Even very slow development of cognitive impairment may be from some other brain condition, such as a tumor.

Testing

Testing is clearly appropriate when confusion has developed. This includes a review of the general medical state and medications, plus the following:

- Brain scan (MRI or CT)
- Blood work, usually a complete blood count, sedimentation rate, thyroid, vitamin B12, and a chemistry profile. The chemistry profile typically includes sodium, potassium, calcium, glucose, creatinine, AST, alkaline phosphatase, albumin, and bilirubin. These assess basic factors circulating in the bloodstream, which may be a clue to some other medical condition (e.g., liver or kidney failure). Clinicians may add other blood tests depending on the medical history.

In certain cases, a spinal fluid examination may also be a part of this workup. It is usually not done if dementia is long-standing, such as being present for more than 2 years. The rationale for a spinal fluid study typically relates to the possibility of an infectious or inflammatory process causing the cognitive impairment. Because the brain floats in spinal fluid, infectious or immune-mediated disorders should generate spinal fluid abnormalities. The lumbar puncture is performed by inserting the collection needle into the low-back region after a local anesthetic deadens the skin where the needle is inserted. The needle punctures the sac containing the spinal fluid; the hollow needle is a conduit through which a small amount of spinal fluid drips out and is collected. Tests run on the spinal fluid include a cell count, as well as measurement of the glucose, protein, inflammatory proteins (immunoglobulin studies), plus whatever else the physician believes is appropriate. If these are all normal, then it is unlikely that an inflammatory or infectious condition is causing the confusion.

Dementia

We should start by defining *dementia*, which can be broadly or narrowly understood. There is no disagreement that dementia implies substantial cognitive impairment. Neurologists stipulate that dementia is characterized by cognitive dysfunction that is sufficient to interfere with activities of daily living. This distinguishes dementia from the lesser condition, *mild cognitive impairment*. In the dictionary definition of dementia, the cognitive impairment can be due to one of a variety of causes, including reversible conditions. In the medical community, the term *dementia* typically has a more narrow colloquial definition, implying a progressive neurodegenerative condition. In this book we will use dementia to indicate cognitive impairment interfering with activities of daily living and due to a progressive neurodegenerative disorder.

DEMENTIA FREQUENCY INCREASES WITH AGING IN THE NORMAL POPULATION

The risk of dementia increases with age, irrespective of PD. The likelihood of dementia in the general population rises substantially after the mid-70s. This jumps dramatically after 90 years of age, when an additional 5–6% of people become demented each year, mostly due to Alzheimer's disease. Thus each of us is at some risk for dementia if we live long enough, regardless of whether we have PD.

THE RISK FOR LATER DEVELOPING DEMENTIA AMONG THOSE WITH PARKINSON'S DISEASE

People with PD are at a higher risk for dementia than the general population. This has been assessed in many studies, with the specific risk depending on how this was ascertained. When dementia was tabulated among large groups of people followed in PD clinics, the prevalence ranged from 11% to 29%. However, this might underestimate the true risk, because the most severely affected people may not be coming to these clinics, especially if they reside in nursing homes.

Investigators have also tabulated PD and PD-dementia in well-defined communities among all inhabitants. This is a more representative number. The prevalence of dementia among these community-based PD patients has ranged from 12% to 41%.

Age interacts with PD to increase the risk of dementia. Younger people with PD tend not to experience substantial thinking and memory problems, at least until they become seniors. Although there are no accurate assessments to allow estimation of the risks by age, the general experience among doctors treating PD is that dementia risks are relatively low among those less than age 65 years. By age 85, the majority of people with PD are found to have some degree of dementia.

WHAT TYPES OF PROBLEMS ARE EXPERIENCED BY THOSE WITH PD-DEMENTIA?

When dementia occurs in PD, the onset is insidious and the progression is slow. Those affected may still be able to function in most respects and may not have to rely on their families, at least for a number of years. Memory is compromised, but typically less than in Alzheimer's disease, where it may be severely impaired. Judgment may be affected and this may have an impact on business decisions. Complex concepts become difficult and multitasking often becomes impossible. Conceptualizing things in three-dimensional space may be especially challenging, which explains why those affected often easily get lost in even slightly unfamiliar surroundings. Personality may change. Previously meticulous people who organized their lives and planned ahead may become careless and apathetic. They may become a little inappropriate in conversations, saying things that previously would have embarrassed them.

People with PD and dementia often experience hallucinations and delusions, discussed in more detail in Chapter 24. Hallucinations imply seeing or hearing things that are not there. In the dementia of PD the hallucinations are almost always visual. Schizophrenics hear hallucinatory voices, whereas those with PD-dementia do not. Instead, people with PD and dementia may see imaginary people, animals, or objects in the room.

Delusions imply false beliefs, such as paranoia, characterized by a sense that someone is conspiring or scheming against them. In PD, delusions often focus on the spouse, a frequent theme being that the spouse is having an affair or is an imposter.

Both hallucinations and delusions may be caused by medications to treat PD. Carbidopa/levodopa, however, is least likely to provoke these and is usually tolerated if used in the absence of other PD drugs. These problems are treatable and are addressed in the next chapter.

THE CAUSE OF DEMENTIA IN PARKINSON'S DISEASE

When dementia occurs, it typically surfaces after many years of otherwise unremarkable PD. This presumably relates to spread of the Lewy body degenerative process. The Lewy pathology is no longer primarily confined to the substantia nigra and a few other brain regions. Rather, the neurodegenerative process proliferates, including extension to the cortex, the seat of intellectual function. These cortical regions do not use dopamine as a neurotransmitter, so carbidopa/levodopa does not benefit cognitive problems.

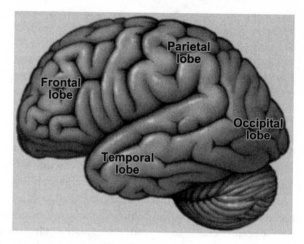

23.1 The thick layer of cortex covers the brain. Higher level cognitive function takes place in these cortical brain circuits. The four major lobes of the cortex are labeled. If dementia is present in PD, these cortical regions prominently contain Lewy bodies.

Figure 23.1 depicts the cortex, which is the thick layer of convoluted brain circuitry that covers the brain from all sides. This is the substrate for higher level cognitive function. The different lobes shown in the figure each process certain aspects of cognition. These cortical regions contain minimal Lewy microscopic pathology during early years of PD. If dementia develops, then Lewy bodies are easily identified under the microscope in these cortical areas.

PARKINSON'S DISEASE WITH DEMENTIA VERSUS DEMENTIA WITH LEWY BODIES

Parkinson's disease, by definition, is not associated with dementia in the beginning of the disease course. If dementia occurs, it is typically years later; the condition is then called *Parkinson's disease dementia*. This contrasts with *dementia with Lewy bodies* (also called *Lewy body dementia*), defined by the concurrent development of parkinsonism and dementia (discussed in Chapter 6). The brain microscopic appearance of PD with dementia is essentially indistinguishable from dementia with Lewy bodies. Whether these reflect the same condition is debated.

To be clear, a little over half of those with dementia with Lewy bodies have a mild degree of superimposed Alzheimer brain pathology. However, this is insufficient to account for the dementia. Some researchers speculate that perhaps the Lewy pathology reaching higher brain levels triggers the Alzheimer changes.

Researchers have developed an arbitrary rule to separate these conditions, relating to when dementia develops. If dementia is present before, during, or within 1 year of parkinsonism onset, this is defined as dementia with Lewy bodies. If dementia develops more than 1 year after parkinsonism onset, this is defined as Parkinson's disease with dementia.

PROCHOLINERGIC MEDICATIONS FOR IMPROVING MEMORY

The available drugs for improving memory enhance the activity of the brain neurotransmitter acetylcholine. Neurons that use this neurotransmitter are termed *cholinergic*. Acetylcholine is contained in brain memory circuits. A region near the base of the forebrain, called the *nucleus basalis*, is enriched with cholinergic neurons, depicted in Figure 23.2. The neurons in the nucleus basalis send cholinergic projections throughout the cortex. Both in animals and humans, depletion of brain acetylcholine impairs memory, whereas facilitating cholinergic neurotransmission does the opposite.

Drugs that facilitate cholinergic neurotransmission may be called *procholinergic*; classes of these medications are shown in Table 23.2. Procholinergic drugs work by inhibiting the breakdown of acetylcholine. Specifically, they block the enzyme acetylcholinesterase, which degrades acetylcholine. Besides improving memory, they may also attenuate hallucinations and delusions. Theoretically, this class of medications should be very effective; unfortunately in practice, the benefits usually are modest.

These procholinergic drugs should not be administered to people with very slow heart rates or major heart rhythm problems without physician approval as they can slow the heart rate. This effect is of no significance to most people, however.

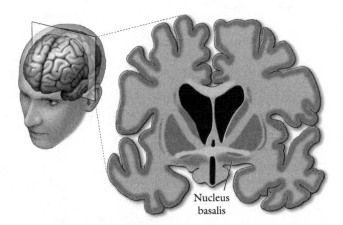

23.2 The nucleus basalis (also called the nucleus basalis of Meynert) contains cholinergic neurons that project widely throughout the cortex. This cholinergic system is important for memory. Drugs that enhance acetylcholine neurotransmission facilitate memory and vice versa.

Table 23.2. Procholinergic Medications to Enhance Memory

Medication	Brand Name	Tablet/ Capsule Sizes	Starting Dose	How to Raise the Dose	Highest Dose
Donepezil	Aricept	5 mg, 10 mg	One 5 mg tablet daily	After about 6 weeks, consider raising to two 5 mg tablets or one 10 mg tablet daily	10 mg daily*
Rivastigmine	Exelon capsules	1.5 mg, 3 mg, 4.5 mg, 6 mg	One 1.5 mg capsule twice daily, with meals	If tolerated, raise the dose every 4 weeks to 3 mg twice daily, then 4.5 mg twice daily, then 6 mg twice daily	6 mg twice daily
Rivastigmine	Exelon oral solution	2 mg/mL	Use dispenser to administer 1.5 mg twice daily	If tolerated, raise the dose every 4 weeks to 3 mg twice daily, then 4.5 mg twice daily, then 6 mg twice daily	6 mg twice daily
Rivastigmine	Exelon patch	4.6 mg; 9.5 mg, 13.3 mg (each per 24 hours)	Apply one 4.6 mg patch and replace each 24 hours	If tolerated, increase after 4 weeks to one 9.5 mg patch replaced every 24 hours, and 4 weeks later, may substitute the 13.3 mg patch	13.3 mg/24 hours
Galantamine	Razadyne tablets	4 mg, 8 mg, 12 mg	One 4 mg tablet twice daily with meals	If tolerated, increase after 4 weeks to 8 mg twice daily, then 4 weeks later to 12 mg twice daily	12 mg twice daily

(continued)

Table 23.2. Continued

Medication	Brand Name	Tablet/ Capsule Sizes	Starting Dose	How to Raise the Dose	Highest Dose
	Razadyne oral solution	4 mg/mL	Use pipette to dispense one mL (4 mg) twice daily	If tolerated, increase after 4 weeks to 8 mg twice daily, then 4 weeks later to 12 mg twice daily	12 mg twice daily
	Razadyne Extended-release tablets	8 mg, 16 mg, 24 mg	One 8 mg tablet daily	If tolerated, increase after 4 weeks to one 16 mg tablet and 4 weeks later to one 24 mg tablet	24 mg daily

*Occasionally, donepezil is increased to 15 mg once daily; higher doses are more likely to cause gastrointestinal side effects. That is why the 23 mg donepezil pill is not recommended.

In the current era, the procholinergic drugs most often selected for memory enhancement are donepezil (Aricept) tablets and the rivastigmine (Exelon) patch. Whereas this class of drugs may cause gastrointestinal side effects (nausea, diarrhea), these two agents seem to be the best tolerated.

Donepezil is initiated as a single 5 mg tablet taken in the morning or bedtime. It may be raised after 6 weeks to 2 of the 5 mg tablets once daily (or one 10 mg tablet). I typically suggest that people then decide whether there has been sufficient benefit to justify continuing. Occasionally, the donepezil dose is raised to 15 mg once daily. A 23 mg tablet of donepezil is now available; however, the additional benefit of this higher dose (versus 10 mg) is modest at best; moreover, it is overshadowed by a markedly increased incidence of gastrointestinal side effects and is much more expensive. The 23 mg donepezil tablet will not be discussed further here.

Rivastigmine (Exelon) is about equally efficacious as donepezil, although no head-to-head clinical trials have been performed. Rivastigmine capsules are more likely to provoke gastrointestinal side effects than the rivastigmine patch (Exelon); hence the patch is preferred. The rivastigmine skin patch dose starts with the 4.6 mg size patch. After 4 weeks, if tolerated, this is graduated to the 9.5 mg patch. These patches are replaced daily. Recently, a rivastigmine patch with a higher dose was introduced, 13.3 mg. This may be tried if the 9.5 mg patch has been tolerated. If there is no benefit after about 6 weeks, the rivastigmine patch may be discontinued.

ANTICHOLINERGIC DRUGS MAY WORSEN MEMORY

Drugs that block brain acetylcholine receptors are termed *anticholinergic*. To put this into context, we just discussed drugs that block the enzyme degrading acetylcholine, which increase cholinergic neurotransmission, or are *procholinergic*. Conversely, drugs that block the acetylcholine receptor inhibit cholinergic neurotransmission, or are anticholinergic. If anticholinergic drugs are able to get into the brain (cross the blood-brain barrier), they tend to worsen memory. These anticholinergic drugs were discussed in prior chapters and are listed in Table 23.1. Note that such medications are commonly used to treat bladder urgency (e.g., oxybutynin/Ditropan), as well as to treat irritable bowel syndrome and related gastrointestinal tract disorders. The scopolamine patch (Transderm Scop) for motion sickness is a potent anticholinergic drug.

The older generation of PD drugs prominently included anticholinergic agents, such as trihexyphenidyl (Artane) and benztropine (Cogentin). These drugs were modestly beneficial for treating tremor and rigidity but did not substantially improve other aspects of PD. These are no longer used in the treatment of PD. Besides memory impairment and provocation of hallucinations, they also have several other troublesome side effects, such as constipation and dry mouth and eyes.

It is common to encounter people who are taking both a procholinergic drug for memory and an anticholinergic drug, often for bladder urgency. Since these tend to work in opposite directions, they should have offsetting effects. It makes sense to use either one or the other, but not both. The anticholinergic bladder drugs are further discussed in Chapter 27.

MEMANTINE (NAMENDA)

The medication memantine (Namenda) was introduced as symptomatic treatment for Alzheimer's disease some years ago. Clinical trials involving people with PD-dementia have also shown modest benefit. This drug has very similar properties to the PD drug amantadine, which we discussed in Chapter 10. Both of these medications mildly block the brain neurotransmitter glutamate (specifically, NMDA glutamate receptors). Amantadine rarely provokes hallucinations, and there have been infrequent cases of hallucinations occurring with memantine. In clinical trials involving people with PD-dementia, memantine was generally tolerated without hallucinations.

Memantine has been available in tablets, extended-release capsules, and an oral solution. It appears that the plain tablets may be discontinued by the manufacturer, now that the extended-release capsules are being marketed. If available, the regular tablets are started in a dose of one 5 mg tablet daily, then a week later raised to twice daily; over the ensuing 2 weeks, they are then raised to 10 mg twice daily. Whether this formulation will be available in generic form in the future is unclear.

The oral solution is provided in a concentration of 2 mg per mL, supplied with a dosing syringe. It is started and escalated in the same dosing scheme as just outlined for the regular tablets; that is, 5 mg once daily up to 10 mg twice daily, raised weekly over 1 month.

The new extended-release memantine formulation (Namenda XR) comes in four capsule sizes: 7 mg, 14 mg, 21 mg, and 28 mg. If tolerated, it can be increased at intervals of at least 1 week, going from the lowest capsule amount (7 mg) to the largest capsule size (28 mg) over 1 month.

DO THE MEDICATIONS USED TO TREAT PD WORSEN MEMORY?

Among drugs for PD, only the anticholinergic medications, such as tri-hexyphenidyl, impair memory, as discussed previously. Very rarely, aman-tadine will provoke a confusional state. Carbidopa/levodopa, dopamine agonist drugs, selegiline, rasagiline, and entacapone do not cause confu-sion or memory impairment, but they may provoke or exacerbate hal-lucinations or delusions. Carbidopa/levodopa is by far the least likely to provoke these problems. Hallucinations and delusions are a separate issue from dementia, although they are much more likely among people with cognitive problems.

SUNDOWNING

Individuals with dementia often have more problems at night, a phenome-non termed *sundowning*. There are multiple reasons for this. With darkness, some of our visual-orienting influences are lost, especially if we are awakened from sleep. The cumulative mental fatigue from a long day may also con-tribute. In addition, there may be something about our internal biological clocks that predisposes to cognitive problems at night. Finally, people with dementia often experience reversal of their day–night cycle, compounding this problem; they sleep during the day and are awake at night. Sedating medicines administered in hopes of inducing sleep may have a paradoxical effect, increasing nighttime confusion.

Sundowning can be a major source of upheaval for the spouse and fam-ily, disrupting everyone's sleep. Treatment strategies tried for sundowning include the following:

- Attempt to establish a normal day–night cycle. Minimize naps dur-ing the daytime (allow one brief nap after lunch). Encourage exercise during the daytime. Establish a consistent daily routine. Do relaxing things in the evening and arousing things earlier in the day. The intent is to entrain the sleep cycle to occur at night.

- For those with PD, nighttime sleep may require adequate doses of carbidopa/levodopa, as discussed in Chapter 20.

- To entrain sleep at night, consider a sleep medication (see Chapter 20). However, this may increase the confused state, so there are no guarantees.

- Avoid the medications listed in Table 23.1 as much as possible, especially in the evening.

- For those awakening during the night, a nightlight may help with orientation. Otherwise, the total darkness of night may add to the disorientation.

- If sundowning includes hallucinations or delusions, then special medications can be used for that purpose, which are discussed in the next chapter.

Note that sundowning must not be confused with REM sleep behavior disorder, which was discussed in Chapter 20. With this phenomenon, people talk in their sleep or act out their dreams, without fully waking up. This is common among those with PD, including those with no cognitive problems. This is treatable, but often requires no treatment.

FINANCIAL, LEGAL, AND SAFETY ISSUES RELATING TO DEMENTIA

People with PD typically have led active and fulfilling lives and may be able to continue doing so for many years, despite PD. With the advent of dementia, certain life changes are necessary. We obviously want to avoid unfortunate business, professional, or financial decisions. It is important to recognize limitations and restructure business and financial dealings so that responsibilities are appropriate to capabilities.

Home safety issues also need attention in those cases where dementia is prominent. Operation of power machinery, cooking (with potential for fire), and similar activities may need to be limited in certain cases. Driving may need to be prohibited.

Nutrition is also of concern in some individuals with dementia. PD, in general, is often associated with weight loss; this may be exacerbated among those with dementia. Forgetting to eat and loss of appetite are frequent accompaniments of dementia and may be further exacerbated if depression is present. If weight loss develops, this should be brought to the physician's attention. A structured diet from a dietitian, food supplements, as well as a daily multivitamin may be appropriate (addressed further in Chapter 30).

FURTHER READING

Parkinson's disease later evolving into dementia complicates the problems and treatment. To specifically address that condition see *Dementia with Lewy Bodies and Parkinson's Disease Dementia* (J.E. Ahlskog; Oxford University Press, 2014).

24

◆ ◆ ◆

Hallucinations, Paranoia, Delusions, and Problematic Compulsive Behaviors

Seeing Things That Aren't There: Hallucinations

Most people with Parkinson's disease (PD) do not experience hallucinations. When they do develop, this is usually later in the course of PD. Medications may be responsible in some cases. These are not necessarily reflective of dementia, and if they develop, this does not necessarily imply that you are becoming demented. Most importantly, hallucinations are treatable.

THE CHARACTER OF HALLUCINATIONS

Hallucinations experienced by people with PD are nearly always visual, that is, they see illusory images. Very rarely, illusory odors may be perceived. The hallucinations of PD do not include hearing voices, which is typical of certain other medical conditions, such as schizophrenia.

In the mildest and simplest form, the hallucinations of PD include spots, bugs, or other small shapes in the field of vision. More troubling are hallucinations of people and animals. For example, hallucinations commonly described include such things as:

- Animals in the yard
- Children playing outside the window
- Family, friends, or strangers sitting in the living room
- Bugs crawling on the refrigerator (or countertop, floor, etc.)

There are countless variations on this theme. Usually they are not perceived as frightening or threatening. These may be fleeting, or persist for minutes or hours. The person experiencing these may or may not have insight to them. If the hallucinations are bugs, bug killer may be compulsively sprayed and the area scrubbed. If children are seen in the bedroom, they may be asked to play outside; when they don't leave, the conversation may get more interesting (hallucinated people usually don't listen!). Sometimes, hallucinated people are incorporated into the day's activities. I recall one senior lady who fixed a large dinner for her friends, only to subsequently realize as she sat down to eat that her "friends" were all illusory.

Delusions and Paranoia

The same underlying factors that cause hallucinations may also provoke delusions and paranoia. *Delusions* are absurd beliefs or ideas that have no basis in fact. In PD, they often involve the spouse, such as suspecting infidelity. For example, a husband may accuse his wife of recently having an affair despite 50 years of marriage. Occasionally, the spouse or other family members are thought to be imposters (so-called Capgras syndrome): "You are not my wife; where is she?" Delusions may have financial implications, with a conviction that some preposterous business idea will be profitable.

Paranoia refers to delusions that are marked by extreme suspicion and a sense of persecution. The paranoid ideation often involves family or friends, perhaps imagining that they are conspiring to steal one's money. The delusion may be quite outlandish, such as the suspicion that the police are spying.

Such delusional ideation can be very disturbing to family members, especially spouses who are the caregivers. The key is to recognize these for what they are. Delusions and paranoia are treated the same as hallucinations, addressed later in the chapter.

Delusions or paranoia are much less common in PD than hallucinations, and they do not necessary occur together. They involve different brain regions. When hallucinations are the sole problem, they often are not very disruptive unless frequent. In contrast, delusional thinking or paranoia markedly challenges family and caregivers. Fortunately, this is much less common than simple hallucinations. Prominent delusions occur primarily among those with PD-dementia; hallucinations are much less likely to be associated with a demented state.

Should the spouse or family confront the person with delusions or paranoia? Should they try to explain reality to them? Generally, you cannot reason with someone in the throes of a psychotic belief. The family or spouse should be reassuring but avoid being too confrontational or argumentative.

What Causes Hallucinations and Delusions in Parkinson's Disease?

Two factors are the primary contributors to these hallucinations and delusions among those with PD:

1. Proliferation of brain Lewy pathology

2. Medications

Occasionally, other medical conditions also play a role, and something as simple as a urinary tract infection may trigger a hallucinatory state. Note that hallucinations or delusions may develop in the absence of any offending drugs or medical disorders, being directly due to the Lewy disorder.

Hallucinations tend to occur when brain regions that process visual images are affected by the Lewy neurodegenerative processes. The visual portions of our brain integrate millions of small stimuli impinging on the retina of the eye. These are ultimately organized into appropriate patterns in the brain, perceived as people, objects, or other figures. This perceptual organization and processing primarily occurs in the occipital cortex, which is located in the back end of the brain (shown in Figure 23.1 in Chapter 23). Lewy neurodegenerative processes may disrupt this visual processing.

Delusions or paranoia reflect the spread of the Lewy neurodegenerative process to brain regions involved in thought and beliefs. Exactly which brain regions are the substrate(s) for these problems is less certain, but likely it is cortex in the front half of the brain.

Medications often are the provocative factor for hallucinations and delusions, and these include the drugs used to treat PD. Of importance, carbidopa/levodopa is the drug least likely to provoke hallucinations or delusions, provided that it is used in the absence of other PD drugs. Thus if hallucinations are problematic, PD is best managed by carbidopa/levodopa alone. The dopamine agonist drugs are a frequent cause of hallucinations and are inadvisable in this situation. The minor PD drugs, such as selegiline, rasagiline, or even entacapone, may provoke hallucinations if added to a stable dose of carbidopa/levodopa. Other medications that are able to enter the brain may also contribute to this problem, especially narcotics and other prescription pain medications, muscle relaxants, and sedating drugs.

Who Experiences Hallucinations?

Fortunately, most people with PD do not experience hallucinations. However, some individuals are predisposed. Hallucinations are more likely with:

- Dementia

- Advanced age

- Long durations of PD

- Certain PD medications

- Anesthesia for surgical procedures (transiently after the surgery)

- Serious medical illness (e.g., pneumonia or other major infections, liver or kidney failure)

  - Minor infections, such as a urinary infection, may exacerbate hallucinatory tendencies

- Blindness

- Severe insomnia with sleep deprivation

Obviously, some of these potential contributors may lend themselves to treatment. These same conditions may predispose to delusional thinking, but much less commonly.

Do Hallucinations Indicate More Serious Brain Disease?

Hallucinations do not necessarily mean that PD is turning into dementia. Sometimes they resolve with the elimination of certain drugs; in other cases, they are transient and relate to some medical illness, surgical anesthesia, or disordered sleep.

Warning: Driving, Power Tools, and Hallucinations

There are some circumstances in which hallucinations are particularly worrisome, especially driving a car. If the hallucinations are exclusively dots or an occasional illusory spider, these may be tolerated. However, if more formed hallucinations are recurring, driving may be dangerous and should be prohibited. The same is true for operating power machinery, such as table saws or farm equipment. Common sense dictates that frequent major hallucinations preclude driving or operating power tools.

Hallucinations or Delusions Caused or Exacerbated by Medical Conditions

Certain medical conditions may provoke hallucination or delusions. Major illnesses, such as pneumonia or other such infections, may be associated with confusional states that include hallucinations or delusions. General anesthesia for surgery may be associated with a postoperative delirium with hallucinations and delusional thought. These are typically self-limited problems that resolve once the underlying medical problem is treated or the effects of the anesthesia slowly abate.

People who are susceptible to disordered thinking may occasionally experience hallucinations or delusions with simple medical conditions such as a urinary tract infection. Unstable medical conditions may increase the susceptibility to hallucinations and such medical disorders should be addressed. Sleep deprivation or untreated sleep apnea may exacerbate tendencies to hallucinations.

If disordered thinking with hallucinations rapidly develops, unexplained by drugs, it would be appropriate to assess general medical issues. A brief history and examination by the primary care physician and routine laboratory tests (complete blood count, chemistry profile, urinalysis) are a good start.

When Should Hallucinations Be Treated?

If one is experiencing only fleeting hallucinations of spots or an occasional bug, these do not demand treatment. However, that may suggest the wisdom of simplifying the medication list, as discussed in the next section. Although spots and bugs are easily ignored, their occurrence could indicate potential for more troublesome hallucinations in the future. The circumstances also influence treatment. For example, if the person is no longer driving, and if PD is otherwise well treated, rare and fleeting hallucinations might be tolerated. Clearly, if formed hallucinations are frequent (e.g., people, animals, large objects), treatment is advisable.

Prominent delusions typically do demand treatment as they often interfere with family and social relationships. However, disagreement between two humans does not necessarily imply that one is delusional (think of political debates).

Eliminating Hallucinations and Delusions Provoked by Medications

If hallucinations or delusions develop, the first step should be to review the medication list, focusing on drugs that enter the brain. This includes PD drugs as well as prescription medications for pain (especially narcotics), muscle relaxants (e.g., cyclobenzaprine, tizanidine), and sedating medications. Table 23.1 in the last chapter lists classes of non-PD drugs that may cause confusion, and these same medications may also contribute to hallucinations or delusions. With the advice of a clinician, these can be reduced and, ideally, tapered off one by one, as tolerated.

Hallucinations are more likely to resolve with a reduction of medications than are delusions or paranoia. However, a focus on drugs is an appropriate early consideration in both circumstances.

PD drugs other than carbidopa/levodopa are frequent causes of hallucinations or delusions (see Table 24.1). If hallucinations are prominent, it may then be wise to gradually eliminate other PD drugs and ultimately use carbidopa/levodopa alone for PD treatment. Which drug should be eliminated first? Obviously, if hallucinations started shortly after a specific medication was recently started, that would be a good candidate for elimination.

Certain PD medications are more likely to have contributed to hallucinations or delusions and those should be eliminated first. Also to be considered is the benefit from the drug, as well as the ease of elimination. With these considerations in mind, the order of medication elimination might proceed as follows:

1. Anticholinergic PD drugs: trihexyphenidyl (Artane), benztropine (Cogentin), procyclidine (Kemadrin), biperiden (Akineton)

2. Rasagiline (Azilect), selegiline

3. Amantadine (if not necessary for control of levodopa-dyskinesias)

4. Entacapone (including transition to plain carbidopa/levodopa if using Stalevo)

5. Dopamine agonists: pramipexole (Mirapex), ropinirole (Requip), rotigotine (Neupro patch)

Table 24.1.   PD Drugs: Risk of Hallucinations and Delusions

Medication	Risk of Hallucinations and Delusions	Comment
Anticholinergic drugs: Trihexyphenidyl (Artane), benztropine (Cogentin), procyclidine (Kemadrin), biperiden (Akineton)	Moderate risk	No longer used to treat PD, with rare exceptions
Rasagiline (Azilect), selegiline (Eldepryl)	Uncommon when used alone, but more frequent in combination with other drugs	Only mildly beneficial for PD and often can be eliminated without substantial deterioration
Amantadine	Mild risk, primarily when used with other drugs	Primary role is to reduce levodopa-dyskinesias; if dyskinesias are not a problem, this may be tapered off
COMT inhibitors: entacapone (Comtan)	Mild risk	Potentiates the levodopa response; usually can be eliminated without major deterioration
Dopamine agonists: pramipexole (Mirapex), ropinirole (Requip), rotigotine (Neupro patch)	Among the currently used PD drugs, these are the most likely to provoke hallucinations or delusions.	In low doses, probably won't be missed. Primarily beneficial in higher doses

The dopamine agonists are listed last, but are often the most culpable. However, they are also more likely to be beneficial for PD than others on the list and will typically require a more prolonged taper.

In the current era, few people are being treated with an anticholinergic drug for PD. This class of medications has a variety of side effects apart from the potential to provoke hallucinations or delusions, such as memory impairment, constipation, and dry mouth and eyes. Hence this class is an obvious first choice for elimination.

The tapering strategy depends on the duration that the medication has been taken; long-term use may require a slower reduction. Certain of these drugs do not need to be tapered because they remain in the body long after discontinuation (e.g., rasagiline, selegiline). Also to be considered is the urgency of the hallucinatory or delusional disorder. With these principles in mind, reasonable tapering schedules are summarized in the following sections; however, these are general guidelines, and the clinician should provide the specific advice. If hallucinations or delusions are seriously disruptive, more rapid tapering may be considered, guided by the response.

TAPERING OFF A PD ANTICHOLINERGIC DRUG

This discussion relates to the four anticholinergic PD medications listed in the previous section (i.e., trihexyphenidyl, benztropine, etc.). If started within the prior 3–4 months, they could be tapered off over about a week. The tapering schedule should be prolonged to about 2–3 weeks if started within the past 1–2 years. If one of these anticholinergic drugs has been taken for years, a more prolonged taper may be necessary, sometimes up to 4–6 weeks. With all of these tapering schedules, this reduction may be speeded up or slowed, depending on the responses and urgency.

ELIMINATION OF RASAGILINE OR SELEGILINE

Rasagiline and selegiline mildly improve parkinsonism by blocking the dopamine degradative enzyme, MAO-B. Once inhibited, reconstitution of brain MAO-B activity requires many weeks (40 day half-life). Consequently, these drugs may be abruptly stopped; they do not require tapering.

AMANTADINE TAPERING

Amantadine is occasionally crucial to the control of dyskinesias, which are the involuntary movements provoked by an excessive response to carbidopa/levodopa (described in Chapter 17). Dyskinesias can always be eliminated by reduction of the carbidopa/levodopa doses. In a minority of people, levodopa reduction results in a return of parkinsonism; this group of people benefits from amantadine. Amantadine reduces dyskinesias without worsening parkinsonism. If amantadine is very beneficial, this drug could be eliminated last. If not being used for dyskinesia control, elimination could be early in this scheme.

Amantadine comes in only one size pill, 100 mg. It is taken in a dose of 1 pill two to five times daily. It may be tapered off by eliminating 1 pill every few days down to zero. However, it often can be tapered off more quickly if necessary.

ENTACAPONE ELIMINATION

Entacapone (Comtan) is not highly likely to cause hallucinations, but occasionally it contributes to this problem. Entacapone comes in one pill size, 200 mg, and is taken with each dose of carbidopa/levodopa. The benefit from this drug is modest and it can be abruptly stopped.

Entacapone is also formulated as Stalevo, which combines 200 mg of enta-capone with various amounts of 25/100 of carbidopa/levodopa. The dosage of Stalevo relates to the amount of levodopa in each tablet. Thus Stalevo-100 contains 200 mg entacapone plus the equivalent of a 25/100 carbidopa/levodopa tablet (i.e., 100 mg levodopa). Similarly, Stalevo-150 contains the equivalent of 1 ½ of the 25/100 regular (immediate-release) carbidopa/levodopa tablets (plus entacapone). To eliminate the entacapone component when taking Stalevo, one may simply revert to the corresponding dose of car-bidopa/levodopa. In other words, if taking Stalevo-150, substitute 1 ½ regular carbidopa/levodopa 25/100 tablets. This will make each carbidopa/levodopa dose slightly less potent than that of Stalevo, which often can be countered by raising the carbidopa/levodopa by a half-tablet each dose. Eliminating enta-capone may also shorten the levodopa response duration by 30–60 minutes, perhaps requiring shortening of the carbidopa/levodopa dosing interval.

TAPERING OFF A DOPAMINE AGONIST

The dopamine agonists—pramipexole (Mirapex), ropinirole (Requip) and rotigotine (Neupro patch)—are often the primary contributors to hallucina-tions and delusions. Higher doses of these drugs taken for many months may require a prolonged taper. Low doses, even if taken for a longer time, can usually be quickly eliminated. A minority of patients on higher doses of a dopamine agonist experience withdrawal (e.g., restlessness, anxiety, irrita-bility, nausea, sweating, depression). This may require a much slower taper.

The tapering schedules provided next are somewhat arbitrary and need to be guided by the responses, with input from the clinician. The schemes that follow are meant to be exemplary and subject to modification. Occasionally, hallucinations and delusions are extremely disruptive and disturbing; in that case, the clinician may suggest a more rapid taper, with close follow-up. Note that pramipexole and ropinirole come in both regular and sustained-release tablets, which are discussed separately, as follows.

> *Pramipexole (regular tablets):* Refer to Table 13.2 in Chapter 13, which provides a dose *escalation* strategy for pramipexole. This may be used *in reverse* to taper off the drug. A conservative strategy would be to decrease the dose weekly, but this may prolong the period of halluci-nations and delusions. If the hallucinations/delusions are problematic, these stepwise reductions could be every 3–4 days. The clinician may need to provide smaller size pills to accomplish this taper.

> *Ropinirole (regular tablets):* Table 13.3 in Chapter 13 provides the dose *escalation* scheme for ropinirole. As just suggested for pramipexole, this scheme may be carried out *in reverse* to taper off the drug. In most cases, these decremental steps for ropinirole may be done every 3–4 days; however, if it seems sensible, the reductions may be made even more rapidly, guided by the response.

Pramipexole sustained-release tablets (Mirapex ER): Refer to Chapter 13, where the recommended schedule is provided for escalating the sustained-release tablet dosage. A conservative scheme would be to reverse these steps every 3–4 days, guided by the response. If tolerated and necessary, this reduction could be done every 2 days. The clinician will need to provide different pill sizes since the sustained-release tablets should not be broken to make smaller doses.

Ropinirole sustained-release tablets (Requip XL): Chapter 13 contains the dose *escalation* schedule that may be reversed to taper off this drug. This schedule from the manufacturer is quite prolonged, and reversal can be done much more quickly. Thus decrements of 2 mg could be made weekly if there is no urgency, but every 2–4 days if necessary. Again, the pace can be changed if the responses suggest that is sensible. The clinician will need to provide different sizes of pills since the sustained-release tablets should not be cut in half to make smaller doses.

Rotigotine (Neupro patch): Chapter 13 also provides an *escalation* schedule for the Neupro patch, which can be reversed to taper off it. A reduction to each smaller patch size can be made every 3–7 days. The clinician will need to prescribe the smaller doses.

If hallucinations or delusions are prominent, the dopamine agonist drug typically must be eliminated and not just reduced. If a withdrawal problem develops, this can be problematic and may require adding a drug to reduce hallucinations and delusions, discussed subsequently.

AVOID ELIMINATING CARBIDOPA/LEVODOPA

Carbidopa/levodopa is the foundation of symptomatic treatment of PD. Unless the parkinsonian symptoms are extremely mild, you should not eliminate carbidopa/levodopa. This medication is necessary to control the parkinsonian symptoms and often does not make a substantial contribution to hallucinatory tendencies if not combined with other PD drugs. It may also be necessary for a good night's sleep, which is important in this context.

Medications for Reducing Hallucinations or Delusions

Among those with PD, few drugs can be used to reduce and eliminate hallucinations or delusions. Nearly all the antipsychotic drugs used by psychiatrists block dopamine receptors and worsen parkinsonism (plus block the effects of carbidopa/levodopa). Drugs to avoid from this class were listed in Table 6.1 (see Chapter 6).

The primary medication used to treat hallucinations or delusions in PD is quetiapine (Seroquel). It does not block dopamine receptors. The only other antipsychotic drug tolerated in PD is clozapine (Clozaril), but this medication has a myriad of potentially serious side effects and is rarely used for that reason.

The acetylcholinesterase inhibitors discussed in Chapter 23 also tend to reduce hallucinations and delusions, although this has not been proven in clinical trials. These include donepezil (Aricept), rivastigmine (Exelon), and galantamine (Razadyne).

QUETIAPINE (SEROQUEL)

Quetiapine is used in high doses by psychiatrists to treat psychosis in such disorders as schizophrenia; usually this is administered on a twice-daily schedule. In PD, much lower doses are typically effective and administered as a once-daily bedtime dose. Quetiapine is very sedating and a single bedtime dose typically facilitates sleep.

Quetiapine is started at a low dose of one-half to one 25 mg tablet shortly before going to bed. How rapidly the dose is raised depends on the degree of urgency. If hallucinations or delusions are quite problematic, it could be raised every 2–4 days by one-half to one 25 mg tablet, guided by the response. The effective dose ranges from 25 mg to 150 mg at bedtime, although occasional PD patients require up to 200 mg at bedtime. Rarely, a small dose earlier in the day is helpful, but the sedating effect will often be apparent. If daytime agitation is a problem, a small dose (e.g., 25 mg) earlier in the day may be used. Quetiapine comes in both 25 mg and 100 mg tablets.

Apart from sedation, quetiapine does not have many side effects. It may contribute to orthostatic hypotension, although this is a modest effect. The U.S. Food and Drug Administration (FDA) has warned about increased mortality with the entire class of antipsychotic medications when administered to people with dementia; however, quetiapine per se does not appear to confer any major risk in that regard, as long as people are not overly sedated from it.

In a perfect world, quetiapine would be started only after potentially offending medications were eliminated and medical conditions treated. However, it may take weeks to taper off these other drugs one by one. If the hallucinations or delusions are very troublesome, it might be sensible to start quetiapine earlier; it can be eliminated later, if that seems appropriate.

CLOZAPINE (CLOZARIL)

Clozapine is a very effective drug for treating hallucinations or delusions but with certain serious side effects. It has the potential to occasionally cause a dramatic reduction in the white blood cell count (agranulocytosis). This is rare but life-threatening when it occurs. When the white count is very low, there is a risk of a serious infection (white blood cells are crucial for fighting infections). This condition is reversible and the white blood count will return to normal when the drug is stopped. However, close vigilance is required when using this medication. The FDA has mandated that a white blood cell count be checked weekly for the first 6 months of clozapine use and less frequently thereafter. Pharmacists may only dispense a week's supply at a time so that low white counts are not overlooked. With clozapine therapy, there is also a very small risk of seizures or potentially serious heart inflammation (myocarditis). This is a highly effective drug for controlling hallucinations and related problems, but it is reserved for the most refractory situations. It is even more sedating than quetiapine and at least as likely to cause orthostatic hypotension.

If used to treat hallucinations in someone with PD, clozapine is typically started with a quarter of a 25 mg tablet in the evening. It can be very sedating, which is why it is started with such a small dose. It can be raised by quarter-tablet increments weekly until the hallucinations have been controlled. Usually it is given as a once-daily or twice-daily dose. Because of the sedation, most of the total daily dose is given in the evening. For those with PD, low doses are usually sufficient to control the hallucinations, typically 12.5 to 100 mg daily. This is in contrast to treatment of schizophrenia with clozapine, where the typical dose is 300 to 400 mg daily.

WOULD A SEDATIVE HELP TREAT THE HALLUCINATIONS?

Family members sometimes inquire if a sedating medication (e.g., Valium) might calm down a loved one who is experiencing hallucinations. This may backfire, leading to increased confusion and perhaps even more hallucinations.

What about Hospitalization?

Usually, hallucinations are best managed outside the hospital. However, if these problems are very disruptive and pose a danger to the person or family, these medication adjustments should be done in the hospital. Most larger communities have a mental health hospital that is well equipped to deal with these types of problems, keeping the person safe and relatively comfortable as treatment proceeds.

Hallucinations and Delusions after Surgery

Confusion and hallucinations for the first day or few days following major surgery is common among seniors with PD. Presumably, this is the consequence of the anesthetics and the metabolic factors linked to the surgery or illness. Narcotic pain medications are notorious for exacerbating or prolonging such problems. Being in a strange hospital room is also disorienting. Often no specific treatment is necessary and the confusion spontaneously subsides.

If postsurgical confusion develops, make certain that the surgical team is reminded that their patient has PD and they should avoid prescribing medications for psychosis that block dopamine receptors. Note that the forbidden drugs listed in Table 6.1 in Chapter 6 are among those often prescribed for postoperative hallucinations and confusion (e.g., haloperidol). Doctors also typically try to minimize narcotics if postoperative delirium occurs.

Newly Developing Pathological Compulsive Behaviors: Gambling, Sex, Spending

Humans do not always behave rationally, and some people engage in risky or troublesome behaviors. Psychiatrists and psychologists have written countless books and papers on this subject. That is not the topic of this section, rather, the scenario addressed here relates to someone with PD who (out of character) begins to focus on gambling, inappropriate sex, or some other inherently rewarding behavior. In most cases, there has been no such prior proclivity, or at least it has not been problematic. These problems typically begin insidiously and continue, often with poor insight or ability to control the behavior. Examples include one or more of the following:

- Gambling, such as at casinos or online; this may involve inability to stop, despite losing thousands of dollars

- Sexual behaviors, perhaps compulsive viewing of pornography, solicitation of affairs, or repeated demands for sex with a spouse many times daily

- Compulsive shopping or spending, such as purchasing many items of the same type with no obvious utility

- Excessive intake of food or other indulgences (e.g., alcohol)

Occasionally, such compulsions involve an excessive amount of time with hobbies, which are less problematic. The common theme of these behaviors is that they are inherently rewarding (at least to some), but have become a central focus for those affected. Sometimes these are done surreptitiously, such as viewing pornography while others are asleep, or sneaking off to a casino. Thus, family members may not become aware of this behavior for months. Once recognized, the family typically reports that these behaviors are out of character and unexpected.

In the context of PD, such newly developing problematic behaviors are almost always due to medications and, specifically, one of the dopamine agonist drugs: pramipexole, ropinirole, or rotigotine. Such behaviors were mentioned as a side effect of these medications in Chapters 10 and 13. It is important for people starting one of these drugs, and for the spouse or family, to be aware of this potential. However, it may be difficult to recognize until it becomes very concerning. In perhaps 80% of those affected, carbidopa/levodopa is also being taken along with the dopamine agonist. However, in my experience, such behaviors are not linked to carbidopa/levodopa if that is the only PD drug.

These behaviors are independent of other aspects of PD or the Lewy neurodegenerative process. They are not due to dementia and may occur early or late in PD. Such behaviors have also occurred when these same dopamine agonist drugs have been used to treat restless legs syndrome in the absence of PD.

Having taken care of many such people with this problem, I have not been impressed that there is a personality type prone to this or any obvious predisposition. Most people taking a dopamine agonist drug do not develop this side effect, although in our clinic, it has been documented in 25% of those on therapeutic agonist doses.

Although the mechanism has been debated, the unique pharmacology of these dopamine agonist drugs provides a compelling explanation. The brain receptors for dopamine have been subdivided into five types, termed, D1 through D5. These culpable dopamine agonists primarily bind to the D3 receptor, with little affinity for the other dopamine receptors, as shown by Gerlach and colleagues in a seminal paper published years ago (in the *Journal of Neural Transmission* [2003] 110:1119–1127). Dopamine D3 receptors are primarily localized to the limbic system of the brain. The limbic system modulates rewards and hedonistic behaviors, which makes this an obvious substrate for problematic behaviors.

Treatment of such behaviors starts with recognition. This must be distinguished from the lesser compulsions and behaviors that humans normally display. An excessive amount of time on the computer or overeating may have other explanations. A lifelong interest in gambling or sexual focus is not explained by a more recently started PD drug. The common-sense criteria for implicating a PD drug and then treating the behavior include the following:

- The behavior started or markedly escalated after beginning a PD medication.

- The behavior seriously interferes with the well-being of the patient, spouse, or family (e.g., monetary loss; risk of arrest or social condemnation).

Once recognized, the family should accompany the affected person to the physician visit—not to accuse, but to present facts. This is not something that family members can unilaterally treat or resolve. They should not be in that position but instead continue to support the affected loved one. The physician should then take responsibility for treatment.

Treatment starts with a review of the medication list, specifically looking for pramipexole (Mirapex), ropinirole (Requip), or rotigotine (Neupro patch). Rarely, other dopamine agonists used outside the United States have also been responsible, such as pergolide or cabergoline. The treatment is straightforward: the agonist must be tapered to zero. We have had experience with other treatment strategies, such as counseling or psychiatric medications; however, it appears that elimination of the dopamine agonist is necessary. In most cases, reduction of the agonist dose is insufficient, but it may be tried if agonist withdrawal symptoms (discussed earlier in this chapter) are problematic. The tapering schedules described in this chapter, with input and appropriate modification from the physician, are the necessary therapy.

Once the dopamine agonist has been eliminated, the behaviors typically do not resolve immediately. This mirrors the onset of the symptoms, which do not begin immediately with starting the drug or raising the dose. Although occasional people note that the behavioral compulsion resolves within a few days after drug discontinuation, others find that weeks or even a few months are necessary for the behavior to abate. Presumably, bad habits are slow to resolve, even when the provocative agent has been eliminated.

Rarely, another PD drug may be responsible for such behaviors, with a few reported cases of this being provoked by rasagiline or selegiline. If a pathological behavior of this type surfaces in the absence of a dopamine agonist drug, it may be sensible to taper off other PD drugs, except for carbidopa/levodopa, and use carbidopa/levodopa exclusively until the situation declares itself.

25

◆ ◆ ◆

Problems with Swallowing, Saliva, and Speaking

Trouble Swallowing

Dysphagia is the medical term for difficulty swallowing. This is rarely a major problem in PD. Even after many years, significant swallowing problems may never develop. If dysphagia is an early and prominent symptom, this may be a red flag for a condition other than PD (e.g., PSP, MSA; see Chapter 6).

Dysphagia in PD is typically due to slowness and hesitancy initiating the act of swallowing. This is analogous to the general slowness of body movement that occurs in PD. Food and liquid tend to pool in the mouth.

Severe dysphagia may lead to pneumonia (infection of the lungs). Normally, swallowed food or liquid passes down the tube-like esophagus to the stomach. However, the passageway to the lungs (trachea) is in front of the esophagus. If swallowing is impaired and food or liquid goes down the wrong pipe, it passes into the lungs. This usually triggers coughing, which is a protective reflex that tends to expel this material. Hence frequent coughing during eating is often a sign of aspiration. *Aspiration* is the medical term for food or liquid inappropriately passing into the trachea and the lungs.

Physicians are able to observe the swallowing function via X-ray techniques. They can administer a liquid that shows up on X-ray, such as barium. Once swallowed, a series of X-rays trace the passage from the mouth into the throat and down the esophagus. If it passes inappropriately into the trachea, this is seen on the X-ray.

TREATMENT OF DYSPHAGIA

Among those with PD, the most effective drugs for dysphagia are the same as those used to treat other aspects of parkinsonism. The most potent is carbidopa/levodopa, and adjusting the dose is the best strategy for improving swallowing problems. Dysphagia may not fully respond to medications; a few simple strategies are also helpful to improve swallowing:

- Sit upright when eating or drinking.

- A slight downward tuck of your head may help the food go down the right pipe. In other words, try to keep your chin down as you swallow (the so-called chin-tuck strategy).

- Don't take large bites or huge gulps. This is especially important when eating food that could get stuck, such as meats; if a big chunk of meat is inadvertently swallowed into the trachea, it could obstruct breathing.

- Slow down your eating.

- If swallowing solids is more of a problem than liquids, you could wash down small bites with a little water.

- Choose foods that are easier for you to swallow. For example, pureed fruits, certain puddings, and creamed dishes are swallowed more easily than tough-textured foods, such as steak, or dry, crumbly foods, like chips or pretzels. Sometimes sticky foods are a problem, such as peanut butter or mashed potatoes.

- Experiment with different temperatures of liquids. For example, most people find that ice-cold liquids are easier to swallow than those that are luke-warm.

- If water or soda pop especially tends to go down the wrong pipe (i.e., the trachea), you could substitute thicker liquids, such as milk shakes or eggnog, or add a thickener. Thickeners are available under brand names such as Thick-it; they can be added to juices to increase the consistency. Recall, however, that milk products contain protein, so milk shakes and eggnog are not good choices to wash down your carbidopa/levodopa.

If dysphagia is a major problem, you may wish to consult a swallowing specialist, who might be a speech pathologist or physiatrist/physical therapist (physical medicine and rehabilitation specialist).

Rarely, swallowing is so severely impaired that nutrition is compromised. In my experience, this is distinctly rare in PD, but it does occur in the parkinsonism-plus disorders discussed in Chapter 6. In that case, a feeding tube may be considered when simpler measures have failed. This often requires only minor surgery with the tube extending externally from the abdomen; this is inconspicuous when covered by a shirt or blouse.

TROUBLE SWALLOWING CARBIDOPA/LEVODOPA

If swallowing carbidopa/levodopa is difficult, you might switch to the orally disintegrating formulation (Parcopa). The pill sizes and colors are the same as those for the immediate-release formulation of carbidopa/levodopa and the doses are interchangeable. These pills dissolve in your mouth; however, the dissolved ingredients still must be swallowed with your saliva. They are considerably more expensive than generic carbidopa/levodopa.

Drooling

Drooling (sialorrhea) is common in PD. It is not due to increased saliva output. Rather, it is a consequence of reduced frequency of swallowing. Normally, we constantly secrete saliva and swallow it unconsciously. This swallowing is automatic. However, automatic movements are generally impaired in PD, such as arm swing, gesturing when talking, or blinking. Thus, like other automatic movements, swallowing frequency is reduced in PD.

In PD, the best treatment for drooling is carbidopa/levodopa in optimized dosage. Just like improvement of arm swing or facial animation with levodopa treatment, the frequency of swallowing increases and, with that, drooling is reduced.

What about medications that dry the mouth? Certain drugs reduce saliva output, specifically drugs from the anticholinergic class, such as glycopyrrolate. However, many people do not like the cotton-mouth feeling associated with inhibiting saliva output.

BOTULINUM TOXIN TREATMENT OF DROOLING

If drooling proves refractory to simpler solutions, botulinum toxin injections may be administered. Typically, botulinum toxin injections are used to relieve muscle spasms, such as occur in dystonia. However, it is also useful in reducing the output of saliva. For this purpose, botulinum toxin is injected into the salivary glands. Saliva output declines a few days after the injections, and this lasts up to a few months. It is uncommon that this is necessary in PD, but it may be needed in the parkinsonism-plus disorders discussed in Chapter 6.

PD Speech Problems

Speaking is typically affected by PD. There are two ways this occurs. First, the precision of speech (articulation) may suffer; this is termed *hypokinetic dysarthria*. This may give speech a bit of a garbled quality. Second, the volume of the voice often declines; this is termed *hypophonia*. Those with hypophonia may comment that they cannot be heard. Making matters worse for seniors with PD is that spouses and friends may have age-related hearing impairment.

WHAT TO DO FOR SPEECH AND VOICE PROBLEMS

Although speech therapy often has a role in treatment (see last section in this chapter), optimizing carbidopa/levodopa dosage is an important initial step. Speaking involves muscle movement, just like walking. When you speak, you are using your lips, tongue, and palate to form words. The repetitive excursions of the chest and diaphragm create airflow generating the voice. These muscles of articulation and breathing may be compromised by parkinsonism, similar to the muscles of your limbs. Just as your limb muscles may be slow and impeded, the same may occur with the speaking and voice muscles. Adequate doses of carbidopa/levodopa are often necessary to improve speech and voice. Thus the same medication principles we discussed in earlier chapters to improve walking or tremor apply to speech and voice.

OTHER SIMPLE THINGS TO TRY

The general principles that apply to the speech problems of PD include the following:

- Speak more slowly. Simply slowing down the rate of speech is often helpful in improving speech intelligibility.

- Speak deliberately. As you slow down, concentrate on precise articulation. Although normal speech is generated without consciously thinking about it, if you concentrate, you can improve the precision.

- Take a deep breath before speaking. This will help insure that you will have a large volume of air to push past your vocal cords.

- Purposely try to speak more loudly than you think is appropriate. People with PD often perceive that they are shouting when simply speaking loud enough to be heard. In other words, feedback of your own voice may cue you to speak too softly.

- Practice your speech in front of a mirror, reciting or reading familiar text, while consciously raising your voice. Shout this out so that someone in the next room could easily hear you with the door closed. Do this to develop a habit of "thinking loud" whenever you speak. For this to be consistently effective, you must practice this on a daily basis; otherwise there is a distinct tendency to fall back on old speaking habits.

There are other practical considerations to improve your intelligibility and communication:

- If your spouse has impaired hearing, as frequently occurs with normal aging, he or she might consider a hearing aid.

- For conversations, seek out quiet rooms. If the TV or stereo is playing in the background, or if others are speaking, the competition from these other sounds may drown you out. Note that hearing aids tend to amplify every sound; if other sounds are present in the room, the hearing aid will also make those louder.

- When dining out, choose quiet restaurants, where tables are not on top of each other and where background noise is minimal.

- Face your friends and family during conversations and hold your head up. Often cues from lips and face, as well as hand gestures, help the communication.

LEE SILVERMAN VOICE THERAPY

Where the measures cited here prove insufficient, consider consulting with a speech therapist familiar with Lee Silverman Voice Therapy (LSVT). This technique incorporates certain of these principles into a rigorous program of speech rehabilitation, designed to raise the voice volume. This has proven beneficial in controlled clinical trials.

The primary strategy of Lee Silverman Voice Therapy is to "think loud" and consciously raise the voice. People undergoing this therapy typically experience marked improvement in the short term. Although encouraged to continue practicing the techniques at home on a daily basis, few people do that. Hence, the benefit tapers off after a few weeks. If planning on engaging in this speech strategy, commit to continuing with the home exercises to maintain the benefit.

26

♦ ♦ ♦

Managing Digestive Problems and Constipation

Background

The autonomic nervous system coordinates gastrointestinal tract motility. The esophagus, stomach, and intestines are essentially a long conduit from mouth to anus, which slowly propels food and liquids through the digestive process. The initiation of digestion occurs in the stomach, whereas digested food products are absorbed into the circulation at the level of the small intestines (jejunum and ileum). At the end of the intestinal system, the colon (large intestine) collects the refuse. Muscles in the walls of this conduit system sequentially contract in a coordinated fashion to slowly move food products at an appropriate rate. The autonomic nervous system is responsible for the initiation and timing of these gastrointestinal muscle contractions. Properly timed and coordinated contractions of these small muscles within the walls of the gut are necessary for normal digestion. These contractions are also necessary for the undigested food products to ultimately be expelled as feces.

The dysfunctional autonomic nervous of Parkinson's disease (PD) tends to impede this process. The normal contractility of the gastrointestinal tract becomes sluggish. This is problematic at both ends of this system. Delayed emptying of the stomach contents may result in bloating or premature fullness while eating. Slowing of colon contractions translates into constipation (see Figure 26.1).

Scientists have identified microscopic evidence of the Lewy neurodegenerative process within the small autonomic nerves controlling gut contractility. This is the same type of microscopic accumulation of alpha-synuclein and related products found within the brain. Involvement of the gut by this Lewy neurodegenerative process may be an early manifestation of PD. Clinical studies have documented an increased risk of later PD among young and middle-aged adults with constipation.

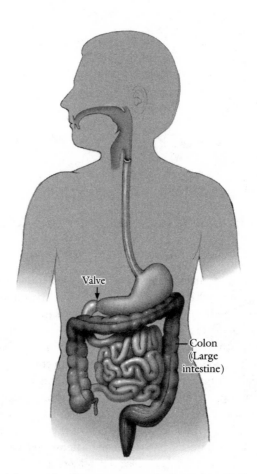

26.1   The stomach has a valve-like narrowing at the far end, restricting passage of foods and pills into the small intestine, but opening when appropriate. The colon (large intestine) is at the end of the gastrointestinal tract, ending in the rectum, with feces expelled through the anus.

CERTAIN MEDICATIONS SLOW GASTROINTESTINAL MOTILITY

Autonomic nerves regulate and coordinate gut contractility, termed *peristalsis*. This occurs via the release of neurotransmitters that activate the intrinsic gut-wall muscles. Certain drugs interfere with this peristalsis by binding to specific neurotransmitter-receptors in the intestinal muscles. This subverts the activity of the autonomic nerves and slows the gut. Two classes of drugs are notorious for doing this:

1. Anticholinergic medications

2. Narcotics

These medication classes are well-recognized causes of constipation and related gut disorders in the general population, but they are especially problematic among people with PD, who are predisposed.

ANTICHOLINERGIC DRUGS

In the gastrointestinal system, the neurotransmitter acetylcholine is released by autonomic nerves to stimulate peristalsis (gut contractions). Drugs that block acetylcholine slow stomach emptying, reduce intestinal peristalsis, and tend to cause constipation.

Anticholinergic drugs were used to treat PD before levodopa was introduced 40 years ago; they no longer are used for that purpose. Currently, the most commonly prescribed drugs from this class are used to reduce urinary urgency. Also, anticholinergic drugs are used to control diarrhea or the loose stools of irritable bowel syndrome. Finally, some of the older drugs used to treat depression have mild anticholinergic properties. These classes of drugs are listed in Table 26.1. If you are taking one of these medications and experiencing constipation, bloating, or other signs of delayed peristalsis, you may consider whether the benefits justify the side effects.

NARCOTICS AND THE GASTROINTESTINAL SYSTEM

Narcotic medications used for pain control are notoriously constipating. These drugs, used to treat pain, in pill or patch form, include the following:

- Codeine (Tylenol #3)

- Hydrocodone (Lortab, Lorcet, Norco, Vicodin, Vicoprofen)

- Oxycodone (Oxycontin, Roxicet, Roxicodone, Percocet, Tylox,

- Hydromorphine (Dilaudid)

Table 26.1. Anticholinergic Drugs That May Induce Constipation or Slow Stomach Emptying

Class of Drug Used for:	Drug
Parkinsonian tremor	
	Trihexyphenidyl (Artane)
	Benztropine (Cogentin)
	Procyclidine (Kemadrin)
	Biperiden (Akineton)
Urinary urgency	
	Oxybutynin (Ditropan)
	Tolterodine (Detrol)
	Hyoscyamine (Levsin, Levsinex, Cystospaz)
	Fesoterodine (Toviaz)
	Darifenacin (Enablex)
	Solifenacin (VESIcare)
	Trospium (Sanctura)
Antidepressants	
	Amitriptyline (Elavil)
	Nortriptyline (Pamelor)
	Desipramine (Norpramin)
	Imipramine (Tofranil)
	Doxepin (Sinequan)
	Trimipramine (Surmontil)
Diarrhea or irritable bowel	
	Atropine (ingredient in a variety of antidiarrheals)
	Hyoscyamine (ingredient in a variety of antidiarrheals)
	Scopolamine (ingredient in a variety of antidiarrheals, as well as motion sickness patch)
	Propantheline (Pro-Banthine)
	Clidinium (ingredient in Librax)
	Dicyclomine (Bentyl)

- Fentanyl (Duragesic patch)
- Levorphanol (Levo-dromoran)
- Methadone
- Buprenorphine (Suboxone)

This is not an exhaustive list of narcotic drugs. If unsure if one of your medications is a narcotic, your pharmacist will be able to answer that question. Note that narcotic pain relievers are often formulated with aspirin, acetaminophen (sometimes abbreviated APAP; Tylenol), or ibuprofen. If the decision is made to eliminate a narcotic drug that has been used for more than a few days, it should be slowly tapered, with guidance from a physician.

DOPAMINE AND THE GASTROINTESTINAL SYSTEM

Dopamine is also a neurotransmitter in the gastrointestinal system, and works in an opposite manner to that of acetylcholine. Hence drugs that stimulate dopamine will tend to slow the gastrointestinal system. This is not nearly as profound an effect as blocking acetylcholine. Although levodopa and the dopamine agonist medications tend to slow peristalsis, this is not very problematic; moreover, stopping these medications is rarely an option.

By the same token, drugs that block dopamine are also used to stimulate peristalsis, such a metoclopramide (Reglan) or prochlorperazine (Compazine). They are modestly beneficial and, more importantly, this class of drugs worsens parkinsonism; they should not be used in those with PD. The single exception is domperidone, which blocks dopamine but does not enter the brain; however, it is not available in the United States.

Treatment

CONSTIPATION

The majority of people with PD are constipated. Constipation reflects poor contractility of the colon (the large intestine). Undigested food products normally accumulate in the colon, which is shown in Figure 26.1. These undigestible food products mix with the normal bacteria that reside there and are the contents of feces. When the colon fails to properly contract, feces tend to back up, which represents constipation.

Constipation is common in the general population, and people without PD can usually have regular bowel movements with simple strategies: intake of fluids, fiber, fruits, and vegetables, and exercise. Among those with PD, these natural remedies are appropriate but often insufficient. Nonetheless, they should be done first:

- Drink adequate fluids, which is about 8 to 10 eight-ounce glasses daily.

- Make certain that your diet includes liberal portions of fruits and vegetables, cooked or raw.

- Include dietary fiber on a daily basis. This includes whole-grain cereals or whole-grain snacks. Also, a variety of high-fiber products are sold as "bulk-forming laxatives" (e.g., Metamucil, Citrucel, Fibercon). These contain fiber ingredients such as psyllium, ispaghula husk, methylcellulose, polycarbophil, bran, or barley malt extract.

- Prune juice may be especially helpful. One strategy is to heat a cup of prune juice in the microwave, similar to heating coffee or tea. Drinking the heated prune juice will tend to stimulate peristalsis.

- Engage in regular exercise.

Stool softeners, such as docusate sodium (Colace), are benign and may also be considered as an elementary component of constipation management. A 100 mg capsule of docusate sodium (Colace) twice daily may help those with mild constipation. Be aware that stool softeners are not laxatives and are minimally beneficial in the context of PD.

WHEN SIMPLE MEASURES FOR CONSTIPATION FAIL

Before considering more aggressive bowel strategies, it is important to establish goals. As a general rule, if you have a well-formed stool at least once every 2 days, that is acceptable. If you frequently go more than 2 days without a bowel movement, additional measures may be appropriate. I recognize that some people would prefer to have a daily bowel movement.

There are many different drugs and strategies for managing difficult constipation. The following discussion is not an exhaustive list of drugs or methods. It reflects my practice; your physician may have other suggestions or strategies. As with any medical treatment, common sense is necessary. If more aggressive therapy provokes diarrhea, cramping, or other gastrointestinal side effects, a revision of the treatment is necessary.

If the simple and natural remedies described previously fail to result in at least one bowel movement every 1 to 2 days, a laxative may be used. Laxatives tend to stimulate colon peristalsis, and there are two basic types, osmotic and stimulant laxatives:

- Osmotic laxatives pass into the colon undigested, and draw water across the intestinal wall (by osmosis). This water expands the colon content, stimulating internal reflexes leading to peristalsis. They also liquefy the stool.

- Stimulant laxatives directly stimulate the muscles of the colon walls to contract (peristalsis). They also stimulate the passage of water into the colon.

If a laxative is going to be used regularly, physicians prefer osmotic laxatives over stimulant laxatives, as these are less likely to irritate the intestinal lining or become habit-forming.

Osmotic laxatives contain one of several basic ingredients that are not digested and pass to the colon, where they osmotically draw in water to stimulate peristalsis and lubricate the feces. These over-the-counter preparations include the following:

- Polyethylene glycol (MiraLAX, GlycoLax, SoftLax, ClearLAX, Osmolax)

- Lactulose (Cephulac, Chronulac, Duphalac, Kristalose)

- Magnesium hydroxide (Milk of Magnesia)

MiraLAX (polyethylene glycol 3350) has become very popular, sold as a powder to be mixed with juice or another liquid. Milk of Magnesia is a very old laxative but should be avoided if kidney failure or severe congestive heart failure is present.

Although osmotic laxatives are preferred for very regular use, stimulant laxatives are effective and acceptable for occasional use. These are also available over the counter and include Bisacodyl (Dulcolax, Correctol) tablets or suppositories, as well as senna (Senokot, ExLax).

Regardless of the laxative chosen, be aware of the potential for impacted stool in the colon to prevent a response to laxatives. This is not likely if bowel movements have occurred every few days; however, if you have gone many days without a bowel movement, then old, desiccated stool may become stuck in the colon and be relatively immoveable. An administered laxative might then provoke painful colon contractions. Not only can the hard stool not be dislodged, but the contractions of the intestine abutting the impaction are experienced as stomach cramps. If this occurs, then a high-volume cleansing enema is appropriate to flush out the impacted stool. Once the colon is cleaned out, laxatives should be effective and tolerated.

Enema kits may be purchased from the drug store. Those with prepackaged small volumes of enema fluid, such as Fleets enema kits, will not be sufficient for the severe impaction problems we are addressing here. You will note from Figure 26.1 the large volume of the colon, which requires a sizeable volume of water to flush it out, perhaps a liter. An appropriate enema kit contains a large receptacle for the fluid and a flexible tube. It may be filled with warm (not hot) tap water. The end of the tube should be lubricated and gently inserted into the anus, with the water allowed to slowly pass into the rectum and further into the colon; holding the bag in the air allows gravity to provide gentle pressure. Obviously, this should be done in the bathroom, so that when the urge to defecate occurs the toilet will be handy. This may need to be repeated if the expelled contents do not contain stool.

Note that severe constipation may be associated with uncontrolled bowel movements manifesting as watery fecal discharge. This seems paradoxical with no formed bowel movements, yet watery diarrhea in the absence of laxatives. This is due to the hard, impacted stool impeding passage of all but watery feces, which leak around it. For this problem, a high-volume, cleansing enema is clearly necessary to clear the colon. Once the colon is opened, the strategies outlined here should work.

IMAGING THE COLON

For most people with PD who are constipated, there is no sinister cause, such as cancer. However, the general rule of thumb is that if there has been a major change in stool habits, the colon should be visualized. This is usually done via colonoscopy. Colonoscopy involves inserting a tube-like endoscope through the anus, which is slowly passed through the colon, allowing the doctor to see inside.

DELAYED OPENING OF THE STOMACH
AS A CAUSE OF NAUSEA OR BLOATING

If the stomach does not empty properly, people tend to experience bloating, nausea, or early satiety (fullness). If such symptoms surface, it is generally advisable to have this evaluated to ensure that there is not some other cause.

There are no medications that effectively treat delayed stomach emptying. The only drug approved for this condition in the United States is metoclopramide (Reglan); however, it blocks dopamine receptors and exacerbates or causes parkinsonism.

Modification of eating habits may help. Fatty foods, oils, or foods in heavy, rich sauces (e.g., heavy cream) tend to slow stomach emptying. Spicy foods, such as marinara sauces, trouble some people, as does alcohol or caffeine. You may try eliminating such foods and beverages one by one, and observe the response.

DELAYED MEDICATION RESPONSES

Slowed stomach emptying may also impede the carbidopa/levodopa response. Note that carbidopa and levodopa are not absorbed from the stomach. Passage into the circulation requires stomach opening and entry into the small intestine where carbidopa and levodopa may enter the bloodstream.

This is illustrated in Figure 26.2. Slowed stomach opening may delay the levodopa response.

How can one speed this up? Recall that filling the stomach triggers internal reflexes that open it. Hence one way to facilitate passage of levodopa into the small intestine is to drink adequate fluids along with your pills. This actually helps in two ways:

1. Fluids tend to expand the stomach, and this expansion will tend to stimulate stomach opening.

2. For the carbidopa/levodopa pill to be absorbed, it must first be dissolved, and fluids are necessary for this to occur.

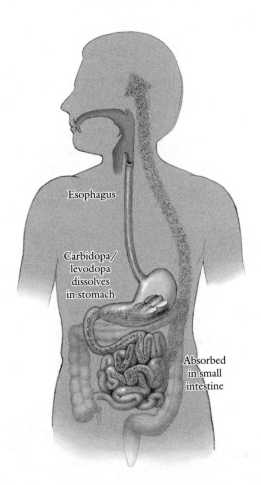

26.2 Swallowed food and pills pass down the esophagus to the stomach. Absorption into the circulation requires stomach opening and entry to the small intestine (jejunum). Carbidopa/levodopa is not directly absorbed from the stomach and must enter the small intestine to reach the bloodstream.

Food may also help open the stomach, but it must be non-protein if ingested with levodopa. Thus dry bread, soda crackers, or half a banana may be tried.

LATER DEVELOPING NAUSEA

Not all nausea is due to levodopa or dopamine agonist drugs. Another cause should be considered if nausea develops long after carbidopa/levodopa and dopamine agonist doses have been stabilized and tolerated.

27

◆ ◆ ◆

Urinary Symptoms

PD may be associated with urinary symptoms relating to bladder control. The autonomic nervous system regulates bladder function, and this may be affected by the Lewy neurodegenerative process. In PD, the autonomic nerves controlling the bladder contain microscopic alpha-synuclein markers of Lewy pathology. These findings are similar to the pathological changes in autonomic nerves controlling the gut, discussed in Chapter 26.

Typically, prominent bladder dysfunction is not an early symptom of PD and may never be a substantial problem. Complicating this matter is the fact that normal aging also impairs bladder function. When bladder symptoms develop, there are appropriate tests, consultations, treatments, and caveats to consider.

Anatomy of the Urinary System

Problems of urinary control reflect bladder dysfunction. Although the kidneys produce the urine, they are not responsible for controlling the urinary stream. The kidneys essentially filter the blood, extracting water and other products that need to be removed. As the kidneys produce urine drop by drop, it passes down tubes to the reservoir that stores the urine. These conduits from kidneys to bladder are called the *ureters* and the reservoir is the *bladder*. When urine is excreted into the toilet, it passes from the bladder

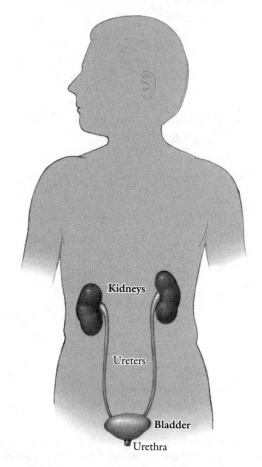

27.1   The kidneys essentially serve as filters of the circulation, maintaining appropriate bloodstream concentrations of crucial biological molecules (e.g., sodium, potassium) and water. Urine is continuously made by the kidneys, then flowing down the ureters to the bladder, which is a urine reservoir. The bladder outlet is the urethra.

through another conduit, the *urethra*. This anatomy is illustrated in the Figure 27.1. When urine within the bladder reaches capacity, the brain is signaled that it is time to urinate.

Normal Bladder Function

The act of urination involves contraction of muscles within the walls of the bladder that squeeze the urine out: the *detrusor muscles*. Coinciding with this is opening of an outlet valve that permits the urine to pass into the urethra. A sequence of autonomic reflexes allows this process to work smoothly. Normally, as the bladder fills, the muscles in the bladder walls are relaxed.

At a certain volume, a reflexive signal is sent to the brain that the bladder is full (and time to go to the bathroom); concurrently, the bladder wall muscles start to tense. The brain reciprocally sends inhibitory signals via the spinal cord and then to bladder nerves that tend to inhibit the bladder muscle tension. Ultimately, when it is time to urinate at the toilet, the brain releases this inhibition and urine flows.

Aging Affecting the Urinary System

Simply getting older may result in urination problems. Aging affects the urinary systems of men and women differently.

Women often develop urinary incontinence in middle age or beyond, primarily due to changes in pelvic musculature, and especially relating to child-bearing. The process of delivering a baby may damage the region around the bladder outlet. In later life this predisposes to incompetence of the outlet valve. The typical symptoms are leakage of small amounts of urine when coughing, sneezing, or laughing. In this circumstance, a poorly competent bladder outlet valve is unable to prevent urine from being expelled when the abdominal wall muscles suddenly contract during coughing or laughing. This is termed *stress incontinence*. If this becomes troublesome, the bladder outlet dysfunction can be surgically corrected.

Men have a different source of bladder symptoms, relating to the prostate. The prostate surrounds the urethra; in other words, the urethra passes through the middle of the prostate gland. In young men, the normal prostate does not compress the urethra and urine passes easily. With aging, the prostate tends to enlarge, sometimes constricting the urethra that passes through it, potentially limiting urine flow. This enlargement of the prostate is a common aging effect and, by itself, is not a sign of prostate cancer.

Normal aging in both genders may also result in more general dysfunction of bladder control, which tends to operate less efficiently as we get older. This may complicate the urinary problems in both men and women.

The Neurogenic Bladder of Parkinson's Disease

Impaired autonomic nervous system bladder control is termed a *neurogenic bladder*, which is the problem that occurs in PD. The neurogenic bladder malfunctions in two basic ways relating to altered contractility of the bladder wall detrusor muscles:

- *Hypoactive*: The bladder wall muscles contract poorly or incompletely.

- *Hyperactive*: Reflexive control of bladder wall muscles is excessively reactive.

Restated, autonomic dysfunction may result in an underreactive or overreactive bladder.

Some with PD have both types of neurogenic bladder. Further complicating this is the possibility of superimposed age-related bladder problems (e.g., male prostatism). These conditions result in a variety of symptoms:

- Hesitancy (impaired initiation of urination; slow stream)

- Incomplete bladder emptying with residual urine after voiding

- Urgency and frequency (need to urinate now! . . . and often)

- Incontinence (leakage; loss of urine control)

- Nocturia (need to urinate at night)

- Enuresis (bed-wetting)

- Urinary tract infections

The different bladder symptoms may suggest the type of bladder problem. However, appropriate treatment requires certain knowledge of the specific cause(s) of bladder malfunction. Guessing about the basis of these symptoms tends to be unreliable, especially considering that more than one type of problem may be present. Urologists are able to conduct special bladder tests to define the problem(s) and treat appropriately (discussed later in this chapter). Before discussing the workup and available treatments, further discussion of these bladder symptoms should provide a useful background.

Hesitancy

Urinary *hesitancy* implies that it is difficult to initiate urination. Besides being hard to start, the flow may be very slow, seemingly taking forever to empty the bladder. Moreover, the bladder may not completely empty, with residual urine left behind (a source of infection).

Hesitancy is typical of male prostate enlargement, constricting the urethra and preventing flow. However, it may also be a symptom of impaired autonomic bladder reflexes—a *neurogenic hypoactive bladder.*

Hesitancy from a neurogenic bladder is due to poor reflexive activation of the detrusor muscles in the bladder walls. The impaired reflexive tensing of these muscles translates into poor contraction during the act of urination. This problem also leads to overfilling, and a full bladder may be sensed too late. If the outlet valve can no longer hold the urine, *overflow incontinence* occurs.

Among middle-aged and older men in general, urinary hesitancy is typically due to prostatic enlargement constricting the urethra and impeding the outflow of urine. Prostatism may not be the primary cause of urinary hesitancy in men with PD. This is a crucial distinction to make, since prostate surgery may convert hesitancy to incontinence if a neurogenic hypotonic bladder is the problem (see later discussion in this chapter).

Incomplete Emptying

When urinary hesitancy becomes more pronounced, it is often associated with a bladder that never fully empties. In other words, after passing urine at the toilet, a substantial amount remains in the bladder, termed the *post-void residual*. This can be problematic in at least a couple of ways:

- Unexpelled, stagnant urine predisposes to urinary tract infections.

- A full bladder that is unable to empty may be uncomfortable or even painful.

In men, autonomic problems causing hesitancy may be additive with the prostate symptoms of aging.

Urgency and Frequency

Urinary *urgency* implies a heightened need to urinate. This is the feeling that we all experience if prevented from going to the bathroom when our bladder is full (e.g., a long car trip with no gas stations in sight). This symptom is typical of a neurogenic *hyperactive bladder*, with an increased tendency for the bladder wall detrusor muscles to contract.

Those with a hyperactive bladder typically experience urgency with only partial bladder filling. This may recur often during the day, termed *urinary frequency*. Note that urinary urgency and frequency may also be experienced by those with urinary tract infections (discussed later).

Incontinence

Urinary incontinence implies inappropriate leakage of urine. There are several ways this may happen:

- Incontinence may occur due to problems of bladder anatomy. Thus leakage may develop if the bladder outlet is damaged by childbirth or pelvic surgery.

- A neurogenic hypoactive bladder may fill beyond the capacity, spilling urine, termed *overflow incontinence*.

- A neurogenic hyperactive bladder with increased bladder reflexes may inappropriately expel urine, termed *urge incontinence.*

Combinations of these problems are not rare among those with PD and require a savvy urologist to sort them out and treat appropriately.

Nocturia (Nighttime Urination)

When the bladder fills to capacity during sleep, an appropriate urge to urinate tends to trigger awakening, termed *nocturia.* Experiencing this once or twice a night is common among seniors. However, this may be exacerbated by several factors, including a neurogenic bladder or bladder anatomy problems (e.g., prostate enlargement).

The tendency for nocturia is increased in poor sleepers. People who sleep soundly tend to unconsciously suppress the urge to urinate until it becomes prominent; only then does this awaken them. Light sleepers are easily awakened by the slightest stimuli, in this case, from the bladder. People with PD who sleep poorly because of insufficient levodopa coverage may be especially susceptible to this problem (see Chapter 20).

Enuresis (Bed-Wetting)

Bed-wetting (enuresis) is not a common problem among those with PD and is rare early in the course of PD. Those with a neurogenic bladder may experience this and require bed pads or absorbant garments at night. Note that sedating medications may exacerbate this problem.

Dysuria and Urinary Tract Infections

Dysuria implies painful urination, often experienced as a burning sensation. This is the most common symptom of a urinary tract infection. Urinary infections are common among those with underactive bladders or from impaired emptying from anatomic causes such as prostate enlargement. Stagnant urine accumulating in an underactive bladder is prone to infection.

If it is painful to urinate, a urinalysis and a urinary culture should be performed. The urinalysis includes examining the urine under the microscope. If bacteria and inflammatory cells (white cells) are present, this suggests an infection. A urine culture is done to identify the strain of bacteria and guide the choice of antibiotic. The culture is less crucial if this is your first urinary infection or at least the first in many years. Those with frequent urinary tract infections often harbor bacteria that are resistant to many antibiotics.

Note that urinary urgency may also be a symptom of a urinary tract infection. Occasionally, the symptoms of urge incontinence will resolve simply with treatment of an infection.

Am I Destined to Experience These Urinary Problems?

Those with PD often do not experience substantial urinary problems beyond those related to aging. Furthermore, when urinary symptoms develop, they may be limited. When problems do occur, however, it is important to sort these out and employ proper treatment.

Urological Assessment of Urinary Dysfunction

The workup of any urinary problem starts with a routine urinalysis. Depending on the symptoms, a urine Gram stain (looking for bacteria under the microscope) plus a urine culture may be performed. If an infection is found, this is treated with antibiotics.

Bladder symptoms beyond a simple infection typically require consultation with a urologist. These specialists are in the best position to characterize a neurogenic bladder and distinguish other factors, such as prostate enlargement or female stress incontinence. Urological tests that they may consider include the following:

- *Residual urine* is measured after routine voiding to assess emptying of the bladder. Normally, the bladder should be completely emptied after urination. Leftover urine provides a nidus for urinary infections.

- *Cystoscopy* is performed to view the bladder and look for anatomic causes of impaired flow. This is done through a scope that allows the urologist to see the bladder wall and urinary passages and to look for pockets of infection, bladder wall cancer, or certain types of urinary obstruction.

- *Urodynamic testing* is done to assess detrusor muscle reflexive responses. Urodynamic studies involve inflating the bladder with water or carbon dioxide to certain volumes and then assessing the bladder reflexes. Such studies can be used to determine whether the bladder is overactive or underactive.

These studies are typically well tolerated.

Medications for a Hyperactive Bladder: Urgency, Urge Incontinence, Urinary Frequency

A hyperactive bladder can be controlled with more than one strategy:

- Anticholinergic drugs

- Mirabegron, which activates the beta-3 adrenergic receptor in the bladder wall that relaxes the bladder muscles

- Botulinum toxin injections into the bladder wall muscles

Note that all of these treatments impede bladder emptying, with potential for incomplete evacuation of urine. Urine left behind is susceptible to infection. This can be assessed with postvoid (after urinating) measurement of urine left in the bladder.

ANTICHOLINERGIC DRUGS

For decades, the conventional treatment for overactive bladders has been medications that block the bladder neurotransmitter acetylcholine: anticholinergic drugs. Acetylcholine is released by nerves that signal the bladder muscles to contract. If these are inhibited, the bladder contractions are reduced, attenuating urgency, urge incontinence, and frequency. Common side effects include constipation, dry mouth and eyes, and blurred vision; it may exacerbate glaucoma. Many of the drugs from this class are able to enter the brain, where acetylcholine blockade may impair memory. The primary medications currently used for hyperactive bladder include the following:

Oxybutynin (Ditropan; Ditropan XL)

Tolterodine (Detrol; Detrol LA)

Solifenacin (VESIcare)

Darifenacin (Enablex)

Fesoterodine (Toviaz)

Trospium (Sanctura)

Other less commonly prescribed anticholinergic bladder drugs include hyoscyamine (Levsin, Levbid, Levsinex, Cystospaz) and flavoxate (Urispas).

No one of these medications appears superior in controlling bladder hyperactivity when doses are optimized. Side effects of these bladder drugs are similar, except for the potential to block acetylcholine receptors within the brain. Acetylcholine is a neurotransmitter in brain memory circuits. Inhibition of brain acetylcholine impairs memory. Recall that the drugs discussed in Chapter 23 to enhance memory (donepezil, rivastigmine, galantamine) promote acetylcholine neurotransmission. Obviously, blocking acetylcholine does the opposite; it tends to impair memory. The only anticholinergic bladder drug that is unable to cross the blood-brain-barrier into the brain is trospium; it has a chemical configuration that makes it impenetrable. Studies in animals suggest that fesoterodine and darifenacin penetrate into the brain but probably do not accumulate; that is, they may not impair brain acetylcholine neurotransmission.

If you are starting an anticholinergic drug for an overactive bladder, it is wise to review the medication list to make certain that you are not already taking a drug from the anticholinergic class, as listed in the previous chapter (Table 26.1). This includes anticholinergic medications for PD, medications for loose stools, as well as certain antidepressant drugs. If you are taking one of these medications, then adding an anticholinergic bladder medication may be redundant.

MIRABEGRON (MYRBETRIQ)

Mirabegron is the first oral drug approved for hyperactive bladders that does not work by blocking acetylcholine receptors. Rather, it activates beta-3 adrenergic receptors in the bladder wall muscles, which reduces their tendency to contract. It does not have the troublesome anticholinergic properties of the drugs just discussed. Perhaps the most common side effect is modest elevation of the blood pressure; however, among those with PD, this is rarely a problem. This seems to be an important addition to the treatment of hyperactive bladder, although at the time of this writing, I have had only limited experience with this medication.

BOTULINUM TOXIN INJECTIONS FOR HYPERACTIVE BLADDERS

Botulinum toxin injections have been used for a quarter-century to reduce excessive muscle contraction states, including dystonias of the feet, toes, or neck. It has gained publicity for reducing wrinkles in seniors, which is does by weakening injected muscles so that they cannot contract to produce wrinkles. More recently, it has been used to reduce the excessive muscle contractions of a hyperactive bladder. For that purpose, it is a last resort, given the substantial expense and the need to repeat this every few months indefinitely. Medications are typically tried before resorting to this procedure.

Strategies for Frequent Awakening to Urinate (Nocturia)

Nocturia is common in middle age and beyond. If nocturia occurs once to twice a night, age may be the cause. However, more frequent trips to the bathroom can sabotage a night's sleep. Factors contributing to nocturia include those listed in this section.

Water balance:
- Drinking liquids in the evening
- Taking diuretics (water pills) later in the day (e.g., hydrochlorothiazide, triamterene, furosemide)
- Drinking coffee, tea, caffeinated soda pop, or alcohol in the evening (all have a diuretic effect)

To reduce nocturia, avoid drinking liquids after supper and empty your bladder just before bed. Confirm that any evening pills are not diuretics.

Light sleep:
- Poor sleep due to inadequate levodopa coverage at night
- Stress or depression
- Chronic insomnia

If parkinsonian symptoms are not controlled during the night, this may result in superficial sleep. Hence any stimulus, including the need to urinate, will tend to cause awakening. This may be treated with adequate nighttime levodopa coverage, which was discussed in Chapter 20. Light sleep for other reasons will similarly make it easier for urinary symptoms to cause awakening. The general strategies for improving sleep quality were discussed in Chapter 20 and apply here, including use of a sleep aid, if necessary.

Bladder dysfunction:
- Urinary tract infection
- Neurogenic bladder
- Prostatism in men

A urological workup may reveal treatable conditions, such as a urinary tract infection. Hyperactive neurogenic bladders may respond to the strategies discussed earlier. Prostate enlargement that impedes urine flow may cause incomplete emptying at bedtime and a full bladder earlier in the night; this is typically treatable.

Treatment of a Distended, Hypoactive Bladder

An enlarged and poorly contracting bladder may be due to either bladder outlet obstruction or a neurogenic (hypoactive) bladder. Among senior men, in general, prostate enlargement is a common cause of bladder outlet obstruction. In men with PD, it is usually not possible to reliably make this distinction without urological assessment.

Symptoms of a hypotonic bladder may include slow or hesitant urination, incomplete bladder emptying (sense of bladder fullness after urinating), or incontinence when the non-contracting bladder overflows. Residual urine in the bladder is a source of urinary infections.

The urological workup typically involves cystoscopy and urodynamics, as described earlier. The workup will also assess the volume of urine left in the bladder after voiding: residual urine.

Effective drugs to stimulate lazy, distended bladders have yet to be developed. The urologist will need to exclude the possibility of obstruction to urine flow, as might occur with an enlarged prostate. However, if no impediment to urine flow is present, drugs are unlikely to be helpful. The urologist can advise about therapeutic strategies apart from medications.

Caveats

Treatment of bladder problems in the context of PD may result in unintended consequences. Earlier in this chapter, we listed common side effects of the anticholinergic bladder drugs, several of which are especially relevant to those with PD, including memory impairment, constipation, and dry mouth and eyes. Urological treatment of prostatism among men with PD additionally deserves discussion.

DRUGS FOR MALE PROSTATISM: BE WARY OF LOW BLOOD PRESSURE

An enlarged prostate may obstruct the flow of urine out of the bladder, resulting in hesitant urination and incomplete bladder emptying. Drugs that block adrenalin (alpha-blockers) are often prescribed to reduce enlarged prostate glands. The medications used for this purpose are as follows:

- Alfuzosin (Uroxatral)
- Doxazosin (Cardura)
- Prazosin (Minipress)
- Silodosin (Rapaflo)
- Tamsulosin (Flomax)
- Terazosin (Hytrin)

These drugs robustly lower blood pressure. As discussed in Chapter 21, a low blood pressure when standing upright (orthostatic hypotension) is common in PD. If orthostatic hypotension is a problem, these medications should be avoided. Note that the erectile dysfunction (ED) drug tadalafil (Cialis) is also chronically prescribed to reduce prostate enlargement. This and the other ED medications tend to lower the blood pressure.

Medications that block androgen effects (5 alpha-reductase inhibitors) are also used to reduce prostate size but do *not* reduce blood pressure. These drugs prevent conversion of testosterone to a more potent metabolite (dihydrotestosterone). Reducing the influence of testosterone reduces the size of the prostate, although this effect occurs slowly over months. These drugs include finasteride (Proscar) and dutasteride (Avodart). They do not lower blood pressure and may be used by those with orthostatic hypotension.

PROSTATE SURGERY

Men with a markedly enlarged prostate that impedes urine flow are typically offered surgery to remove the obstructing prostate tissue. This might include surgical resection with a procedure termed transurethral resection of the prostate (TURP). More recently, laser destruction of obstructing prostate tissue has been commonly employed. In general, these procedures go well, but the exception is among those with a neurogenic bladder, where urinary hesitancy can be converted to urinary incontinence. This relates to impairment of the normal valve function at the bladder outlet following this surgery. Urologists usually are aware of this potential problem and will factor this into a surgical decision. However, they may overlook it if they are not aware that you have PD; hence inform them.

28

♦ ♦ ♦

Sexual Dysfunction, Estrogen, and Menstrual Cycles

Sexuality

In the general population, sexual desire and performance begin to decline in middle age in both men and women. Although this reflects the natural cycle of life, there may be contributing factors such as depression, stress, or medications. Despite the universal interest in sexual function, limited treatment options have surfaced to combat this mid-life sexual decline, especially for women. Sexual dysfunction can be frustrating or embarrassing, with potential to impair marital and partner relationships. Parkinson's disease (PD) adds yet another factor that compromises sexual function. The goal of this section is to put these problems into context, recognizing the therapeutic limitations.

Male Impotence Is Universal

Impotence implies difficulty with sexual performance, that is, problems achieving and maintaining an erection, which normally should lead to ejaculation and organism. Before we consider factors that can disrupt sexual performance, we should recognize that occasional impotence is common. This is not something that only a few men experience; it can, and does, happen to even the most macho guys.

Men are at their sexual peak during their teenage years and and a few years thereafter. With passing decades, not only does the urge for sexual gratification decline but also the ability to perform. Hence, as males pass beyond the years when sex dominates their thoughts, occasional impotence is fairly common. We need to accept this, just as we are stuck with the joint pains that never bothered us when we were young, or the middle-aged requirement for reading glasses.

PSYCHOLOGICAL ISSUES

Any man who is depressed, anxious, stressed, or distracted will be at an increased risk of impotence. Appropriate treatment of these problems is an important first step in treating impotence.

MALE PERFORMANCE ANXIETY

Sexual acts come naturally. You cannot "will" an erection; the harder you consciously try, the more the erection is sabotaged. For men who have experienced impotence, this tends to become a focus during subsequent sexual engagements. "What if this happens again?" "I need to do something to avoid this embarrassment!" If this is the foremost thought in your mind as you begin the sexual foreplay, you will be doomed. Like a quarterback who throws an interception, you must not take this experience to your next play. Forget about it and move on. All men will experience this on occasion. You can't dwell on it. Unfortunately, this is easy to say, but harder to do.

MEDICAL CONDITIONS AND MALE IMPOTENCE

A variety of medical problems (besides PD) can cause impotence. These problems become more common as we age.

Any disorder that leads to atherosclerosis (hardening of the arteries) increases the likelihood of impotence. This is because blood circulation to the penis is a critical component of erections; it is engorgement of blood within the penis that makes it firm and elongated. Diseases or conditions that lead to atherosclerosis may impair circulation to the genital organs. Predisposing conditions include the following:

- Diabetes mellitus
- High cholesterol
- Smoking

- Uncontrolled high blood pressure
- Normal aging

These factors do not cause impotence directly or immediately; however, after years, they contribute to atherosclerosis, and this may then be a factor in circulatory problems within the genital organs. Unfortunately, once atherosclerosis develops, it tends to be irreversible. However, with attention to these risk factors, it may stabilize; compensation is possible if not too advanced.

Any major illness or disease of the internal organs may be associated with impotence. Thus liver, kidney, heart or lung failure, or major infectious illness (e.g., pneumonia, kidney infections) make sexual performance problematic. Endocrine disorders may also be associated with impotence, such as untreated thyroid disease.

Certain neurological diseases besides PD are also associated with impotence, including multiple sclerosis, peripheral neuropathy, and spinal cord conditions. Disorders resulting in chronic pain also make sexual performance difficult.

Long-standing substance abuse may ultimately result in impotence. This is especially common among alcoholics.

TESTOSTERONE

The male hormone testosterone obviously is critical to male sexual performance. It is uncommon for this to be the primary cause of impotence, however. Furthermore, treatment with testosterone-like substances does not reverse impotence except for those occasional men in whom the measured blood testosterone levels are very low; even then, there are no guarantees. Hence, although you might think testosterone supplementation would be a good treatment for problems with erections, it typically is inadequate unless your doctor identifies a deficiency. Even when testosterone treatment is administered to those with low levels, impotence may not be cured, since other problems are often contributing.

Testosterone treatment runs the risk of encouraging the growth of prostate cancer that might otherwise have been indefinitely dormant. In fact, treatment of prostate cancer involves blocking the effects or release of testosterone. If diagnosed with prostate cancer, you should not receive male hormone replacement therapy.

MEDICATIONS (OTHER THAN PD DRUGS) AND IMPOTENCE

Many medications of all types have the potential to cause male impotence. The list is too long to enumerate here. Many of these drugs will cause this only occasionally. This list includes a variety of medications that lower the blood pressure and treat chronic pain, muscle relaxants, antihistamines, water pills (diuretics), cancer treatments, and many psychiatric drugs. Some or all of these may be critical to your health. However, it is appropriate to have your physician review your list to determine if any drug is particularly likely to be responsible. If such a drug is identified, your physician can tell you whether it is safe to stop it for a few weeks to determine if this was the offending agent. If impotence only became a problem after starting a new drug, this medication may be the culprit. Note that "recreational drugs" may also impair impotence, including narcotics, marijuana, and alcohol.

The selective serotonin antidepressant medications (SSRIs) used to treat depression are sometimes blamed for reduced libido or impotence (see Chapter 22). This may be true in some cases, but in others, as they effectively treat depression, sexual function secondarily improves. Untreated depression blunts sexual desire and function.

PARKINSON'S DISEASE AND IMPOTENCE

Parkinson's disease may predispose affected men to impotence. This is not to say that everyone with PD is impotent. However, PD increases this risk. As previously discussed, PD is associated with autonomic nervous system dysfunction, which may result in bladder difficulties, constipation, or orthostatic hypotension. Since sexual functioning is also regulated by the autonomic nervous system, it also is susceptible.

PD MEDICATIONS AND MALE IMPOTENCE

The drugs administered for PD are sometimes blamed for impotence. However, I suspect that the opposite is often true. In other words, adequate treatment of parkinsonism with carbidopa/levodopa may actually facilitate sexual performance. Undertreatment may be more likely to result in impotence, although this is an area that has not been adequately studied.

Interestingly, following the introduction of levodopa therapy, several publications reported an increased sexual appetite among those newly treated. Initially, this was thought to represent a true aphrodisiac effect. However, it later became apparent that the improved sexual performance was likely the consequence of regaining the ability to move. As best we know, Levodopa has no substantial aphrodisiac effect in men without PD.

DOPAMINE AGONISTS AND PATHOLOGICAL SEXUAL BEHAVIORS

To this point, poor sexual performance and reduced libido has been the topic. Since the discussion has shifted to PD drugs, we must briefly digress and address the opposite problem: compulsive, excessive sexual behavior. The dopamine agonist drugs pramipexole, ropinirole, and rotigotine uniquely have the propensity to provoke excessive sexual behavior in a minority of people. From the reports coming to me, these drugs do not improve potency, but but rather generate compulsions to engage in pornography, extra-marital affairs, unreasonable and repeated demands for sex, and consorting with prostitutes. Affected people often have poor insight and are unable to control these urges. These often are very much out of character for that person. These drugs may also provoke compulsive gambling or other pathological behaviors, as discussed in Chapters 10, 13, and 24. Treatment requires tapering off the offending agonist drug.

Now back to treating poor libido and impaired sexual function.

SIMPLE STRATEGIES TO IMPROVE MALE SEXUAL PERFORMANCE

For normal sexual function, the dopamine deficiency state of PD should be adequately treated with carbidopa/levodopa. Undertreatment resulting in prominent residual parkinsonism seriously challenges sexual performance.

Sexual performance may be impossible if in a parkinsonian off-state. If levodopa off-states are prominent and recurring, time the carbidopa/levodopa doses so that an on-state is present during love-making.

Among the myriad of other factors that may sabotage sexual functioning, some are beyond our control. Things we can address to enhance sexual desire and performance include the following.

- Treat psychological and psychiatric problems; if issues are weighing heavily on your mind, sexual performance will suffer.

- Learn to forget previous potency problems.

- Work with your physician to treat any active medical problems.

- Do all the right "health" things:

  1. Exercise regularly.

  2. Get enough sleep.

  3. Drink enough fluids.

  4. Consume no more than modest amounts of alcohol (alcohol may impair potency).

  5. Avoid obesity.

- Have a physician review your medication list for drugs that could be contributing to impotence.

- Discuss any potency concerns openly with your partner, who may be able to help by way of additional stimulation techniques and more patient expectations.

- Recognize and respect your partner's role as it changes with the advent of your PD. Your partner may be taking on added work and burdens that make it more difficult to find the time and energy to be sexually receptive.

- Engage in sex in a relaxed environment without time constraints. Set aside a period of time for this rather than trying to squeeze it in before work in the morning or at other times when you are hurried. Also, things may go better if you don't defer it until late at night when you are starting to become tired.

Although this list is for male impotence, many of these common-sense strategies are relevant to women with PD as well.

WHEN SIMPLER STRATEGIES DON'T WORK: DRUGS FOR ERECTIONS

If you have done all the right things and failed erections are still a problem, you may be a candidate for a phosphodiesterase-5 inhibitor, better known as

- Sildenafil (Viagra)

- Vardenafil (Levitra, Staxyn)

- Tadalafil (Cialis)

- Avanafil (Stendra)

These medications will not change sexual appetite but rather have a specific effect on penile blood flow, helping to achieve and maintain erections. An erection will not be achieved with these alone; sexual stimulation must also be employed.

The instructions to physicians for this class of drugs indicate that they may be taken with or without food. However, a high-fat meal may reduce the rate of absorption and delay or inhibit the effect.

It appears that the durations of the effect of sildenafil, vardenafil, and avanafil are similar, lasting around 4–6 hours (some sources report up to twice that duration in some men). Tadalafil is unique, with a 36-hour effect. Avanafil acts most quickly, allowing for administration as soon as 15 minutes before intercourse, compared to 30–60 minutes for the other drugs in this class.

Sildenafil (Viagra) Dosage

The usual dose of (Viagra) is a single 50 mg tablet taken approximately 30–60 minutes before intercourse. Those over age 65 years should start with a 25 mg dose, subsequently raised to 50 mg if necessary. The highest recommended dose is 100 mg; this should be tried only if lower doses fail and only on a subsequent day. Only one dose is advisable per day. This drug comes in three pill sizes: 25 mg, 50 mg, and 100 mg.

Vardenafil (Levitra, Staxyn) Dosage

The starting dose for vardenafil (Levitra) is a 10 mg tablet taken about an hour before intercourse. If you are over age 65, start with 5 mg, but with the option of trying 10 mg the next time. Don't take more than one dose in a day. The maximum dose is 20 mg daily. Four pill sizes are available: 2.5, 5, 10, and 20 mg.

Vardenafil is also formulated in a tablet that dissolves on the tongue and swallowed with saliva, marketed as Staxyn. It comes in one tablet size, 10 mg, taken about an hour before sexual intercourse. The maximum dose is 1 tablet per day.

Tadalafil (Cialis) Dosage

This drug is similar to the other medications, except for a longer duration of effect, lasting up to 36 hours. Thus, it is not necessary to time the dose with respect to intercourse. When used in anticipation of sexual intercourse, the usual dose is 10 mg, but half this dose for those over age 65 years. As with the other drugs from this class, only one dose per 24 hours is advised. Three pill sizes are available: 5, 10, and 20 mg, with the maximum dose of 20 mg per day.

Tadalafil may also be used once every day, in which case a lower dose is advised, starting with 2.5 mg daily, with the option of raising it if necessary to 5 mg daily. Urologists sometime prescribe daily tadalafil for prostate enlargement that impairs urinary flow; the dose recommended for that purpose is 5 mg per day.

Avanafil (Stendra) Dosage

This drug has been marketed as quickest acting. The starting dose is 100 mg, taken about 15 minutes to 30 minutes before intercourse. The dosing range is 50 to 200 mg once daily. There are three tablet sizes: 50, 100, and 200 mg.

CAUTIONS FOR THOSE STARTING ON A PHOSPHODIESTERASE-5 INHIBITOR

This class of ED medications tends to lower blood pressure, with effects lasting around 4–6 hours for all, except tadalafil, which has a 36-hour effect. This is a concern for those with PD who are prone to orthostatic hypotension. A drop in the blood pressure following a dose of one of these medications may manifest in one of two ways:

- The lowered blood pressure may occur only when you get up, such as when going to the bathroom. This is typical of the orthostatic hypotension occurring in PD, where the blood pressure drops with standing, but is satisfactory when lying or sitting.

- The blood pressure may drop to low levels even when lying down, causing faintness. Furthermore, sexual performance may suffer, since low blood pressure sabotages erections.

Before taking the first dose, it might be wise to check the lying and standing blood pressures, doing this when levodopa is working (on-state). Remember that levodopa and the dopamine agonists will reduce blood pressure for up to a few hours after each dose (orthostatic hypotension). If your pressure readings are around 90/60, this suggests a risk of even lower values with the addition of a phosphodiesterase-5 inhibitor drug.

If you have a serious heart problem, especially angina (chest pain due to impaired blood flow to heart muscle), avoid these drugs unless your physician approves. These medications should not be used if your heart condition requires you to take a nitrate drug (i.e., nitroglycerin, isosorbide), although your doctor may allow exceptions. These medications should generally be avoided if serious liver or kidney disease; with physician approval they may be allowed, but in lower doses. People with sickle cell disease or retinitis pigmentosa should not take these medications.

Rarely, use of one of these drugs will be associated with sudden vision or hearing loss. If that occurs, immediate medical evaluation is advisable (e.g., emergency room). Another rare side effect is an erection that does not go away; medical attention is recommended if this persists beyond 4 hours.

A number of minor side effects may also develop with use of these drugs and are not worrisome. These include changes in color vision or visual acuity, facial flushing, nasal congestion, nausea, or headache.

BEYOND PHOSPHODIESTERASE-5 INHIBITORS

The other options for men with inability to obtain erections are more complicated and require consultation with an urologist. The urologist may first assess the quality of erections by overnight measurement; men tend to get erections during sleep, which can be measured with a special device. Treatment options from the urologists include the following:

- Administration of a medication into the end of the urethra at the tip of the penis (i.e., into the orifice at the end of the penis—the same orifice from which urine passes). This is done with a small applicator prior to sexual activity. When this dissolves into the penile tissue, it causes an erection.

- Injection of a different medication into the base of the penis via a small needle prior to sex. This sounds painful but is actually well tolerated by most men, resulting in an erection lasting several minutes to hours.

- Use of a special vacuum tube that is placed over the penis, resulting in increased blood flow and an erection. A rubber band–like ring is then placed at the base of the penis, which traps the blood and allows the erection to be maintained.

The first two of these options may occasionally result in side effects, so they are typically initially tried in the urologist's office to make certain everything goes smoothly.

Surgery is also an option for treatment of impotence. Penile implants surgically placed into the shaft of the penis are generally of two types:

- Semi-rigid rods that result in a permanent erection (they can be easily bent backwards to conceal this in one's trousers).

- Inflatable implants that can be pumped to achieve the erection when appropriate. The actual pump is surgically placed in the scrotum and the reservoir with the air for inflation is implanted in the abdomen. These are all well concealed.

Obviously, these implants will not precisely duplicate a natural erection.

Female Sexual Function

There is a wealth of medical literature on male sexual dysfunction, including impotence caused by chronic neurological disease. However, much less has been written about the influence of neurological disease on female sexual function. Only in recent years has the effect of PD on female sexual functioning received any attention in the medical literature. Moreover, women are generally reluctant to discuss sexual functioning with their physicians, especially if the physician is male. Male physicians managing PD are reluctant to ask their female patients about sex; rather, they tend to focus on more elementary problems of PD, such as tremor and ability to walk. Hence sexual functioning is usually ignored. I plead guilty as well to this shortsightedness.

It is difficult to draw any broad conclusions about the effect of PD on female sexual function, because what has been written is either anecdotal or has focused on small numbers of women. Furthermore, some form of sexual dysfunction occurs in the majority of middle-aged women without PD (e.g., reduced libido, lack of orgasm, pain with intercourse, tightness or dryness of the vagina). Hence, female sexual dysfunction cannot all be blamed on PD. In limited published studies, women with PD do experience reduced desire for sex and reduced orgasm, and often complain of vaginal tightness, dryness, or pain. To what extent these problems were specifically linked to PD is unclear; normal aging is also associated with such symptoms.

What can women with PD do to enhance their sexual desire and function? There are no aphrodisiacs that will magically turn you into a sexual animal. The best we can do is address general issues that might improve sexual function.

First, female sexual responsiveness is maximal when there are no distractions, stressors, or any physical pain or discomfort. Extrapolating from that, it makes sense that female sexuality will be optimized if parkinsonian symptoms are adequately treated. Undertreatment may be associated with akathisia (inner restlessness; inability to get comfortable); stiffness, painful cramps other sources of pain, or frank anxiety. These problems can easily sabotage sexual enjoyment and function. Hence appropriate treatment of PD should benefit sexuality.

Second, psychological depression should be treated. Depression is notorious for contributing to sexual dysfunction and poor libido in the general population. Those with PD are at an increased risk for depression, and this is important to recognize and treat (see Chapter 22). Parenthetically, the selective serotonin reuptake inhibitor (SSRI) drugs are commonly used to treat depression but may reduce libido and sexual function in some people. A psychiatrist can advise about the best medication choice if this issue is of concern.

Third, if experiencing vaginal discomfort, pain, tightness, or dryness during intercourse, discuss this with your internist or gynecologist. Besides the obvious water-soluble lubricant (e.g., K-Y Jelly), they might also recommend an estrogen cream. Daily use of an estrogen cream applied to the vaginal area increases the natural suppleness and lubrication. Also, discuss with your sexual partner the need to increase the time of foreplay to allow the natural lubrication to develop.

Finally, timing is often critical. Although sexual activity goes best when spontaneous, you can sometimes plan ahead and create the proper time for sex that fits with your biological and parkinsonian cycles. First, libido diminishes when tired. Hence midnight trysts may not be the optimal time for some individuals. Second, if your response to carbidopa/levodopa fluctuates, make certain that you are in a levodopa on-state at the anointed time. If you lapse into a levodopa off-state, this will disrupt performance and enjoyment.

Effects of Menstrual Periods and Estrogen on Parkinsonism

Estrogen and progesterone are the two major female hormones. Before menopause, the blood levels vary with the menstrual cycle. Blood estrogen levels especially correlate with a variety of subjective symptoms among all women. A plummeting estrogen level just before and during menstrual periods is associated with the myriad of symptoms that have been termed *premenstrual syndrome*.

Women with PD may be especially susceptible to the effects of estrogens. Among those who are premenopausal with regular periods, the response to their PD drugs (especially carbidopa/levodopa) may decline just before and during their menses. This decline in the response correlates with low estrogen levels. This doesn't happen in every woman, but it occurs frequently. The key is to recognize the pattern. If you do, then a medication strategy can be employed. You may need to plot the pattern for a few menstrual cycles to be certain.

WHEN CARBIDOPA/LEVODOPA FAILS TO KICK IN DURING CERTAIN TIMES OF THE MENSTRUAL CYCLE

If you are able to identify a monthly menstrual pattern when carbidopa/levodopa does not kick in, higher individual doses may be tried during this time. Recall that the response to levodopa tends to be all-or-none. If carbidopa/levodopa fails to work during certain times of the menstrual cycle, small increments of each dose should put you over the response threshold. Usually, dose increments of a half-tablet of the 25/100 immediate-release formulation should be helpful. Try this for several doses. If still insufficient, you can raise the dose again by another half-tablet. Note that this relates to each carbidopa/levodopa dose and not the total daily dose. Once that time of the month is over, return to the prior carbidopa/levodopa dosing scheme.

"MY LEVODOPA EFFECT DOESN'T LAST AS LONG DURING MY MENSES."

If carbidopa/levodopa kicks in adequately during menses but the effect does not last long enough, then don't change the size of the doses. Rather, shorten the interval between doses to match the response duration. Obviously, if you shorten the interval between doses, you will need to add an extra dose or two each day so that you are not uncovered at the end of the day. Once the problematic time of the menstrual cycle is passed, revert back to the previous dosing scheme.

POSTMENOPAUSAL ESTROGEN REPLACEMENT THERAPY

Will estrogen therapy (e.g., Premarin, Estrace) affect PD and the response to PD medications? It will probably not have any major impact on parkinsonian symptoms or the response to carbidopa/levodopa. If anything, it likely will improve your response to PD medications. Any decision to start estrogen therapy should be made on other grounds.

29

♦ ♦ ♦

Other Treatment Problems: Swelling, Skin Rashes, and Visual Symptoms

Several other conditions are common in Parkinson's disease (PD) and require treatment other than carbidopa/levodopa and related drugs. In this chapter, three such problems are discussed: swollen legs, certain specific skin rashes, and visual distortions or blurring.

Swollen Legs

Swelling of the legs is common among seniors, and the likelihood increases with age. For reasons to be addressed below, those with PD may be more susceptible. Sometimes the swelling is mild and unimportant. However, it could also be a sign of a medical condition that requires attention. Before addressing specific causes and treatments, background information is necessary.

The medical term for swelling is *edema*. Leg edema typically relates to problems of veins. Recall that *arteries* carry blood from the heart to the rest of the body; after the oxygen and nutrients have been extracted, blood flows back to the heart via the *veins*. If blood flow is impeded in leg veins, fluid (water) tends to leach out into the surrounding tissues. In fact, this may occur if there is resistance to the flow of venous blood anywhere between the leg veins and the heart. Thus a clot in a leg vein may cause leg edema, as would a failing heart that cannot keep up with the necessary pumping of blood.

Edema may also occur if there is excessive fluid in the body or if the veins have been damaged and are leaky. Some types of leg edema are more important than others. First, we should discuss more concerning causes of leg swelling

URGENT: ONE SWOLLEN, TENDER LEG

A blood clot in a leg vein causes swelling due to the impaired flow. The increased pressure in the vein behind the clot causes leakage of fluid into the surrounding leg tissues. This backed-up venous blood distends the affected veins, resulting in tenderness and aching pain. Such leg vein blood clots are termed *thrombophlebitis* and nearly always affect just one leg.

Thrombophlebitis is potentially life-threatening, due to the potential for the clot to dislodge and travel in the vein to the lungs, termed *pulmonary embolism* (plural, emboli). Massive pulmonary emboli may prevent blood return to the lungs, which could be fatal. Hence people with leg thrombophlebitis must have this condition recognized early in the course and treated. Treatment typically involves a major blood thinner (anticoagulant).

The diagnosis of leg thrombophlebitis starts with proper suspicion. If one leg becomes swollen and tender, this must be brought to the attention of the clinician. A simple ultrasound study of the leg veins can then be done to determine if there is indeed a clot.

In the context of PD, those who are chronically sedentary are more prone to leg thrombophlebitis. This is due to pooling of blood in leg veins, pulled there by gravity when seated with the legs hanging down. It is harder for blood to flow uphill, which is the case when seated with the feet on the floor. Although the uphill flow also occurs when standing venous blood flow is facilitated by the leg muscle contractions during walking. Obviously, many adults with office jobs spend much of the day sitting and rarely experience this problem. However, prolonged and recurrent sitting without activating the leg muscles is one factor among others that may lead to thrombophlebitis. Slowly moving blood, which pools in the feet and legs, clots more easily. Strategies for reducing this particular risk factor include elevating the legs to about the level of the heart (allowing gravity to assist venous blood flow), as well as frequent breaks from sitting with short walks.

Clues to thrombophlebitis, rather than some other less worrisome cause of leg swelling, include the following.

- *Affects one leg*: More benign forms of leg swelling typically involve both legs, whereas thrombophlebitis almost always affects only one leg.

- *Recent onset:* A single swollen leg that developed in the last few days or weeks should raise suspicions.

- *Pain*: The swelling is often, but not always painful, usually in the calf. This is in contrast to most other causes of leg swelling, which are painless.

- *Tenderness*: The distension of the veins and perhaps the swelling in surround tissues makes the calf tender when gently squeezed.

If these clues surface, have a low threshold for being urgently evaluated by a physician. If an urgent appointment cannot be arranged, go to the emergency room. If newly developing shortness of breath is experienced, this is even more urgent and rapid transport to the closest emergency room is advisable.

SERIOUS, BUT NOT URGENT CAUSES OF LEG SWELLING

Major internal organ failure may be associated with leg swelling, typically both legs. This is common in congestive heart failure and may be suggestive of cardiac decompensation; that is, the heart is unable to maintain adequate pumping function and blood is backing up in the veins. Edema also may occur in kidney failure due to impaired clearance of fluids and solutes by the kidneys. Physicians typically can sort this out with a history and examination, often complemented by blood tests or a simple imaging study (e.g., ultrasound of the heart, called an *echocardiogram*). Most people with PD and leg swelling have more benign reasons for the edema.

PARKINSON'S DISEASE: COMMON AND LESS SERIOUS CAUSES OF LEG SWELLING

Leg swelling among those with PD usually has less worrisome causes, provided that it involves both legs and is painless:

- Inactivity (with dependency of legs)

- Incompetent veins

- Treatment of orthostatic hypotension with salt

- Dopamine agonist drugs

We will consider each of these, recognizing that often more than one factor plays a role.

Inactivity (Dependency of Legs)

Those with PD may be less active, especially if undertreated with carbidopa/levodopa. As discussed earlier, the more you sit with your legs down, the more the blood tends to pool in the feet and legs, pulled there by gravity. Over the course of the day, tiny amounts of fluid seep from the veins, causing the edema. Leg swelling is common in any neurological disorder in which walking is compromised and people spend most of the day sitting. Strategies for minimizing this include elevating the leg when seated (to the approximate level of the heart) and taking frequent, short walks.

Incompetent Veins

With normal aging, the leg veins lose elasticity, tending to become baggy and often leaky. This is the opposite of what happens to arteries with aging. Arteries tend to narrow because of arthrosclerosis, whereas veins become dilated as they age. In some cases, previous clots in the leg veins (thrombophlebitis) damage these veins. These damaged veins tend to dilate and leak. Knee-high compressive hose are often used to reduce this tendency.

Treatment of Orthostatic Hypotension with Salt

Orthostatic hypotension is a drop in blood pressure occurring when standing, discussed in Chapter 21. The first line of treatment is salt and fluids, sometimes in combination with fludrocortisone, which facilitates sodium (salt) retention. This treatment may cause leg swelling, although it usually is minimal, unless some other factor is at play, such as congestive heart failure.

Dopamine Agonist Medications and Leg Edema

The dopamine agonists pramipexole, ropinirole, and rotigotine cause leg swelling in a minority of treated patients. The mechanism for this is unclear. If you are taking one of these drugs and experiencing minor leg edema, this can be ignored. Occasionally, however, I encounter people on a dopamine agonist with massive leg swelling that is not responding to aggressive edema treatment. Improvement then requires tapering off the agonist.

Amantadine and Legs

Amantadine is typically used to treat levodopa-induced dyskinesias when levodopa dose reduction is not tolerated. Amantadine may cause mild swelling, but more often reddish or purple discoloration of the legs in a fishnet pattern (livido reticularis). This is not a serious problem and does not require eliminating this medication.

TREATMENT OF CHRONIC PAINLESS SWELLING OF BOTH LEGS

We have already alluded to several simple strategies for reducing leg edema when it is not due to thrombophlebitis or to heart or kidney failure. These may be summarized as follows:

- *Salt restriction*: Reducing salt intake is usually an initial strategy for edema treatment, although this may not be feasible if orthostatic hypotension is a problem.

- *Elevate your legs*: Raising the feet to the level of your heart will allow gravity to assist flow in the leg veins while seated. Note that a low footstool will not be high enough.

- *Avoid prolonged sitting*: If you have a sedentary job, periodically get up and walk around. The muscle contractions in your legs during walking tend to pump blood and reverse pooling in your feet. If forced to sit, such as on an airplane, consciously contract the muscles in your legs.

- *Wear compressive hose*: Knee-high compressive hose constrict the leg veins and limit swelling. When purchased, make certain that they are the proper fit; if they are too loose, they won't help. Also, avoid compressive leg bands, such as rubber bands, to hold your stockings up; these will impede blood flow in veins. Be cognizant of the fact that the compressive hose recommended to treat orthostatic hypotension (Chapter 21) require thigh or waist length; to treat leg edema, knee-high hose are appropriate.

- *Diuretics (and a note of caution)*: Physicians often prescribe a diuretic (water pill) to treat swelling, for example, HCTZ (hydrochlorothiazide), triamterene (in Dyazide), or furosemide (Lasix). These drugs induce the kidneys to excrete sodium (salt) and water. However, if you have a tendency toward orthostatic hypotension, diuretics may cause decompensation; that is, diuretics lower blood pressure. Avoid water pills if you have orthostatic hypotension.

Fluids, per se, are not the primary cause of edema, since water without sodium (salt) is excreted by the kidneys. Salt (sodium) in tissues draws in water by osmosis and tends to hold it there. Hence the treatment of swelling typically focuses on reducing sodium intake.

Skin Rashes

SEBORRHEIC DERMATITIS

Seborrheic dermatitis is the hallmark rash of PD and was common before the advent of levodopa. In the current era with carbidopa/levodopa availability,

I rarely encounter this among people I see with PD. Likely, the impaired mobility from advancing PD in the pre-levodopa era compromised self-care and personal hygiene. However, seborrheic dermatitis is not just a hygiene problem, and rigorous washing is not the simple answer once this occurs.

Before we discuss this further, we should define terms. *Seborrhea* is oiliness of the skin. Usually, seborrhea occurs where the skin's oil glands are most dense, especially the face and scalp, as well as regions of skin folds, (e.g., armpits).

Those with seborrhea may develop seborrheic dermatitis. *Dermatitis* is a general term implying inflammation of the skin. In other words, the oiliness of the skin predisposes to an inflammatory reaction. Seborrheic dermatitis is marked by redness and scaling, in addition to the oiliness. This occurs especially over the face, where the reddened, flaky skin is most apparent on the sides of the nose, eyebrows, eyelids, and over the ears. In the scalp, it tends to generate large dandruff-like flakes. Seborrheic dermatitis may also occur in the skin-fold regions where there is a high density of oil glands: arm pits, under the breasts, the groin and buttocks.

THE CAUSE OF SEBORRHEIC DERMATITIS

There are several factors that contribute to the development of this skin condition. Obviously, the oil (sebum) from skin oil glands is a factor and may act as an irritant if left on the skin. Also, it may interact with microscopic skin organisms to generate irritative products. The yeast *Pityrosporum ovale* (also termed, Malassezia) appears to play a central role in the development of seborrheic dermatitis. This yeast is a normal inhabitant of human skin, but under the right conditions, it causes or contributes to this problem. Medications that reduce levels of this yeast, such as ketoconazole or terbinafine, are effective treatments.

TREATING SEBORRHEIC DERMATITIS

If the rash is on the face or scalp and fits the description just given, this could well represent seborrheic dermatitis. If your physician agrees, you could proceed with a course of treatment. If there is doubt, or if treatment proves unsuccessful, a dermatologist should advise.

There are a variety of treatment agents for seborrheic dermatitis, and we will not cover each and every one here. Rather, we will provide limited suggestions; if your physician prefers other agents, defer to those suggestions.

TREATMENT: SEBORRHEIC DERMATITIS
OF THE SCALP, BROWS, AND OTHER HAIRY REGIONS

- Try simple things first. Shampoo two to three times per week with preparations containing either selenium sulfide (e.g., Selsun Blue) or zinc pyrithione (e.g., Head and Shoulders). A product containing a higher concentration of selenium sulfide (2.5% vs. 1%) is also available by prescription. Allow these medicated shampoos to remain in contact with the scalp/face for 5–10 minutes. You could do this by washing, rinsing, and then washing again. In between, use regular shampoo on a daily basis. For milder cases, especially where dandruff is more of the problem than redness, this strategy may be sufficient.

- For more troublesome cases, especially if redness is present, an anti-yeast shampoo containing 2% ketoconazole (e.g., Nizoral) is appropriate. Leave it on for about 5 minutes and apply this two to three times weekly. You may continue to use the shampoos cited in the previous paragraph two to three times weekly, with a regular shampoo the other days. You may also apply the ketoconazole shampoo to your face. This product requires a prescription, although a 1% ketoconazole shampoo is available over the counter and might be effective. Improvement will take 2 to 4 weeks. Once the dermatitis is controlled, you could continue using this once weekly to prevent a recurrence.

- Low-potency steroid (corticosteroid) lotions, gels, or creams are typically an important component of treatment. These are available over the counter as 0.5% or 1% hydrocortisone preparations. They suppress the redness (inflammation). They may be applied daily and even up to three times daily if that seems necessary.

- In addition to the medicated shampoos cited earlier, a 2% ketoconazole cream may also be necessary to eradicate the yeast. Apply this daily after shampooing. It is available either alone or with hydrocortisone, 0.5% or 1%.

- A good alternative to the ketoconazole cream is a cream or gel containing 1% terbinafine (Lamisil), which is available over the counter. It is applied once to twice daily.

TREATMENT: SEBORRHEIC DERMATITIS OF THE FACE AND OTHER NON-HAIRY AREAS

- Washing with a medicated soap is an integral component of treatment. You may choose to wash your face and other affected areas with the same medicated shampoo you use for your hair (see previous discussion). For the face, a bar soap containing zinc pyrithione is available (ZNP soap) and may be used with the same general guidelines described earlier for the hair. You may use this soap or shampoo daily.

• After washing, apply a 2% ketoconazole cream (Nizoral) to the affected areas and reapply later in the day. If you have much redness and inflammation, you may use a ketoconazole preparation that also contains 0.5% or 1% hydrocortisone. Allow up to 4 weeks for a response.

• As mentioned, an excellent alternative to the ketoconazole cream is terbinafine (Lamisil), sold over the counter as a 1% cream or gel. As with ketoconazole, apply this twice daily.

Are there any serious side effects that one could encounter with these skin treatments? Typically not, but if it seems that the agent(s) you are using is causing irritation or in some other way making the problem worse, abandon that treatment and have a dermatologist review treatment. Rare individuals are allergic to sulfites and may experience a reaction to ketoconazole. If you suspect a sulfite allergy, don't use this unless your physician approves.

RASHES CAUSED BY MEDICATIONS FOR PD

Although the drugs for PD may cause side effects, rarely do they cause skin eruptions or true allergic reactions. There are two exceptions:

1. Amantadine frequently causes discoloration of the legs with a mottled (chicken wire pattern) purple or red appearance, sometimes with mild swelling. It is not dangerous, and if it does not bother you it is acceptable to continue taking amantadine.

2. Carbidopa/levodopa in the 25/100 immediate-release formulation may rarely cause a rash. Importantly, the rash is *not* from either the carbidopa or levodopa, but rather from the yellow food coloring used in the preparation of this particular pill. The other carbidopa/levodopa preparations are formulated with different color additives and these may be used instead: immediate-release 10/100, 25/250 (both blue), sustained-release 25/100 (pink or gray), and 50/200 (tan or gray).

If you are allergic to yellow dye and wish to start carbidopa/levodopa, use the same schedules shown in Chapter 12, but substitute the 10/100 tablets for the 25/100 tablets. These have the same levodopa content and hence the same potency; they can be used interchangeably. There is less carbidopa with the 10/100 formulation and, consequently, a greater possibility of nausea. If nausea develops, add one 25 mg supplementary carbidopa tablet (Lodosyn; orange pill) with each 10/100 pill; this effectively converts the dose to 35/100. See also the discussion of supplementary carbidopa in Chapter 12. Recall that if nausea is not experienced, the amount of carbidopa may be ignored.

DISCOLORED LEGS DUE TO INCOMPETENT VEINS

Leg veins may become damaged and incompetent with aging, especially with prior leg blood clots. Damaged veins may result in slow leakage of fluids and blood products into the leg tissues. When this occurs on a chronic basis, these products may discolor the skin, sometimes resulting in a low-grade inflammatory reaction; this has been termed *stasis dermatitis*. The skin discoloration typically has a brownish appearance and is often distended by the leg swelling. This bronze or brown discoloration is the clue to this process. Sometimes varicose veins are prominent as well. If this has induced a prominent inflammatory reaction, there may also be redness and scaling of the skin, sometimes with weeping sores.

There is no quick and easy treatment of this problem. The typical strategies include the following.

- Avoid prolonged standing.

- When sitting, elevate the legs to the level of the heart.

- Wear compressive hose fitted to the size of your legs when up and about; take these off at night when in bed.

- If you are obese, attempt to lose weight.

- If there is a prominent inflammatory component, an over-the-counter corticosteroid cream may be applied two to three times daily for a few weeks. For more troublesome problems, a higher potency prescription topical corticosteroid is often employed.

If there are open sores, a dermatology consultation is advisable. People with stasis dermatitis are prone to reactions from creams and salves, especially antibiotic ointments. Hence the treatment may become complex.

Water pills (diuretics) are typically a mainstay of treatment to reduce leg swelling. However, those prone to orthostatic hypotension (low blood pressure when standing) should use diuretics sparingly, if at all. The standing-up blood pressure should be checked before starting a water pill and periodically rechecked after. If you are starting a diuretic and if feeling light-headed, this is a clue to a low blood pressure (see Chapter 21).

DRY SKIN

Dry, flaky skin is a common age-related problem among seniors. Chronic sun exposure in prior years is a contributor. In northern climates, the dry heat from furnaces in the wintertime exacerbates this problem. Those frequently exposed to solvents or detergents (including homemakers doing the dishes) will be even more prone to this in the exposed areas.

Dry skin can be treated with a variety of measures. Common-sense strategies include the following:

- Avoid exposure to solvents and detergents as much as possible. Use protectant gloves if necessary. Although frequent hand-washing with soaps also dries the skin, certain bar soaps are less problematic, including Aveenobar, Purpose, and white Dove soap.

- Religiously apply a moisturizer immediately after washing and perhaps again later in the day. These are more effective when the skin surface is still slightly damp after bathing. The moisturizer prevents evaporation of the water that has been absorbed from the bath, preventing the skin from drying out. A range of moisturizers may be found in the drugstore, such as CeraVe, Keri, Lubriderm, Moisturel, and Nivea. Certain thicker formulations remain in place longer but are messier, such as Eucerin, Aquaphor, and various petroleum products (variations on Vaseline).

If you have more than dry skin, with redness and swelling, then have your doctor evaluate this.

Visual Symptoms

PD will not cause you to lose your vision. Although researchers have identified subtle visual conditions among those with PD, these do not translate into meaningful problems. For example, minor abnormalities of color vision have been found in PD patients. Also, the retina of the eye is mildly altered in PD, documented with special ophthalmological testing called *optical coherence tomography*.

Impaired vision affecting people with PD primarily occurs due to age-related eye conditions. This deserves further elaboration.

COMMON CAUSES OF IMPAIRED VISUAL
ACUITY AMONG SENIORS

With aging, vision declines in a variety of ways. Since most people with PD are middle-aged and older, these age-related eye problems are relevant. First, background information on normal eye structure and function is appropriate. Visual acuity requires each component of the eyes to be working optimally. These components include the following:

- *The pupil*: This is the aperture in the front of the eye that lets in the light. Just like the aperture of an automatic camera, the pupil enlarges or constricts, depending on the amount of ambient light.

- *The lens*: This is just behind the pupil and focuses the light appropriately on the back of the eye (i.e., on the retina), just like the lens of a camera. The lens refocuses as we shift our gaze from near to far.

- *The vitreous*: This is the water-like fluid that is contained within the eye. The image focused on the retina passes through this clear fluid.

- *The retina*: This is analogous to the film in a camera. The lens focuses the light rays on the retina, which registers that image. The image on the retina is then transmitted to the brain. Transmission from the retina is via the ophthalmic nerve to lower brain centers and ultimately to the visual cortex (occipital lobe).

These eye components age to variable degrees, sometimes affecting visual acuity. The usual conditions that may affect vision during normal aging include the following:

- *Fixation of lens shape*: Through early adulthood, the lens shape automatically changes, allowing us to easily shift focus from far to near and vice versa. By middle age, the lens loses this flexibility—the primary reason for requiring reading glasses in mid-life.

- *Floaters*: Debris may collect in the vitreous fluid producing spots that "float" in the visual field. Usually, these are benign; however, if massive, this could be a sign of bleeding in the retina and warrant evaluation by an ophthalmologist.

- *Macular degeneration*: This is a degenerative condition of the retina that may develop later in life; it may seriously impair vision when advanced.

- *Cataracts*: This aging change causes clouding of the lens; this is treated with surgical resection of the affected lens.

All of these conditions are common among those with PD, but no more common than among the general population of the same age.

GLAUCOMA AND PD MEDICATIONS

Glaucoma is an eye condition characterized by the pressure inside the eye rising above normal. If the pressure is sufficiently high on a chronic basis, this may result in damage to the retina. The anticholinergic drugs listed in Table 23.1 (Chapter 23) tend to increase the intraocular pressure; those with glaucoma should be wary of this and discuss it with their ophthalmologist. Theoretically, carbidopa/levodopa could worsen glaucoma, but this has not been the general experience. If you have glaucoma and take carbidopa/levodopa, inform your ophthalmologist, who can monitor your eye pressure.

DOUBLE VISION

Seniors occasionally develop double vision (diplopia). Diplopia may have a variety of causes, warranting evaluation by an ophthalmologist and sometimes by a neurologist. Often no specific cause is identified. It is unclear whether people with PD are more susceptible to double vision.

The cause for double vision, in general, is loss of normal eye alignment. Our two eyes normally see things in parallel. Each eye focuses on the same image and these images are superimposed in the brain. Normally, the overlap in the brain is precise and we perceive one image. However, if the parallel eye alignment is lost, the images deviate from one another. When this occurs, our brain perceives two images—double vision.

If the eye deviation and double vision are constant, it can sometimes be corrected with a prism in your eyeglasses. A *prism* is an asymmetrically thickened lens that bends the path of light rays. By measuring the degree of the eye deviation, a prism can be fashioned that realigns the visual images in parallel. An alternative strategy involves obscuring one lens of your eyeglasses by taping over it (perhaps with opaque tape); then you will be using only one eye and, hence, see only one image.

Occasionally, medications may provoke double vision. Primarily this is with sedating drugs, such as muscle relaxants, prescription pain medications, or anti-anxiety drugs (see Table 19.2, in Chapter 19). The timing of diplopia should be a clue, such as when it develops shortly after starting a new medication or resolves when a drug has not been taken for many hours.

VISUAL BLURRING

A wide of factors may blur vision, including excessive tearing (which ironically can be triggered by dry eyes; see next section), cataracts or other eye conditions; also dirty eyeglasses should not be overlooked. Medications may also cause visual blurring or reduced acuity, especially the anticholinergic drugs listed in Table 23.1 (Chapter 23). Anticholinergic medications affect the function of the lens and pupil of the eye.

PROBLEMS OF THE OUTER EYE: DRY EYES, EXCESSIVE TEARING

People with PD blink less than normal. Blinking serves a purpose. It lubricates the surface (cornea) of the eyes, preventing drying. A slowed blink rate results in reduced lubrication. As a consequence, the eyes may dry out, causing them to feel irritated. If this is a minor problem, simply applying artificial tears several times daily may be helpful (e.g., HypoTears, Refresh). Also, if parkinsonism is poorly controlled, optimizing carbidopa/levodopa will also help, as this should raise the blink rate toward normal.

Paradoxically, excessive tearing may occasionally be a consequence of dry eyes. The reduced blinking of PD that causes eye dryness reflexively triggers tears. Furthermore, because of the reduced blinking, the tears tend to pool on the lower eyelid, overflowing. Tearing may be so pronounced as to run down the face. For lesser problems, optimized carbidopa/levodopa dosing to increase blinking plus use of artificial tears may be effective. For more troublesome conditions, ophthalmologists are able to treat this by placing plugs in the tear ducts; with the reduction in normal tears, artificial tears are used as a substitute.

INVOLUNTARY EYE CLOSURE (BLEPHAROSPASM)

People with PD occasionally develop involuntary closure of the eyes, termed *blepharospasm* (*blepharo* = eye lid). Blepharospasm is a dystonia, meaning an involuntary spasm or muscle contraction. Hence it is analogous to other forms of dystonia occurring in PD, such as dystonic curling of the toes or foot inversion.

In its mildest form, the blepharospasm of PD manifests as increased blinking. When more severe blepharospasm, the eyes may tend to involuntarily stay closed. Anything that irritates the eyes, especially drying of the eyes, will exacerbate this problem.

Blepharospasm is not common among those with PD, and when I have encountered it, it most often has been associated with levodopa off-states, or when parkinsonism is insufficiently treated with carbidopa/levodopa. It may also be seen in those who have a parkinsonism-plus disorder, most notably progressive supranuclear palsy (see Chapter 6).

Treatment of blepharospasm is along two lines. First, an ophthalmologist should evaluate the eyes to determine if an inflammatory eye condition is present, or whether there has been any subtle injury to the outer surface of the eye, the cornea. Dried or inflamed eyes will tend to reflexively close. Excessive dryness of the eyes should be treated, and the ophthalmologist can address whether there is an injury to the cornea. If the ophthalmologist excludes a primary cornea disorder, control of parkinsonism with carbidopa/levodopa should be optimized, since this eye dystonia may be a symptom of PD. If blepharospasm occurs only during levodopa off-states, then these fluctuations should be treated as discussed in Chapter 17. On the other hand, if parkinsonism is generally doing poorly, blepharospasm may be one component, requiring more aggressive carbidopa/levodopa treatment across the board (see Chapter 12).

Uncommonly, blepharospasm could be a manifestation of an excessive levodopa response. If it occurs only when the levodopa effect is present (on-state) and goes away several hours after a dose, then this is likely. Similarly, if blepharospasm is present only during times of levodopa dyskinesias (i.e., levodopa excess), it likely is from an excessive levodopa effect. If you think it is being directly provoked by carbidopa/levodopa, you can test this by skipping a carbidopa/levodopa dose. If the blepharospasm is absent when you have not taken carbidopa/levodopa for 6 hours or so, a reduction in the levodopa dose should be considered.

Finally, for those who cannot control blepharospasm with simpler measures, botulinum toxin injections are appropriate. It is administered via a tiny needle and weakens muscles at the site of the injection. The effect typically lasts 2 to 4 months. For treatment of blepharospasm, botulinum toxin is injected into the muscles surrounding the eyes responsible for eye closure. This procedure is typically done by either an ophthalmologist or neurologist. This should be reimbursed by Medicare, Medicaid, and health insurance.

HALLUCINATIONS

Seeing things that aren't there occurs in PD, often provoked by medications. This is a problem of brain visual perception centers, rather than the eye, although severe vision loss predisposes to hallucinations. We discussed hallucinations in Chapter 24.

PART TEN

◆ ◆ ◆

Nutrition, Exercise, Work, and Family

30

♦ ♦ ♦

Diet, Vitamins, Nutrition, Osteoporosis

Do I Need a Special Diet?

In general, those with Parkinson's disease (PD) do not require dietary changes. If you have a well-balanced diet, that is sufficient. You should also avoid obesity, since carrying extra body weight compromises movement and gait. To maintain a stable body weight, your caloric intake should match your energy expenditure. If you eat more, then additional exercise is necessary.

Whereas PD per se does not require major dietary changes, people with short-duration levodopa responses may need attention to dietary protein and the timing of meals, as discussed in Chapter 17. To reiterate, if the carbidopa/levodopa dosing interval is less than 4 hours, some of the carbidopa/levodopa doses will fall close to meals and be inhibited by dietary protein; recall that amino acids compete with levodopa for transport into the brain. Chapter 17 addressed strategies for working around this problem. Note, however, that protein is an important constituent of our diets, and at least one meal daily should contain protein sufficient to meet the daily requirement.

Homocysteine and Levodopa Therapy

Homocysteine is a metabolic byproduct of certain biochemical reactions in the body and can be measured in the bloodstream. High levels of homo-cysteine have been consistently associated with an increased risk of strokes, heart attacks, and dementia. The risks are relatively small but statistically significant. Researchers continue to debate whether high homocysteine concentrations directly cause these problems or whether this is simply an association. General clinicians treating strokes and heart attacks often do not measure homocysteine levels in their patients because of uncertainty of whether this is of clinical (causative) importance. Nonetheless, the associations have been well documented.

Numerous studies have documented the tendency for carbidopa/levodopa treatment to elevate homocysteine concentrations. This occurs because the metabolism of homocysteine and levodopa use certain of the same cofactors: folic acid (folate), vitamin B12, and vitamin B6. In some (but not all) carbidopa/levodopa-treated patients, there may not be enough of these three vitamins to fully metabolize both levodopa and homocysteine. If the levodopa metabolic pathway borrows these vitamins from the homocys-teine pathway, homocysteine levels may rise.

It has long been known that elevated homocysteine levels in the general population normalize with administration of relatively large doses of folic acid and vitamins B12 and B6. This is also an effective treatment if the cause of high homocysteine concentrations is due to carbidopa/levodopa.

Clinicians prescribing carbidopa/levodopa who are concerned about homocysteine could simply order a homocysteine blood test. If levels are elevated, they could be treated, and if normal, then not treated. Of course, the problem for these clinicians is that a one-time measurement may not be sufficient. Any subsequent increase in the daily levodopa dose might further challenge these biochemical pathways. In other words, someone with an ini-tially normal homocysteine level but later taking more carbidopa/levodopa doses should then have homocysteine retested. This situation could become complicated.

My personal solution is to treat everyone taking carbidopa/levodopa with the vitamin supplement conventionally prescribed for elevated homocysteine levels. I am unsure if the potential compromise of homocysteine metabolism by carbidopa/levodopa is clinically important, but I do not wish to take any chances. This prescription medication contains high levels of three vitamins in a single pill:

Folic acid (folate)—2.5 mg

Vitamin B12—1–2 mg (1000–2000 mcg)

Vitamin B6—25 mg

The vitamin concentrations may vary slightly among the different brands, but they are essentially interchangeable. There is no true generic, so the prescription is written with one of the brand names, such as Folbic, Folgard, or Folbee. A prescription for this is necessary, since the concentrations are much higher than those available over the counter.

There is no risk of overdose with either folic acid (folate) or vitamin B12 (also called cyanocobalamin); these are safe in even very high concentrations. Very high doses of vitamin B6 (pyridoxine) can be toxic, but with doses more than 10 times higher than in these prescription vitamins (i.e., 25 mg of vitamin B6 is not close to being dangerous and is safe even if combined with a multivitamin).

Most neurologists do not prescribe a folic acid–vitamin B12, B6 supplement to their carbidopa/levodopa-treated patients. However, since this is a benign medication, few would object.

Osteoporosis and Calcium Metabolism

The density of our bones decreases as we age. Bone mass severely lost through this process is termed *osteoporosis*. When osteoporosis occurs, bones become susceptible to fracture. This is typically the underlying process when seniors fall and fracture a hip.

Calcium is the primary element that is critical for bone strength. Separate from the importance to bone structure, calcium is required for many important metabolic processes. Blood levels of calcium are tightly controlled by various internal regulatory mechanisms. A constant blood level of calcium is critical for normal physiology.

Our body's storehouse of calcium is located within our bones. If blood levels of calcium are low, the body's regulatory mechanisms pull calcium out of bones. This can lead to osteoporosis. Studies indicate that many Americans over the age of 50 receive inadequate amounts of dietary calcium. Obviously, this deficiency may contribute to osteoporosis and fracture risk.

VITAMIN D

The absorption of calcium from our diet takes place in the small intestines, and vitamin D is required for this to be done in an efficient manner. Once ingested, vitamin D is biochemically modified to make it a more effective. One important step in this processing of vitamin D requires skin sunlight exposure. Sunlight striking the skin is part of the natural process that converts vitamin D into a metabolically active form. Although not a lot of sun exposure is required, many adults in our culture spend little time outside, especially in northern climates with long winters.

Studies suggest that many with PD have suboptimal vitamin D intake and metabolism. Hence people with PD may need slightly more vitamin D than average.

LACK OF EXERCISE PROMOTES OSTEOPOROSIS

Inactivity also promotes calcium reabsorption from bone. This renders bone less dense, and therefore more prone to fracture. Hence those with PD who have curtailed their physical activities may be especially susceptible to osteoporosis.

OSTEOPOROSIS RISK IS INCREASED IN PD

To summarize, those with PD tend to be prone to the development of osteoporosis for several reasons:

- Osteoporosis occurs with aging, and PD is most common among seniors.

- A sedentary lifestyle, as may occur in PD, facilitates development of osteoporosis. Physical activity is necessary to maintain bone strength.

- Reduced outside activities with little sun exposure limits the metabolic conversion of vitamin D to the fully active form.

- Those with PD who treat orthostatic hypotension with increased salt intake tend to reciprocally excrete calcium in the urine.

DETECTING OSTEOPOROSIS

Osteoporosis is without symptoms until a bone fracture occurs. It may be suspected from x-rays, but is routinely assessed with a particular type of bone scan called a *bone density study* (dual-energy x-ray absorptiometry, or DEXA scan; DXA scan). Bone density scans are relatively painless. A substance is injected by vein that binds to bones. This injected substance has a radioactive marker that is detected by the scanner and provides an index of bone mass and strength. The radioactivity exposure is minimal and of no consequence.

There are three general categories of bone integrity: normal, osteopenia, and osteoporosis. *Osteoporosis* implies reduced bone strength with substantial risk of breaking with trauma. *Osteopenia* is a lesser degree of bone weakness intermediate between osteoporosis and normality. Treating clinicians are able to consult tables or websites that provide risks of fracture in relation to the bone density values.

PREVENTION OF OSTEOPOROSIS

Because the development of osteoporosis is without symptoms, it is wise to take early preemptive measures. This includes adequate daily intake of vitamin D and calcium, plus exercise.

The advice for daily intake of vitamin D and calcium varies slightly depending on the source, but a sensible recommendation for all adults middle-age and older may be summarized:

Vitamin D: 800–1,000 units daily

Calcium: 1200 mg of *elemental* calcium daily

The vitamin D and calcium may come from a variety of sources, including diet, vitamin pills, or supplements. Note that one multivitamin tablet usually contains 400 units of vitamin D, as does drinking a quart of milk. Vitamin D is routinely measured by a blood test, and this may help guide the intake.

Why is "elemental" calcium specified in these recommendations? The amount of calcium is measured in two different ways, which specifies the method being used. Calcium in pill form is attached to another substance, such as gluconate, phosphate, lactate, or carbonate (e.g., calcium gluconate). Unless "elemental" calcium is specified, the measurement may include both calcium and the substance to which it is combined; in other words, it may relate to the total compound of calcium plus carbonate or calcium plus gluconate. The term *elemental* indicates that only the element calcium is being specified. The recommendation of 1,200 mg elemental calcium implies calcium measured by itself, and not with the other ingredient (e.g., carbonate, gluconate, etc.). When looking for the calcium content on pill labels, look for "elemental calcium," which may be buried in small print. If only "calcium" is specified, that likely relates to the total amount of both calcium and the attached molecule (i.e., carbonate, gluconate, etc.).

Individuals prone to kidney stones should consult their physician. Many kidney stones contain calcium, and if they do, these guidelines are not appropriate. Note that the content of kidney stones can be analyzed to determine the ingredients and guide the treatment.

MILK

Milk is a good source of calcium and vitamin D. However, milk is also a source of protein, which may inhibit levodopa from entering the brain. This is not a problem if carbidopa/levodopa doses are not taken at the same time as milk ingestion, similar to the guidelines for protein meals.

TREATMENT OF DOCUMENTED OSTEOPOROSIS

When bone density scans reveal osteoporosis, the administered treatment goes beyond simple calcium and vitamin D supplementation. Medications called *bisphosphonates* may be prescribed, which increase bone density; there are both oral as well as intravenous formulations. This includes drugs such as alendronate (Fosamax), ibandronate (Boniva), risedronate (Actonel), and zoledronate (Zometa; Reclast). Drugs that directly interact with calcium metabolism are also used, such as calcitonin nasal spray (Miacalcin, Fortical) or the parathyroid hormone analog teriparatide (Forteo). A relatively new drug, denosumab (Prolia), is a monoclonal antibody that targets and inhibits the cells that break down bone (osteoclasts). Treatment may also include the administration of an estrogen in certain postmenopausal women, for example, raloxifene (Evista).

Occasionally, one of these drugs may be recommended for someone in the osteopenic category (i.e., the intermediate category between normal and osteoporosis). This may be sensible for those who are at risk for falls.

Supplements, Multivitamins

The medication lists of seniors in my neurology clinic typically include a long array of over-the-counter supplements and vitamins. There is a huge market for a variety of dietary supplements and these are aggressively advertised. Although most of these are benign, many are expensive and have no proof of benefit. Furthermore, the medication list often becomes so lengthy and complicated that important prescription medications are overlooked. To rephrase Einstein, medication lists should be kept as simple as possible, but not simpler. In other word, maintain drugs with a clear and proven purpose and eliminate the rest. I can assure you that your doctor will greatly appreciate this, since long drug lists make it challenging to keep things straight.

We have already addressed vitamins and supplements that have a clear purpose: calcium, vitamin D, and a folic acid/vitamin B6/vitamin B12 supplement (for those taking carbidopa/levodopa). If you have no major gastrointestinal disease and eat a well-balanced diet and have a stable body weight, you should not need other dietary supplements. If you use a multivitamin for the 400 units of vitamin D in each tablet, that is reasonable to maintain. However, the other ingredients in a multivitamin are easily obtained through your diet. Those individuals with major gastrointestinal disorders, cancer, or liver or kidney failure or who have undergone bariatric (weight reduction) surgery or weight loss may need certain additional vitamins or supplements, and a physician should then advise.

ANTIOXIDANT VITAMINS

For years, antioxidant supplements have been advised for nearly every medical condition. To put this into context, consider the body's oxidation chemistry. Obviously, oxygen is fundamental to life. Countless oxygen reactions are ongoing in every cell of our body—that is, oxidation. Scientists know that excessive oxidation can damage cells. However, oxidation reactions are so crucial and ubiquitous that there are many natural biological mechanisms in our cells that protect against excessive oxidation. Any serious insult to cells does tend to unleash oxidative mechanisms that are involved in degradation and disposal of damaged cellular components or the cells themselves. This is important to the well-being of our organs and the repair processes. Many cellular checks and balancing mechanisms modulate these oxidative mechanisms. There is speculation, however, that such oxidation may contribute to disease states. This is theoretically defensible, but without evidence that antioxidant drug interventions provide benefit in this complex process.

Antioxidant medications for PD were prominently advocated a quarter of a century ago. This enthusiasm led to a major, controlled clinical trial at that time, assessing the response to large doses of the potent antioxidant vitamin E (the DATATOP trial, listed as the first entry in Table 9.1 in Chapter 9). The enthusiasm for such antioxidant treatment waned when the trial results revealed that 1 year of high-dose vitamin E was no better than placebo (sugar pill). Since then, no other antioxidant strategies have been demonstrated to provide benefit to those with PD in controlled clinical trials.

COENZYME Q10

In the first edition of this book, a small clinical trial of coenzyme Q10 administered to people with PD was discussed. The rationale for this trial related to the fact that coenzyme Q10 is a cofactor in an important biological pathway in mitochondria. Notably, mitochondria tend to be dysfunctional among those with PD. In that trial, coenzyme Q10 doses of 300 mg and 600 mg were no better than placebo, whereas PD patients administered 1,200 mg daily fared significantly better than placebo treatment. In the interim, two randomized, long-term, clinical trials with many more PD subjects failed to show coenzyme Q10 benefit. These included comparable doses (1,200 mg daily) as well as higher doses (2,400 mg daily). Hence, it appears that the book is now closed on coenzyme Q10 treatment of PD.

ONE MORE THING: VITAMIN B6 (PYRIDOXINE) AND CARBIDOPA/LEVODOPA

When levodopa therapy was first introduced in the 1960s, it was administered as levodopa, alone, without carbidopa. At that time, it was recognized that levodopa metabolism in the circulation could be accelerated by administration of vitamin B6 (pyridoxine), reducing levodopa effectiveness. However, research documented that this no longer occurred with the addition of carbidopa to make carbidopa/levodopa. Despite this recognition decades ago, admonitions still occasionally surface advising elimination of pyridoxine supplements (vitamin B6) if one is taking carbidopa/levodopa. This advice can be ignored.

31

♦ ♦ ♦

Exercise, Physical Medicine, and Physical Therapy

Aerobic Exercise

We have no drugs proven to slow the course of Parkinson's disease (PD). However, a compelling argument was made in Chapter 9 for ongoing aerobic exercise as a strategy that may slow PD progression. Beyond that, there is also substantial evidence for aerobic exercise having anti-aging benefit, tending to counter age-related loss of muscle, bone, and brain volume. Exercise also tends to counter atherosclerosis (hardening of the arteries). Atherosclerosis increases the risks of strokes, heart attacks, and dementia (small artery atherosclerosis appears to add to dementing processes). Finally, exercise is good medicine for treating depression and is crucial to countering the weight gain common in later life.

Aerobic exercise is physical exercise that tends to increase your pulse, cause you to perspire, and tire you out—vigorous exercise. This should be a central strategy for countering not only PD but also aging.

A discussion of ongoing vigorous exercise is timely for all in our society, where much of what we do is passive. Many of our jobs are performed at desks or standing behind counters, with little expenditure of physical energy. Our recreation has become increasingly passive, focused on television, computers, and electronic games. Our Western culture is paying a price for this couch potato lifestyle, with a striking rise in obesity as well as the secondary negative health consequences. This passivity translates into increased rates of diabetes mellitus and risks of heart attacks and strokes. Moreover, the complications of normal aging are exacerbated by this easy lifestyle. Osteoporosis is accelerated by lack of physical activity, with consequent hip fractures. As we age, our muscles tend to lose their strength and bulk (sarcopenia), and this is exacerbated by lack of physical activity. Our tendons and ligaments lose their elasticity with age, and a sedentary life style increases the symptoms of stiffness and aching. The old adage "if you don't use it, you lose it" is an irrefutable fact relevant to aging. Graceful aging requires that we all stay physically (and mentally) active to preserve our bodies as best we can.

Parkinson's disease is inextricably tied to aging. It usually starts in middle age or beyond and parallels the aging process; the longer you have PD, the older you get. Thus, people with PD need to fight both their disease and normal aging. It turns out that vigorous exercise is a key element in both of these battles.

Aerobic exercise instruction is generally not within the domain of physical therapists, even though they likely favor such exercise and should be in a position to advise. Unfortunately, medical reimbursement does not cover aerobic exercise training. Hence, this is something that must be self-initiated.

Physical trainers can be quite helpful, although their fees will be an out-of-pocket expense. They can identify exercise schemes tailored to individual needs and with appropriate escalation of the workload. Frequent scheduled appointments with a trainer can additionally reinforce exercise habits (it is easy to drop out after a few weeks).

As mentioned in Chapter 9, a discussion with your primary care physician prior to starting a vigorous exercise program is often advisable. Heart or lung conditions or orthopedic problems may require modifications or limitations. Such limitations can then be communicated to the trainer.

Crucial to engagement in aerobic exercise in PD is optimization of carbidopa/levodopa dosage. In the last 20 years, a school of thought has emerged that advises very conservative use of this medication, including "saving it for later." Unfortunately, saving it for the future may put people at risk for an increasingly sedentary lifestyle, which can be very difficult to reverse (i.e., if you don't use it you lose it). Moreover, there is no evidence that levodopa responses can be "saved" for later; likely, this translates into lost opportunities. It is important to maintain mobility and the capacity for exercise, which often requires adequate carbidopa/levodopa dosage. Hence the advice in Chapters 12, 15, and 17 should be considered a prelude to engagement in our vigorous exercise routines.

Forms of vigorous exercise are myriad and many cost nothing. Unless you have marked imbalance or major orthopedic problems, simple walking is an excellent exercise. Ideally, the walking would be at a brisk pace. However, start more slowly if that seems appropriate. Later you can set goals for walking speed and distance. For those with good legs and balance and no cardiopulmonary disease, a 3-mile walk three to four times a week would provide an excellent exercise routine.

Not to be overlooked are routines around the house, such as walking behind a lawnmower (not a riding mower), raking leaves, shoveling snow, digging holes for tree-planting, and any project that makes you tired and sweaty.

Exercise equipment in the home or basement also provides an excellent outlet. This might include an exercise bicycle or rowing machine, which can be used in the sitting position. Treadmills are also a good choice, if the moving platform does not put you at risk for a fall.

Seniors often have outdoor recreational exercise options such as golf or pickleball. Unfortunately, golfers are often encouraged to use carts, negating the exercise benefits.

Most communities have health clubs, YMCAs or YWCAs, and gyms, with an array of exercise equipment. This typically includes various exercise machines that can be used in the sitting position (important if there is poor balance). Resistance exercises, such as weight-lifting, are extremely beneficial for maintaining muscle strength, which tends to diminish with age. These exercises can be done sitting, as can those with the resistance machines (e.g., Cybex). One can transform these resistance exercises into aerobic routines by reducing the weight (resistance) to values that can be performed 15–20 times before tiring, and then quickly moving to the next exercise without resting.

Health centers often have swimming pools that can be used to swim laps. Swimming the length of the pool back and forth is an excellent form of aerobic exercise. Note that formal water exercise routines typically have a different purpose than aerobic exercise; simply stretching and toning in water does not translate into aerobic exercise.

Aerobic exercise tends to make people hot, sweaty, and tired and to raise the heart rate. These parameters suggest that the exercise is sufficiently vigorous, tending to make us fit. However, these parameters do not necessary relate to all aerobic exercises or all people. Thus, swimming laps is not associated with sweating, but is a superb aerobic exercise. People taking a beta-blocker for hypertension, such as atenolol, metoprolol, or propranolol will be unable to raise their heart rates (a common measure of exercise vigor); however, that does not indicate absence of exercise benefit.

One key element of such aerobic exercise routines is to choose activities that you will maintain. It doesn't help in the long run to exercise fanatically for 6 weeks, get bored, and then give it up. Often, switching from one type of exercise activity to another is a good way to maintain interest. For example, if you belong to a health club, you may elect to ride an exercise bicycle for several weeks, then switch to a rowing machine and perhaps add weight training. If that starts to get old, you might swim laps, or join an appropriate aerobics class. Finding an "exercise buddy" who partners in such exercise activities often helps maintain these good habits.

If you have been leading a sedentary lifestyle, start your exercise program slowly, with limited immediate goals. Exercises that are onerous tend not to be continued. It is easy to talk yourself out of exercising. However, as you acclimate to your new program after a few weeks, push yourself a little and increase the exercise goals. Part of the fun of exercise is seeing yourself reach new heights. However, this is never immediate, and you need to be patient. Remember that life is a marathon, not a sprint.

A Second Form of Exercise with Different Goals

Distinct from aerobic exercise are strategies focusing on developing good motor patterns, improving balance, and increasing flexibility. This approach complements aerobic exercise but has quite different goals and distinctly different methods. Physical therapists have the primary responsibility for instructing people in these routines, and this therapy is medically reimbursable, although not indefinitely.

REFERRAL TO A PHYSICAL THERAPIST FOR BALANCE TRAINING, STRETCHING, AND IMPROVING MOTOR PATTERNS

The benefits from a physical therapy referral depend on the needs and limitations of the individual PD patient. For example, many in my clinic are still very capable of going for walks, raking leaves, playing golf, and going to the gym. I usually do not refer these people to physical therapy, but rather encourage active engagement in a variety of physical routines that can be incorporated into their usual activities. Raking leaves on a gentle slope is not only good aerobic exercise but also provides a form of balance training. Playing golf or tennis tends to facilitate good limb range of motion and helps one to maintain adequate balance.

By contrast, those with PD who are becoming more compromised do indeed benefit from referral to a physical therapist. At larger medical centers the referral is often to the Department of Physical Medicine and Rehabilitation (PMR). This is a specialty in medicine that focuses on the practical needs of people with disabilities, both compensatory strategies and rehabilitation. PMR physicians typically oversee a team of physical and occupational therapists, with the treatment tailored to each patient's needs. They design the physical therapy routines used by the therapists, advise about gait aids (e.g., canes, walkers, motorized scooters), and suggest modifications in the home to assist activities of daily living (e.g., grab bars in showers or by bath tubs).

The exercise strategies employed by physical therapists typically include routines to improve balance, such as practicing standing on one leg (with proper assistance). They also focus on maintaining a good range of motion. The limb rigidity of PD frequently benefits from ongoing range-of-motion exercises and stretching to improve flexibility.

Physical therapists also may instruct in so-called BIG therapy. The rationale is to increase the amplitude (size) of movements. People with PD tend to take short strides when walking; arm swing is attenuated; voluntary movements fall short of normal. Such problems can consciously reversed by thinking about making exaggerated, or "big," movements. This parallels the so-called LOUD speech therapy of LSVT (Lee Silverman Voice Therapy), where those with a soft voice are encouraged to project their voice (talking loudly). These strategies work, although they require ongoing attention to this task.

Ask your therapist if there are any other resources in your community that would be appropriate. For example, Tai Chi classes that enhance flexibility and balance may be available through community centers, YMCAs, and other such centers.

Exercise Issues Unique to Parkinson's Disease

TIPS RELATING TO LEVODOPA DOSING TO FACILITATE EXERCISE

For those with longer-standing PD and fluctuating levodopa responses, there are a few principles you need to know to make exercise go as smoothly as possible:

- Exercise goes best when you are in your levodopa on-state. When the effect has worn off, it is hard to exercise and stretch.

- If you have a narrow margin between carbidopa/levodopa doses causing dyskinesias versus being underdosed, you will exercise best if slightly overdosed despite dyskinesias. Obviously, severe dyskinesias will not be tolerated.

- When exercising, your levodopa effect will not last as long. For example, if you normally experience a 3-hour levodopa response, it may only last 2 hours when vigorously exercising. So take your carbidopa/levodopa doses at appropriately shorter intervals during exercise.

Remember that energy levels are highest and fatigue least during levodopa on-states.

ORTHOSTATIC HYPOTENSION, DIZZINESS, AND EXERCISE

A minority of people with PD experience symptoms from orthostatic hypotension, as was discussed in Chapter 21. This problem of a low blood pressure when being upright translates into light-headedness and, if the blood pressure is very low, risk of fainting. Among susceptible people, this problem surfaces after each carbidopa/levodopa dose; that is, carbidopa/levodopa tends to lower the standing blood pressure for 3–4 hours after each dose.

Symptoms of orthostatic hypotension sometimes develop during vigorous exercise. Exercise generates body heat, and the body normally dissipates heat by dilating skin surface blood vessels. Such dilatation of the vasculature tends to exacerbate orthostatic hypotension.

If you feel faint when exercising, have someone check your blood pressure and pulse at that time. If your systolic blood pressure is less than 90, then the faintness is due to too low a blood pressure. Don't try to continue with the exercise (we don't want you to faint). Treatment was discussed in Chapter 21. Remember that this tends to be a problem in the erect position (standing, walking, running). If this is a persistent problem despite treatment, you might be able to engage in sitting exercises, such as with a rowing machine.

It is also important to check your pulse if you feel faint, because a problem of heart rate could also be the cause. If your rate is very slow, such as less than 40 beats per minute, this should be semi-urgently discussed with your physician. Exercise will normally raise your heart rate, but among those middle-aged and older, it should not rise much above approximately 160 beats per minute. If you feel faint and your heart rate is much greater than that, this also needs to be addressed by your physician.

Physical Therapy Strategies for Certain PD Problems

MOVEMENT FREEZING

Most people think of a cold day when the word *freezing* is used. Those with PD use the term quite differently, to address the momentary paralysis of movement due to parkinsonism. In the vernacular of PD, "frozen gait" relates to an inability to take a step; the feet are stuck in place as if magnetized to the floor. Such freezing may also affect hand movements and sometimes speech. However, it is the frozen gait that is most common and deserves special comment.

People with gait freezing typically experience this in specific circumstances. Notoriously, it occurs when taking the first step; they cannot get started. However, once that first step is taken, they usually are able to continue walking. Once stopped, freezing recurs. Turning around or turning corners also provokes freezing. Turning in place is done with many short steps rather than a smooth pivot. Walking through doorways typically provokes freezing, even when the door is wide open without impediments. Stressful situations or walking in crowds also exacerbates this tendency. With severe gait freezing, people may become stuck in place and require help to restart walking.

Carbidopa/levodopa often effectively treats gait freezing. However, a minority of people cannot control their freezing despite maximum adjustment of carbidopa/levodopa dosage. Presumably, this relates to the Lewy neurodegenerative process extending into brain motor control circuits that do not use dopamine for a neurotransmitter.

Why should your feet initially become stuck to the floor, and then seconds later be able to walk normally once that first step is taken? This presumably relates to the fact that the brain has separate motor control circuits for initiating walking and maintenance of walking. This act of gait *initiation* seems to be especially susceptible to the effects of PD.

Treatment of gait freezing starts with addressing carbidopa/levodopa dosage. This includes identifying the optimum dose; if there are fluctuations, the dosing interval should match the levodopa response duration. Rarely, freezing occurs with excessive doses of dopamine agonists; however, I have encountered this in only three or four people over my 30+ years of practice.

For those with gait freezing despite optimal carbidopa/levodopa dosage, certain physical therapy tricks may be helpful. The theoretical intent is to use your conscious brain to substitute for the malfunctioning brain circuits that program gait.

Initiating walking is an unconscious act, just like swinging your arms when you walk. People with PD tend not to swing their arm(s), but they can if they think about it. Although arm swing is not crucial to walking, this illustrates how one can adapt. Thus, if the brain's unconscious arm-swinging circuit doesn't work properly, you can use a conscious brain motor circuit to override this. In other words, think about swinging your arms, and they will swing.

Similar to consciously swinging your arms during walking, you can make a conscious effort to initiate walking when your feet are frozen. It requires thinking the right thought to do this. Simply thinking about walking is ineffective. You need to think about a different leg movement that will unleash that first step. Once you get started, then walking typically can continue (the brain area that *maintains* walking then takes over). This process starts with a pause, at which time you need to mentally envision a specific movement of one leg. Here are a few tricks that physical therapists might suggest to successfully take that first step:

- Swing one leg forward. Think about simply swinging the leg, rather than walking. Start with a long leg swing that will place that leg far in front of you (but not so far that you will fall).

- Try goose-stepping. This was the marching gait of German soldiers. They would stiffly lock their knees and march by taking long, stiff steps. Envision what they looked like and keep this thought as you take your first step.

- Think about a drum major's marching step, raising one leg straight up off the ground before placing it forward. Envision that same movement when you get stuck.

- Think about a drill sergeant's marching cadence: "one-two, one-two, one-two. . . ." You might even count out loud. This might get you started and help you mentally envision a marching step.

- Thinking of a certain musical tune may be helpful. For example, a gliding first step may come more easily if you hum "Blue Danube" in your mind and imagine a ballroom dancer gliding in that same way. A boogie or rock-and-roll tune that brings a dance step to mind may also work.

- Find a target on the floor and step on it. Sometimes people imagine they are stepping on a fly on the ground in front of them. Look for an imaginary fly on the floor and try to crush it; this may get your gait started.

- A variation on this involves using a laser pointer to create a target to step on. If you point the laser light 1 to 2 feet on the floor in front of you and then think about stepping on that tiny lighted spot, this may get you going. Laser pointers are used by professors and lecturers and may be purchased at bookstores.

- A special laser pointer that attaches to a walker and projects a line forward on the floor may be especially helpful for some people; this is commercially available and your physical therapist may know where this may be obtained.

This is not an exhaustive list but is meant to illustrate the concept of mental imagery to get you going. You are left to your own creative ideas about what strategies might work best for you. The idea is to have some mental image that you can call upon repeatedly throughout the day. When you freeze, momentarily relax (pause), think that thought, then go.

FALLS

Early in PD, imbalance is minimal or nonexistent. With PD progression imbalance may slowly develop and, if prominent, result in falls. Normal aging also contributes to this problem; after age 80, many of us easily lose our balance. Imbalance sufficient to cause falls does not develop in all those with PD; however, if you live long enough, it probably will be an issue sooner or later.

Falling is one PD symptom that does not respond to carbidopa/levodopa or any other medication. PD medication adjustments should be tried if imbalance and falls are occurring, but the best we can do is speed up compensatory leg movements that help counter loss of balance.

A physiatrist or physical therapist is important when imbalance becomes a problem. They can address several factors that lend themselves to treatment:

- *Avoiding situations that put you at risk for falling.* Falls often occur when distracted or when trying to do two things at once. When on your feet, it may be necessary to avoid thinking about other things or engaging in other tasks. Walking while carrying heavy items (e.g., grocery bags) may challenge balance mechanisms. Since falls often occur when changing positions or postures, the therapist may work with you to pause when changing positions and consciously think about using proper body mechanics. If gait freezing seems to provoke falls, then the strategies outlined earlier are appropriate.

- *Muscle weakness and deconditioning.* If you have been leading a sedentary lifestyle and your muscles have weakened as a consequence, they will be less able to compensate for minor missteps during walking. Maintaining muscle strength is important in compensating for imbalance. Depending on your general medical condition and other factors, your physiatrist may even recommend a weight-training program.

- *Exercise as a component of a weight loss program.* Obesity exacerbates problems of imbalance. If you carry around an extra 50 or 100 pounds of fat tissue, it is that much harder to overcome minor imbalance, potentially leading to falls. Weight loss requires both dieting plus calorie-burning exercise.

- *Balance training.* Balance exercises do help. However, a balance exercise program must be designed that meets both your needs and your capabilities. As you make gains, the goals can be increased as you work with your therapist.

- *Gait aids.* As already mentioned, there are a variety of aids that compensate for imbalance, but they are not appropriate or necessary for everyone. Depending on your specific problem, a physiatrist or physical therapist will choose what meets your needs, from a walking stick or cane to a wheeled walker.

- *Optimizing the home to avoid trips, falls, and injuries.* Physiatrists look at the big picture and will consider the things in your home that might exacerbate the tendency to fall, such as throw rugs or slippery floors.

They also can advise about minor home modifications, such as grab bars where you might be stepping over impediments (e.g., bathrooms, or the step from the garage to your house). Certain aspects of your home may also need to be considered, such as hard floors or sharp furniture corners, which put you at an increased risk for injury if you do fall; these are modifiable.

If imbalance and falls are present, you should pay special attention to related discussion in Chapter 30, where we discussed osteoporosis prevention. Obviously, strong bones are especially critical if your balance is impaired.

"STAND UP STRAIGHT!"

PD often results in a stooped posture. Sometimes this is written off to normal aging or incorrectly attributed to osteoporosis. However, just as tremor, rigidity, and bradykinesia are due to changes in brain motor control mechanisms, so, too, is a stooped posture. PD medications usually only partially improve posture. Physical therapy strategies may be helpful.

THE CAUSE OF STOOPING

Our spinal column is made up of a series of vertebral bones, stacked one on top of another, similar to a tower of children's building blocks (see Figure 31.1). Each vertebral bone is shaped like a short oil drum and separated from the adjoining vertebrae by cushioning discs. This tall column of vertebral bones and discs is surrounded by muscles, which stabilize it, as illustrated in Figure 31.1.

The configuration of the spinal column is primarily regulated by the muscle contraction of the surrounding *paraspinal* muscles. The brain normally adjusts the tone in these muscles so that we stand erect and tall, but also with a little curvature at our neck and lumbar regions (termed *lordosis*). The computer code for this is imprinted in the motor control area of your brain; there, the signals to the supporting muscles are unconsciously generated for a normal posture. Voluntary bending and twisting of our trunk and neck is accomplished by appropriate contraction of these spinal muscles. These volitional trunk and neck movements are accomplished through other brain motor control regions that program our routine movements.

Among those with PD, malfunction of the unconscious programming of the spinal muscles causes stooping. Rather than resulting in an erect posture, these muscles may revert to a default motor program, resulting in a flexed (stooped) posture. Unless severe, the capacity for voluntary movements of the trunk is at least partially preserved (i.e., you can bend and flex your trunk and neck).

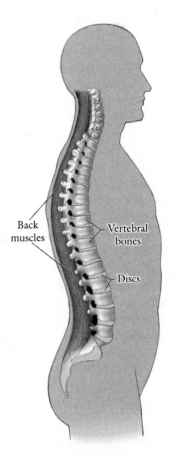

31.1   The normal spine is not perfectly straight, but rather is concave at the neck and lumbar regions (lordosis); an opposite (convex) curve is present at the mid-spine (thoracic spine). The longitudinal paraspinal muscles along the spine are appropriately contracted to generate this alignment.

This is analogous to other involuntary and unconscious movements that suffer in PD, such as arm swing and facial animation. Those with PD can stand up straight, swing their arms, and frown their faces. However, unless they think about it, the posture tends to become stooped, arm swing diminishes, and facial animation dampens.

The physical therapy strategy for countering this is to consciously think about pulling your shoulders back and standing straight. Your spouse may have already told you to do this (perhaps too often!). For this strategy to be effective, you need to constantly think about it. When distracted, there is a tendency to revert to the stooped pattern. Nonetheless, you can train yourself to stand straighter if you focus on this. Unfortunately, with long-standing parkinsonism, these spinal deformities may become more fixed.

STOOPED POSTURES AND LOW BACK PAIN

A stooped posture is probably not the primary cause of low back pain in most people. However, if you have a tendency toward lumbar pain, stooping may contribute. Note what your back muscles must do to maintain the trunk in the forward, stooped position. This forward posture requires the lumbar muscles to pull against gravity to keep you from doubling over on yourself. Such overworked muscles begin to ache after awhile. If you have an inherent tendency toward low back pain, this will add to it. Compare that to the work required if you are standing up straight. When standing erect, your vertebrae are resting one on top of another (see Figure 31.1); in that position, the supporting muscles of the back don't need to do much work, other than stabilize. The body's entire center of gravity is over the feet. Compare that to the spine that is programmed by the brain to stoop forward.

Rare individuals with PD develop more profound dystonic deviation of the back or neck. This might manifest as a pronounced tilt, rotation, or flexion of the trunk or neck, with dystonic contraction of the paraspinal muscles locking this posture into place. This condition has proven very difficult to treat and is not responsive to carbidopa/levodopa or any of the PD medications. Botulinum toxin injections are often employed, but this too may not prove very helpful.

32

◆ ◆ ◆

Family, Friends, the Workplace, and Caregivers

Should I Keep My Diagnosis a Secret?

Should the diagnosis of Parkinson's disease (PD) be disclosed to friends and family? Clearly, your spouse or partner must not be kept in the dark. Disclosure beyond that, however, is a personal choice and depends on the circumstances. Let's think about some of the factors that should be weighed in this decision.

If your PD is well-controlled and you are experiencing no compromise of activities, it is not necessary to reveal the diagnosis outside of your spouse or partner. For some, the symptoms in the first year or two are so minimal that no medications are required. Once treatment is necessary, carbidopa/levodopa is typically very effective in controlling the symptoms and signs. Hence parkinsonian signs may not be obvious to others.

For some, it is important to talk about the PD diagnosis with friends, and sometimes clergy or therapists. Not everyone easily comes to grips with their disrupted sense of infallibility and immortality. If the mental burden weighs on your mind, then by all means, share this with appropriate friends and family. Talking about things that bother us helps make peace with ourselves and confront our shortcomings. Conversely, if the recognition of a neurological disorder can be accepted, it may be better to downplay the illness and focus on the positives in life. As we age, "stuff happens," and successful aging necessitates accommodating and moving on.

Should you disclose the diagnosis to your boss or coworkers? It is quite acceptable to keep this secret, provided that the signs of PD are not obvious and work performance is not compromised. An argument for nondisclosure is that this avoids being defined as a PD patient. If parkinsonism is beginning to interfere with work or workplace interactions, it may be advisable to make the diagnosis known. This may allow reduced workplace demands or other accommodations. Similarly, for social, community, or volunteer activities that challenge your capacity to engage, disclosing the diagnosis allows appropriate reduction of these commitments.

Reduced Energy May Necessitate Reduced Demands

Even when PD is otherwise well controlled, there is often a decline in energy and stamina. Carbidopa/levodopa, as well as other medications, is often insufficient to return energy levels to their previous baseline state. If you have been a high-energy, go-getter, doing three things at once, you may not be able to keep up as you once did. At the very least, multitasking tends to be compromised after a few years of PD. The expectations of friends, family, and employer may need to be reduced. Disclosing that you have PD is a good excuse for turning down yet another committee or volunteer job.

Workplace Decisions

Parkinson's disease does need not to force you into retirement. Many with PD have worked for years after the diagnosis was made. Obviously, the demands and requirements of work are a factor. A cardiac surgeon or a jet pilot has little margin for error, and rather minimal problems may force them to the sidelines. On the other hand, most jobs in the workplace are compatible with PD, at least in the milder stages. My view is to continue working as long as you are able to comfortably meet the demands of your occupation. In general, we are all happier and most fulfilled when busy and challenged with responsibilities.

To continue working, optimize your PD medications, most notably carbidopa/levodopa. It's OK to limit PD medications if you are functioning well. However, if your job is suffering, it is a mistake to arbitrarily avoid carbidopa/levodopa in hopes of saving the best responses for later. Your carbidopa/levodopa responses are not bankable; failing to take advantage of them results in lost opportunities. Deferring carbidopa/levodopa so that it will work best later is like trying to save your youth.

Physical Challenges to Continuing in the Workplace

If your job is more physical than mental, PD symptoms will provide a greater challenge. Climbing ladders, walking on roofs, or heavy labor are not possible indefinitely if you have PD. Problems with walking, balance, or slowness may force you into more sedentary work, to seek disability, or to retire. It is important to recognize this in a timely fashion if there are any safety concerns.

Long work days or frequent overtime also challenges those with PD, recognizing that fatigue and reduced work capacity often accompany PD. This can be partially reversible with carbidopa/levodopa treatment of parkinsonism and insomnia, as well as treatment of depression. However, the chronic fatigue that occasionally is prominent in PD may be difficult to completely eradicate.

PD also tends to interact with normal aging to exacerbate aches and pains in our muscles and joints that may make it difficult to do physical tasks. These can be challenging for those without PD who reach middle age and have jobs with high physical demand; the addition of PD to the problems of aging joints and limbs may force an occupational change. Recall, however, that pain from any source will be increased if undertreated with carbidopa/levodopa.

Actually, I see many farmers, carpenters, and skilled laborers in my practice who keep up with the demands of their work, at least for several years. Hence PD can indeed be compatible with physically demanding jobs, although not in every case.

White Collar Work

Sedentary jobs without physical demands are more compatible with PD. However, a variety of problems may make even sedentary occupations difficult:

- Fatigue or reduced energy

- Reduced dexterity, compromising writing or computer keyboarding

- Inability to do two things at once, multitasking

- Reduced ability to handle stress (stress is inherent in every job)

- Softer voice, making it more difficult to communicate

- Slowed thinking (bradyphrenia), paralleling slowed movements

- Cosmetic issues, such as a prominent tremor or dyskinesias that distract you or your customers

- Walking problems, making it difficult to travel on business

- Unpredictable off-states that immobilize

- Disrupted nighttime sleep, resulting in daytime drowsiness

Thus no job is safe from PD, although with optimum medical treatment it may be possible to limit these problems. Again, if your job is being compromised, take full advantage of carbidopa/levodopa therapy and ignore suggestions to withhold or limit treatment.

Disability and Retirement

If the demands of work are beginning to exceed your capabilities, it may then be time to consider disability or retirement. Before proceeding, you will need to discuss this with at least three people:

- Your doctor, to make certain that you have not missed some therapeutic opportunities that might make you better able to cope

- Your employer, who may be able to modify your job to better accommodate your needs

- Your spouse, and perhaps others in your family, since this will result in a shared lifestyle change

Disability status is not automatic with the diagnosis of PD. You will need a physician's statement on the appropriate paperwork to qualify. However, if your doctor is able to document disability from PD, it is unusual for the disability to be disallowed.

Your Rights

What if you believe that your job performance has not suffered from PD, but your employer disagrees and is threatening to fire you? What recourse do you have? You obviously need to consult an attorney to obtain the correct advice. However, we can summarize the basic legal doctrines that bear on this matter. The federal statute that covers this is the Americans with Disabilities Act, and most states also have similar laws on the books. If your parkinsonism is sufficiently advanced to compromise activities of daily living and is confirmed by a medical opinion, you should be covered by these statutes. Those who meet these disability criteria cannot be fired just because they have a disability. It is incumbent upon your employer to make reasonable accommodations to allow you to do your job. However, you, the employee, must also be able to perform the essential functions of your job, with or without these accommodations. If you can't perform them despite these accommodations, and if your employer cannot reassign you to another job, then you can be let go. Hence, you are protected to a certain degree, but you also need to be able to meet reasonable work standards.

If you are fired, where can you plead your case? You may file a complaint with the Equal Employment Opportunity Commission. You do not need an attorney to do this, but the chances of success increase with the help of a knowledgeable employment attorney. Another avenue is via the Department of Human Rights in your state, which may be consulted for advice.

Late in Parkinson's Disease: Providing and Accepting Care

Many with PD do well for years and the stress on the family is never substantial. Unfortunately, this is not true in every case. Moreover, the problems of aging eventually become superimposed, becoming apparent in the late 70s and beyond. There may come a time when family, and especially your spouse, becomes a crucial and necessary part of your care. The good news is that PD is treatable; we typically can keep people active and ambulatory for many, many years. The bad news is that sooner or later, we all get old, and PD adds to the burden of aging.

Some people cringe at the thought of having to depend on someone else. "I don't ever want to be a burden on my wife (or husband, or children)!" We typically go through our lives with a self-image of strength and independence; we can do anything necessary for our families and ourselves. We have been the pillars and the caregivers. Now the tables have turned. What an embarrassment! What a humiliation!

It seems to me that this is a very shortsighted perspective. We are looking at the natural cycle of life. Most people who live long enough will develop some condition later in life that requires help. Even if you are in the peak of health, you can still fall, break a hip, and be stuck in a wheelchair. These are things we cannot change; they have been written in our genetic codes. We live our lives as best we can, but when the time comes for us to get old or develop illnesses, we need to accept this.

Depending on others is not all bad for either the afflicted person or the caregiver. Some of the best love stories have come through my clinic. These will never be recorded in literature, but this devotion of a partner to their spouse could be the stuff of best-selling novels. I have been the witness to husbands who bring their frail parkinsonian wives to the clinic, attending to their every need and treating them like they were the 16-year-old beauty queens of 60 years ago. I have been humbled by wives who fawn over their ailing parkinsonian husbands, even though they no longer are the handsome athletes who won their hearts in their youths.

The cycle of life also ties children to their aging parents. There is a beauty to this cyclic process. Think about the mother who stayed up countless nights nursing her baby, then worrying and sacrificing as she lovingly raised her child to adulthood. For children to be able to return that love as a caregiver later in life can be very fulfilling and enriching.

Becoming a caregiver is often no small task, and my point is not to trivialize the work and sacrifice. However, it can be rewarding and enriching, and we shouldn't lose sight of that.

Caregiving

PD is a progressive condition; after 10 to 20 years, many lose at least some of their independence. Furthermore, since this is a disease that typically starts later in life, the problems of aging are superimposed. Hence, with passage of time, it is often critical to have someone who can help with the activities of daily living. For many, only limited assistance will be necessary; for a minority, the need for help will be extensive. The family, especially the spouse, typically becomes the major caregiver. If the necessary assistance is not substantial, this may be an easy transition. Unfortunately, that is not always the case.

The Challenges and Stresses of Caregiving

Entire books have been written about caregiving. Caregiving issues are not restricted to PD, since there are a multitude of disorders that chronically compromise lives, especially later in life. PD is so heterogeneous that you cannot predict what caregiving requirements, if any, will ultimately be necessary. However, let us consider a few basic principles that apply primarily to spouses (occasionally children) who are challenged with an intensive caregiving relationship. If you are in the role of the caregiver and this necessitates a major commitment of your time and energies, you should give some thought to the following.

- *What you are doing is heroic.* Recognize this and don't take your efforts for granted, even if everyone else does (including your spouse with PD). In your quiet moments, recount the things you have done for your loved one that day and congratulate yourself. None of us are required to become caregivers. We are free to abandon that person if that is our choice. Those that stay and fight the battle are special human beings. Keep that in mind.

- *Don't expect many words of thanks or any outward signs of reward.* What you are doing may require a huge sacrifice of your time and effort. Yet in chronic, ongoing relationships of this type, a "thank you" is rare. However, with each kind thing you do, the loving bond grows stronger and stronger; this is the unspoken reward.

- *Roles are invariably reversed in caregiver relationships, and sometimes this is a source of stress.* Men who are used to managing the finances or driving the family automobile may resent relinquishing these tasks to their wives. Women who took pride in their homemaking may complain about the bland food now cooked by their husband or the lack of cleanliness of the house. In caregiving situations, new roles are borne, and this needs to be recognized.

- *Don't expect perfection in the caregiving role.* The person with PD will come up short on some tasks, and that needs to be accepted. Roll with the punches and accept what you have.

- *Don't forget to look around and see the beauty in the world.* Enjoy the morning sunlight and the birds singing. Appreciate the leaves in the fall and the sunsets in the summer. It is too easy to get carried away with all the responsibilities of caregiving and forget those things that can bring us a moment of joy.

- *Maintain your own interests and make time for them.* Don't make caregiving a 24-hour-a-day task. Set aside time for the things that you need as necessary perks in your life. Caregiving can be a long road, and you should not ignore yourself.

- *If your caregiving requirements are intense, program regular respites into the schedule.* Get away for a few hours every day, if possible, or at least two to three times weekly. Don't feel guilty about this. It may seem inappropriate to go out and play golf for a few hours when your spouse is stuck at home. However, this is OK. You need time for you! This is necessary to cope with the demands of caregiving. If your loved one has problems staying alone, seek community resources to help with this, such as senior centers or perhaps someone hired for this purpose. Don't be reluctant to hire caregiving help.

- *Maintain relationships with friends and community.* There is a tendency to abandon these relationships as we get bogged down with the responsibilities of the day. If your life becomes restricted to the person we are caring for, we lose perspective and it's easy to get discouraged. We need friends and other relationships to keep going.

- *Have someone you can talk to when your life becomes too stressful.* This may be a close friend or other family member; it could be clergy. Sometimes it is hard to be objective when we are stuck in our own little world. Most of us occasionally need others to talk to or to allow ventilation; this is necessary for our own sanity and to maintain a broad perspective.

- *It's OK to get angry at your loved one.* Caregiving relationships are necessarily challenging because of the limitations of that person with advanced PD. Frustration is an integral part of these relationships. Accept your anger when it occurs, and don't feel guilty about this. However, avoid carrying that anger, as that will be detrimental to both of you in the long run. If you can't shake the anger, then find someone to talk to about this.

- *Get enough sleep.* PD often results in poor sleep for not only the patient but also the sleep partner. All sorts of things may occur during the night, ranging from acting out dreams (REM sleep behavior disorder) to the repeated need to urinate. It is common for the person with PD to keep a spouse or family up at night. A sleep-deprived caregiver will find coping even more difficult. If your loved one with PD is keeping you awake, there are strategies for improving his or her sleep; these have been discussed in previous chapters. Be certain that your physician addresses these as best as possible.

- *Address your own physical and mental needs.* Caregivers are not immune from illness. They also need annual medical examinations. When you go for this annual exam, this will also provide one opportunity to bring up your own mental health. Caregivers get depressed, and for good reason; their life has taken an unanticipated and demanding turn. Depression may need to be treated; this is not a sign of weakness.

- *Live one day at a time.* There is a tendency to worry about the future and ruminate about things over which we have no control.

Caregivers may also benefit from local PD support groups. Most communities have such groups where caregivers may share their experiences.

PART ELEVEN

◆ ◆ ◆

Surgery and Procedures for Parkinson's Disease: Present and Future

33

♦ ♦ ♦

Deep Brain Stimulation (DBS) and Other Brain Surgery for Parkinson's Disease

In the current era, deep brain stimulation (DBS) is the primary and predominant brain surgery used for treating Parkinson's disease (PD). It evolved from brain *lesioning* surgery that was first directed at PD or tremor well over 50 years ago. Brain lesioning implies destruction of a small area of brain. Properly placed lesions can stop tremor, improve parkinsonism, and prevent levodopa dyskinesias. Presumably, effective lesions interrupt reverberating tremor circuits or reset balance in motor control systems.

Both the lesioning and DBS surgeries for PD have targeted brain regions that are wired in series with the dopaminergic nigrostriatal system:

- Globus pallidus (pallidum)
- Subthalamic nucleus

If used specifically to abolish tremor, the thalamus is targeted. These brain nuclei are shown in Figure 33.1. Since surgical lesioning was the forerunner of modern DBS, we will begin our discussion with those procedures, as they provided the initial rationale for DBS.

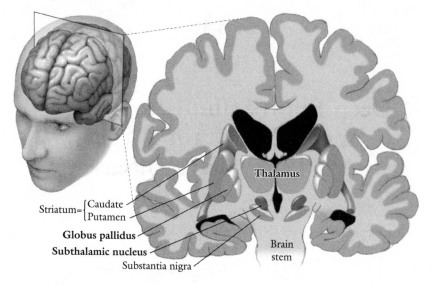

Striatum=$\begin{cases}\text{Caudate}\\\text{Putamen}\end{cases}$

Globus pallidus
Subthalamic nucleus
Substantia nigra

Thalamus

Brain
stem

33.1 The primary nuclei of the extrapyramidal motor system are shown. Surgery for Parkinson's disease or tremor typically targets specific nuclei within this circuitry: thalamus, globus pallidus (pallidum), or subthalamic nucleus.

Lesioning Procedures

Effective surgical lesioning of the brain requires precise localization of this destructive lesion. The procedures are named on the basis of the targeted brain area. *Thalamotomy* implies destroying (lesioning) a small area of the thalamus; *pallidotomy* similarly implies lesioning a region within the pallidum. Neither the entire thalamus nor the whole pallidum is destroyed with these lesioning procedures; rather, only a very specific small portion of these nuclei is damaged.

Correct location of the lesion target is crucial, and this is especially challenging because the targets are deep within the brain, precluding visual guidance. A misplaced lesion may not only fail to benefit, but might cause new and troublesome symptoms from unintended brain damage.

Why should destroying brain tissue improve PD? After all, the symptoms of PD are due to loss of brain cells; why wouldn't a surgical lesion to the brain add insult to injury? A simple explanation lies in the complex interplay of brain circuits. The brain has many interconnected regions that work in concert and provide checks and balances on one another. Some components of circuits facilitate certain movements, and this is counterbalanced by other components that inhibit these movements. If one component is lost, as is the case with PD (i.e., loss of the nigrostriatal system), there may be a shift toward too much activity in another component of the system. Hence, a small destructive lesion in the right place may help reset balance in the circuitry. Our understanding of these circuits and their precise interactions is very rudimentary, and we can only explain the effects of these lesions in these very general terms.

Lesioning can be done in a variety of ways. The most common technique involves inserting an insulated wire with an exposed tip to the targeted brain area. The tip is heated for a brief time (typically about a minute) to a certain specified temperature. This cauterizes (destroys) a small amount of tissue in a concentric circle around that site. Hence, a small hole is created in the brain. There are other ways in which lesioning has been done, but cauterization is the method currently employed by most neurosurgeons.

In the 1950s and 1960s, brain lesioning was frequently performed as treatment for PD. With the advent of levodopa therapy, they were performed much less frequently and only for very specific reasons, such as thalamotomy to treat tremor.

A resurgence of interest in lesioning procedures surfaced during the 1990s, when pallidotomy was reintroduced as surgical treatment for PD. Surgical destruction of a limited region of the globus pallidus (pallidum) proved to be very effective in terminating levodopa-dyskinesias. As discussed in earlier chapters, a small minority of those with PD are unable to benefit from carbidopa/levodopa unless the dose is raised into the dyskinesia range; pallidotomy effectively controls that problem. Pallidotomy also had other benefits directed at parkinsonism. With the advent of DBS some years ago, pallidotomy was largely abandoned.

Lesioning procedures are usually done on only one side of the brain. Surgeons quickly recognized that lesioning both sides of the same brain region (e.g., globus pallidus) tended to cause problematic motor effects. Since the right brain controls movement in the left body and vice versa, surgeons typically choose the more affected side of the body to treat.

Deep Brain Stimulation (DBS)

Deep brain stimulation evolved from these lesioning procedures and has supplanted them. DBS was borne of the recognition that tremor could be terminated, and parkinsonism improved by electrically stimulating specific brain sites through the exposed tip of an insulated wire (electrode). This proved to be at least as effective as lesioning. This procedure allowed for ongoing modulation of the effect through adjustment of the stimulating parameters. In contrast to lesioning procedures, DBS can safely be done on both sides of the brain (i.e., bilaterally).

Initially, thalamic DBS was used to treat tremor and was found to have more consistent and persistent benefits than thalamotomy. DBS was then extended to PD, targeting the pallidum (the target for pallidotomy) or the subthalamic nucleus. The subthalamic nucleus had previously been considered as a target for lesioning, but initial experience revealed potential for involuntary (dyskinetic) movements. With DBS targeting the subthalamic nucleus, the effect could be fine-tuned to avoid such dyskinesias. Currently, the subthalamic nucleus is the most commonly used DBS target for PD, although certain clinical characteristics may convince the surgeon to target the thalamus or pallidum. For tremor without other symptoms (e.g., essential tremor), the thalamus is the usual target.

The mechanism of the DBS effect was initially attributed to inhibited firing of neurons at the tip of the electrode (conceptually similar to reversible lesioning). The DBS stimulation is typically administered with very high–frequency pulses (e.g., 130–185 cycles per second, i.e., hertz), and it was thought that such high frequencies inactivated the neurons at the electrode tip. More recent studies have suggested that the mechanisms are not that simple, and ongoing research is directed at understanding this phenomenon.

The advantages of DBS over lesioning are threefold:

1. There is less damage to normal brain tissue (although some damage does occur via insertion of the electrode).

2. Adjustments of the stimulation parameters allows optimization of the effects, both initially and later.

3. DBS can safely be done on both sides of the brain, in contrast to lesioning.

Note that adjustments of the DBS parameters are made with a programming device that does not require direct contact with implanted pulse generator (much like a TV remote control). However, a relative downside of DBS compared to lesioning is the implanted electronic gadgetry and wires.

DBS Surgery from the Patient Perspective

DBS sounds simple, but it is quite complex, given the need to precisely place the electrode tip at the brain target, with little margin for error. Moreover, this electrode placement is simply the first stage (albeit most important). Implanting the stimulating electrodes is an all-day undertaking for the patient.

The usual procedure starts with placement of the head frame; one typical head frame is depicted in Figure 33.2. This is done under mild sedation and with local anesthetics. The head frame must be firmly attached to the skull, since it provides reference points for precise placement of the brain electrode. Usually it is held in place with small bolts or pins (it cannot be allowed to move). It has a three-dimensional coordinate system with markers that

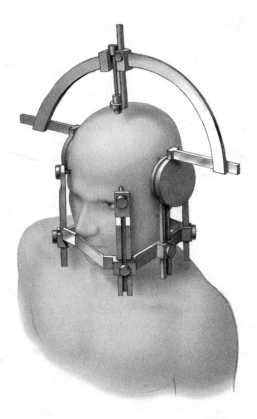

33.2 An example of a head frame used for DBS surgery. Such frames contain no metals that would be incompatible with the magnetic fields used in brain MRI. Markers on the frame provide reference points in three-dimensional space.

are detected during subsequent brain scanning (usually MRI). It allows the surgeon to convert the anatomy of the brain into a three-dimensional grid system. With this head frame in place, any given brain site can be specified in numerical coordinates (e.g., X millimeters from the midline, Y millimeters from a reference point in the front-to-back plane, and Z millimeters in a top-to-bottom plane). This is termed *stereotactic* brain surgery.

Next a brain scan is performed with the head frame in place. Usually, this would be done with MRI (magnetic resonance imaging), although it could be performed with CT (computed tomography). In both cases, a computer integrates the scanned brain images with the markers on the special head frame. With this, the computer is able to provide exact three-dimensional coordinates for any given brain locus. The coordinates are with respect to specific points on the head frame.

Once the brain scan has been done, the patient is moved to the operating room for the actual surgery. Mild sedation and pain-relieving medications are used, but not full anesthesia; the surgical team needs the person awake when the electrode has been placed and trial stimulation is administered. Deep anesthesia would prevent the surgical team from monitoring brain cell electrical activity or assessing the preliminary effect of the stimulation on parkinsonism or tremor.

Once on the operating table, a small (dime-sized) hole is made in the skull, exposing the brain. Many surgeons then record brain electrical activity as a recording electrode is lowered into the brain. This recording electrode picks up the normal electrical activity of brain cells in the region of the exposed electrode tip. The pattern of brain cell activity provides clues to the surgical team about the location within the brain. Sometimes several passes of this recording electrode are made to confirm the target. The recording electrode is ultimately withdrawn. With knowledge of the proper coordinates, the final step is to implant the deep brain-stimulating electrode into the designated site. For most people with PD, electrodes are implanted on both sides of the brain (e.g., in both right and left subthalamic nuclei); hence this electrode placement procedure is repeated. Each permanent stimulating electrode is attached to a wire that will later be connected to the stimulating unit, termed the *implantable pulse generator* (*IPG*). Implantation of the IPG typically is done with general anesthesia in a second surgery.

Parenthetically, if *lesioning* were being performed, the procedure would be similar up to this point. The lesioning electrode is inserted and properly positioned at the targeted site. The electrode tip is heated for the predesignated time, and then the outcome is evaluated. A member of the surgical team assesses certain aspects of parkinsonism (e.g., tremor, rigidity, etc.) to determine the effect of the lesion. The lesion may be enlarged, depending on what is learned from this assessment. Once satisfied, the surgeon withdraws the lesioning electrode, the scalp is sewn, and the surgery completed.

To complete deep brain stimulation surgery, the IPG and connecting wire(s) must be surgically placed, and general anesthesia is used. Often this is performed a day or several days after the brain electrode placement (the first stage). The IPG device is implanted just below the collar bone/clavicle and the wire connections are tunneled under the skin. The implanted device is shown in Figure 33.3. Once healed, the only visible evidence is the bulge of the IPG under the skin, below the clavicle (similar in appearance to that of a heart pacemaker), plus the small, dime-sized divot in the skull where the electrode was inserted; the latter is visible only among those who are bald.

Often the surgeon will defer turning the stimulator on immediately after the surgery because the stimulation parameters are expected to be unstable until a few weeks elapse. Hence there is no immediate benefit. However, sometimes the small lesion from the electrode insertion provides transient benefit even without stimulation (much like a lesioning procedure).

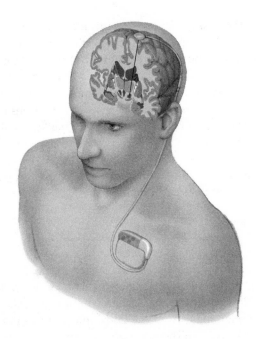

33.3 The figure depicts the stimulating electrode tip within the subthalamic nucleus connected to the implantable pulse generator below the clavicle (collar bone). Both the wiring and pulse generator are under the skin. Once healed, the path of the wire is not visible. When disrobed, the implanted pulse generator produces visible elevation of the skin, similar to a cardiac pacemaker.

Programming the DBS Parameters

The programming of the DBS device is typically deferred until several weeks after the surgical implantation. In the interim, the patient is home, managing parkinsonism with medications alone. Upon subsequent return to the DBS clinic, the programming is done as an outpatient.

The implantable pulse generator shown in Figure 33.3 is the source of the electrical stimulation delivered to the electrode tip within the brain. This pulse generator is programmed with an external device sending radiofrequency signals that can vary the stimulation parameters. The pulse generator electrical current originates from an internal battery with a life span of about 4–5 years; when it starts to lose power, minor surgery is necessary to replace it. Patients are given a magnetic switch that allows the stimulator to be turned off and on; the actual stimulation adjustments, however, are done by the DBS clinical team. Currently in development is an IPG with a rechargeable battery.

Programming the stimulation is complex, with a variety of parameters that can be modified. The electrode within the brain has four separate stimulation sites and the device can be programmed to stimulate from (or between) any of those four. Also, the electrical signal parameters can be adjusted in numerous ways to produce the best response. This includes changing the frequency of the stimulation, which is typically set to fire at a very rapid firing rate (about 130 to 185 stimulation bursts per second). The stimulation is measured in volts and this reflects the stimulation intensity; it is initiated with low values, ultimately raised to between 2 and 5 volts, guided by both benefit and side effects. As the voltage intensity is slowly raised, medications may be reduced.

When DBS for PD was first introduced, some medical centers tried slowly eliminating all PD medications. However, it subsequently became recognized that certain PD drugs needed to be maintained, albeit in lower doses, to provide the best outcomes. Often, all PD drugs except for carbidopa/levodopa are markedly reduced or eliminated.

DBS Down the Road

The neurostimulating units have proven to be reliable. However, the wires connected to the units have been known to break or erode through the skin, albeit very infrequently; this requires minor surgical repair. As with any implanted foreign material in the body, infections can occur; these also are uncommon. However, if the brain electrode becomes infected, it often is necessary to remove it.

Usually, once the initial programming of the IPG has captured a favorable response, no further adjustments are necessary for long intervals. Later, if there is a decline in parkinsonian control, adjusting the stimulation parameters may restore the lost benefit.

Published experience with DBS for PD indicates that the beneficial effect is sustained over years. However, the natural history of PD is one of slow progression and DBS does not alter that course. Hence clinical parkinsonism scores are worse after 5–10 years, compared to the first year after DBS; this reflects PD progression rather than loss of the DBS effect. When the Lewy neurodegenerative process spreads beyond the dopaminergic pathways, DBS loses its impact. The exception is tremor control, which is usually sustained regardless of whether it has been levodopa-responsive.

Who Are Candidates for DBS?

A minority of people with PD are appropriate candidates for DBS surgery. Why not offer surgery to all with PD? There are several reasons.

- Brain surgery is *not* low risk.

- Not all problems linked to PD respond to surgery (only tremor and levodopa-responsive symptoms).

- Medical treatment is quite beneficial in most cases.

Some have advocated for DBS treatment very early in PD. This argument needs to be balanced against the following:

- Surgical risks, albeit small

- The possibility that technological advances will allow more effective surgical strategies in the future

- Recognition that medications are nearly always necessary after DBS to effectively treat all symptoms

There is no evidence that DBS slows the progression of the Lewy neurodegenerative process. The utility is solely for symptomatic treatment, similar to PD medications.

Factors Increasing the Likelihood of Surgical Complications

Certain factors increase the risk of complications with DBS surgery:

- *Dementia.* Cognitive impairment may worsen with any brain surgery, including DBS for PD. Most surgeons will not offer DBS to those experiencing substantial problems of thinking and memory.

- *Advanced age.* This is a relative, rather than an absolute, contraindication, and published reports have documented successful DBS surgery in people in their early 90s. However, surgical risks tend to increase in advanced seniors. First, general medical complications are more likely in older ages, such as heart attacks, strokes, and pulmonary emboli. Second, the brain slowly shrinks over a lifetime; brain cells and connections are lost due to the aging process. As a consequence, there is less brain "reserve"; incidental brain damage during surgery is less easily compensated. Thus surgical teams are more cautious in offering DBS surgery to people beyond 80 years of age.

- *Other serious medical problems.* A variety of medical conditions outside the brain may make these surgeries too risky, including failure of major organs, such as heart, liver, kidneys, or lungs. Bleeding problems or requirement for blood thinners obviously increases the risk of a brain hemorrhage during surgery. Blood thinners can be briefly stopped and alternative anticoagulant "bridging therapy" can be used around the time of surgery; however, this is not without additional risks.

Symptoms Favoring DBS Surgery

Symptoms responsive to levodopa therapy are expected to respond to sub-thalamic nucleus or pallidal DBS. Symptoms that fail to respond to levodopa (despite aggressive carbidopa/levodopa dosage) will not respond to DBS (except for tremor, which usually can be controlled with DBS regardless of the cause or levodopa response). Obviously, physicians would like to have a surgical option for people not benefitting from levodopa; unfortunately, DBS fails in that regard. Clinicians have recognized that DBS is not substan-tially better than your best levodopa response.

Two specific PD problems are especially benefitted by DBS:

1. Fluctuations in the levodopa response, with prominent levodopa off-time, despite appropriate medication adjustments (This especially includes people with a levodopa response of 3 hours or less. Such brief responses make it difficult to stay in a levodopa on-state, especially with the inhibitory effect of meals.)

2. Levodopa-induced dyskinesias (involuntary movements) that are severe or disabling and that cannot be eliminated by lowering the levodopa doses without unacceptable parkinsonism

Note that tremor typically responds dramatically to DBS regardless of the levodopa response. This is the sole exception to the rule that DBS only ben-efits levodopa-responsive symptoms. If tremor is the most troublesome prob-lem and cannot be controlled with medications, DBS is a good option. This is true for any tremor, whether due to PD or not. Thus, tremor secondary to a traumatic brain injury, essential tremor, or other causes should respond to DBS. For tremor as the sole problem, the thalamus is typically targeted.

Of note, subthalamic nucleus DBS does not *directly* reduce dyskinesias, unlike pallidal stimulation. Subthalamic nucleus DBS tends to reproduce the levodopa benefit, which allows a reduction of levodopa doses; levodopa reduction translates into much less dyskinetic movement.

What if you have not responded to carbidopa/levodopa because you have trouble tolerating it (e.g., due to nausea or orthostatic hypotension)? Obviously, this does preclude subthalamic DBS surgery. If the diagnosis of PD seems certain but carbidopa/levodopa is not tolerated, DBS is an option. However, intolerance to carbidopa/levodopa can be a red flag for one of the parkinsonism-plus disorders discussed in Chapter 6; these do not respond to DBS.

A comment about orthostatic hypotension is in order. Troublesome orthostatic hypotension causing faints and near-faints tends to be driven by carbidopa/levodopa. In such susceptible people, the standing blood pressure typically plummets for a few hours after each carbidopa/levodopa dose. Subthalamic nucleus stimulation allows a reduction in the carbidopa/levodopa doses, which should allow the blood pressure to be maintained at more normal levels. Note that multiple system atrophy is commonly associated with troublesome orthostatic hypotension and does not respond to DBS (see Chapter 6).

Symptoms not Helped by These Surgeries

It is important to recognize DBS limitations. Certain problems often associated with PD that are not expected to benefit include the following:

- Dementia (may make it worse)
- Hallucinations, delusions (may worsen at the time of surgery)
- Psychological problems (depression)
- Urinary or bowel symptoms
- Fatigue
- Sexual dysfunction

The common denominator of symptoms responsive to DBS is response to levodopa.

Non-motor PD Symptoms

A variety of non-motor symptoms occur in PD. Those that are levodopa-responsive may also respond to DBS, albeit less predictably than motor symptoms. Thus anxiety, insomnia, or pain that improves with carbidopa/levodopa often responds to DBS; however, ongoing carbidopa/levodopa treatment is often necessary to experience the most the benefit. Non-motor symptoms that are not levodopa-responsive typically do not improve with DBS. Speech and voice disorders usually do not improve, and these sometimes worsen following DBS.

Which Brain Target for DBS?

DBS may target the subthalamic nucleus, globus pallidus (pallidum), or thalamus. Currently, the most common target for PD treatment is the subthalamic nucleus. However, comparative trials suggest that pallidal DBS provides similar outcomes. The thalamus is only used for those whose sole or primary problem is tremor.

A second consideration is whether to perform the DBS surgery on one side or both. Most people with PD experience motor symptoms on both sides of the body, hence implantation on both sides of the brain is appropriate. However, some with PD have motor symptoms primarily on only one side of the body; for them, DBS targeting only the opposite brain side is a consideration (recall that the left brain controls the right body and vice versa). Implanting the DBS electrode on one side does not preclude later surgery on the other side. Added factors that might favor one-sided DBS include advanced age or other surgical risks.

Which Medical Center Should Do the DBS Surgery?

Brain surgery has little margin for error. DBS surgery is complex, best done with the most modern equipment and experienced surgical teams. Smaller medical centers usually do not offer DBS surgery because of the considerable investment in staff and equipment. This surgery is typically done at referral centers where the DBS demand keeps the surgical team well-practiced in their art. For many patients, this translates into travel to a more distant medical center.

The DBS support staff are important components of the team and contribute to the success of the DBS program. Typically, a neurologist will do the initial screening to determine if the person is indeed a good candidate for DBS. This often will include observation in the office before and after a dose of carbidopa/levodopa to determine levodopa responsiveness. Those with Parkinson look-alike conditions such as progressive supranuclear palsy or multiple system atrophy need to be recognized, since they are unlikely to benefit from DBS (see Chapter 6 for a discussion of these parkinsonism-plus disorders). The screening goes beyond parkinsonism, with assessment of cognitive function, psychological stability, and patient expectations.

Following the surgical implantation, neurologists and nurses who are part of the DBS team take responsibility for programming the implanted pulse generator and adjusting PD medications. The most seamless care occurs when the medical center involved with the surgery is also responsible for longer-term care. Some DBS teams will decline to do the stimulator programming unless there has been involvement from the beginning, including the surgery.

In the current era, there are a number of medical centers in North America that have an excellent track record in performing DBS surgery. In a perfect medical world, published statistics would help PD patients choose centers with the best record. However, these data are not available, and even if they were, the results could be easily manipulated or misinterpreted. For example, an "excellent outcome" might differ from one medical center to another. Some centers with greater morbidity might be accepting more complex patients.

Risks to DBS Surgery

Brain surgery carries risks. The implanted electrodes must pierce the overlying brain before reaching the ultimate implantation site in the subthalamic nucleus, pallidum, or thalamus. Small hemorrhages may occur. The implanted electrode is a foreign body and can become infected. The devices may malfunction or the wires may break. Fortunately, among properly selected people, the serious risks are relatively small. For example, in one recently published series of about 300 PD patients receiving pallidal or subthalamic nucleus DBS surgery, adverse events were infrequent (and nearly identical in the pallidal and subthalamic groups): 7–8% developed surgical site infections; DBS device problems occurred in 1–3%; brain hemorrhages developed in 1–2%; suicidal depression occurred in about 1% in each group. Mental confusion was documented in about 20% in each group; although this was not discussed in the published report, it likely represented the transient confusional state that is common among people with Lewy body disease undergoing surgical anesthesia. Of note, the surgeries were all done by experienced DBS surgical teams after careful selection of appropriate surgical candidates.

Side effects due to the stimulation per se can be controlled by adjusting the stimulation parameters. Usually this can be done without compromising the stimulation benefit.

Lesioning, Including Ultrasound-Guided Lesions

Occasional people might prefer lesioning rather than implanted electrical gadgetry and thus opt for thalamotomy or pallidotomy. These procedures were commonly done until the advent of DBS and now are rarely performed. Conventionally, this has been done as described earlier in this chapter, with an implanted electrode tip heated for a brief time to cauterize the targeted brain tissue.

Recently, brain lesioning with focused ultrasound has gained attention. Ultrasound commonly used to treat painful joints and muscle does not damage tissue because the transmitted energy is very low. However, ultrasound energy can produce tissue damage if sufficiently intense. To produce a brain lesion with focused ultrasound, multiple ultrasound beams from many sites around the head are focused at the target deep within the brain (e.g., thalamus). The energy from each individual ultrasound beam is too low to damage tissue. Where the many beams converge, the additive energy destroys a small area of brain tissue, that is, the lesion occurs only at the site where the beams overlap.

This approach requires similar technical strategies as conventional lesioning procedures to precisely locate the intended brain target (e.g., thalamus). The challenge is proper localization; there is no margin for error when brain lesioning is done. At present, this approach is a work in progress.

34

♦ ♦ ♦

Experimental Treatments: Fetal and Stem Cell Implantation, Neurotrophic Hormone and Gene Therapy, Vaccines and Immunotherapy

The lay press frequently promises that the cure for Parkinson's disease (PD) is near, capitalizing on ongoing molecular biological discoveries. Researchers, however, recognize that human biology is extremely complex. Theoretically promising treatments reported in cultured cells or animal models often fail when translated to human disease.

A variety of molecular strategies have been proposed for PD, including cell implantation or infusion of genes into the brain, as well as targeted activation of immune mechanisms. Many of these approaches are under active investigation; not all will work, but hopefully, at least one will prove efficacious.

Optimistic reports in newspapers typically need the PD treatment strategy placed in proper biological context. Ideally, the treatment would be based on a clear understanding of the cause of PD. Unfortunately, we do not know the cause. Hence, some of the new-era treatments are trial-and-error endeavors.

Stem cells or gene therapy are not the cure for all medical diseases, although the lay press might lead one to that conclusion. Judging the promise of each of these therapeutic strategies requires an understanding of the therapeutic modality, the specific goal (e.g., restoring degenerated dopaminergic neurons) plus the biological context. Since cell therapy for PD with fetal or stem cells has been center stage for a number of years, this perhaps deserves our initial attention.

Background: Cell Therapy with Fetal or Stem Cells

Stem cell and related cell therapies have been proposed for many diseases that would benefit from restoration of new healthy cell lines. Replacement of diseased liver or heart tissue with immature cells capable of developing into new liver or cardiac tissue is a highly promising work in progress. This makes good intuitive sense for those internal organs that are primarily composed of one cell type that performs a stereotyped set of functions. For example, liver cells (*hepatocytes*) have specific biological activities that do not substantially differ from one hepatocyte to the next. If damaged liver tissue was replaced by new hepatocytes, liver function theoretically should be restored. Similarly, congestive heart failure due to weakened heart muscle could theoretically be treated with replacement cardiac muscle cells to restore strength.

Published articles addressing stem cell therapy usually mention PD as a prototypic neurological disorder lending itself to such cell transplantation. Although this is true in a narrow sense, PD is not that simple. The assumption underlying such cell transplantation is that replacing the lost dopaminergic nigrostriatal neurons will effectively treat or even cure PD. Thus stem cells genetically programmed to become dopaminergic neurons and implanted into the striatum could provide an ongoing source of dopamine. Unfortunately, this rationale is based on a limited view of PD and overlooks the poorly treatable problems that develop after years of PD; importantly, these are not dopamine based. Currently available treatments for dopamine-based symptoms are reasonably effective: carbidopa/levodopa and related medications, plus deep brain stimulation (DBS). While dopamine neuron replacement could theoretically restore dopamine function more smoothly and efficiently, it will not provide meaningful benefit beyond what is already available; this ignores the poorly treatable problems that surface after some years. Crucially needed are effective treatments for non-dopamine-based conditions: PD-related dementia, autonomic dysfunction (e.g., urinary incontinence, orthostatic hypotension), and levodopa-refractory motor symptoms. Does restorative cell therapy provide hope for treating such (non-dopamine-based) problems? To address this question, it must be placed in a broader context.

THE CHALLENGES OF ADVANCING PD

Why do people with long-standing PD continue to experience progressive disability despite treatment with levodopa and related drugs, and DBS? Although normal aging makes a minor contribution, the substrate for this problem relates to the progression of the Lewy neurodegenerative process well beyond the dopamine neurons. Unfortunately, most of these nondopaminergic symptoms have limited effective treatment (e.g., cognitive impairment/dementia). This includes certain parkinsonian symptoms that are poorly responsive to levodopa, such as falls and sometimes gait freezing; frequent falls and other levodopa-refractory motor symptoms imply Lewy body involvement of nondopaminergic motor systems. Although we can do well for many years treating dopamine-based symptoms, the next major therapeutic breakthrough will need to address more than dopamine problems.

THE BIGGER PICTURE

The evolution of PD spans decades, as outlined in the Braak staging scheme (discussed in Chapters 3 and 8). This reflects a slowly progressive spread of the Lewy neurodegenerative process. The earliest symptoms—constipation, REM sleep behavior, or loss of the sense of smell—are not dopamine based but do not cause important disability. When PD is recognized and diagnosed years later, the dopaminergic motor symptoms and signs are the central features. This intermediate stage, which reflects loss of the dopaminergic nigrostriatal system, persists for years and is quite treatable with carbidopa/levodopa, plus related drugs and DBS. At that time, the primary problems are dopamine based, and disability is minimized by available treatment options. Major disability remains limited until the Lewy neurodegenerative process spreads well beyond the nigrostriatal system and into non-dopamine substrates. Then, treatment starts to fail, and new treatment options are seriously needed.

Thus PD is appropriately conceived as much more than a dopamine deficiency disorder, even though dopamine replacement treatment is so effective for many years. The poorly treatable disability that surfaces after years of otherwise typical PD reflects the Lewy neurodegenerative process invading non-dopamine brain regions to cause dementia, dysautonomia (e.g., urinary incontinence, orthostatic hypotension), and levodopa-unresponsive movement symptoms. This occurs to variable degrees in different people, but rarely are those with long-standing PD left with only dopamine deficiency problems. (The exceptions are some of the very young-onset parkinsonism patients, whose condition started before age 30 years; they may have a pure dopamine neurodegenerative disorder.)

Implications for Treating Parkinson's Disease with Stem Cells

If considering stem cell restorative therapy to address the problems of PD, the specific brain circuits that we wish to restore must be specified. As just discussed, if simply targeting dopamine systems, restorative therapy will fail to address the most challenging problems affecting those with advancing PD. Note that much of the publicity given to stem cell and related therapy for PD aims at restoring dopamine function.

This begs the question of whether stem cell therapy could reconstitute the non-dopamine brain circuits lost to Lewy neurodegenerative processes. Might impaired cognition be restored, or levodopa-refractory imbalance and falls be reversed? To do this, the vast arrays of non-dopamine brain circuits would need to not only be restored but also rewired. If this sounds complicated, consider how the brain became wired in the first place.

DEVELOPMENT OF THE BRAIN

The brain is far more complex than the most sophisticated computer conceived by scientists. It contains at least 10 billion neurons, and many of these individual neurons have thousands of connections with one another. These connections are the wiring circuits, conceptually like a computer circuit. As we learned in Chapter 2, connections to distant areas in the brain are made via axons, which are the wire-like extensions from neurons (see Figures 2.1 and 2.2 in Chapter 2). Axons transmit signals to other neurons and may extend long distances throughout the brain (and spinal cord). For example, a primary neuron located in the cortex (outer layers of the brain) may send an axon all the way to the bottom of the brain (the brain stem) or down to the spinal cord. Moreover, there may be many connections along this path. Not all brain neurons, however, have long projections. Some interact only with neurons in their own region, but perhaps with thousands of connections.

The receiving end of the neuron is equally complex. Recall that signals from neuron to neuron are transmitted through synapses, where a neurochemical such as dopamine is released (see Figure 2.2, Chapter 2). The receptors for this neurochemical signal are often located on dendrites, which are the wire-like extensions from the cell body. These dendrites do not travel long distances like axons; however, they may form extremely complex networks. For example, a single neuron in the cerebellum may receive 150,000 synaptic connections through its dendrites.

The picture we are painting is that of very, very complex brain wiring. Not only are there perhaps 10 billion neurons, but many interact with one another by way of thousands of synaptic connections.

This complicated brain did not happen all at once. It slowly was built in the mother's womb (although brain development also continues through the early years of life). It is in the womb that the fundamental brain wiring is formed. This occurs through a complex cascade of events. In this cascade, each step depends on the previous one. Initial immature cells divide in the center of the brain to form neurons, and these new neurons then migrate outward. The areas in the middle of the developing brain where these cells replicate are called *germinal zones*. In these germinal zones, neurons destined to be located in distant areas of the brain are being formed. These newly formed cells then physically move outward (migrate) to their ultimate destination. Certain classes of neurons go first, then another type of neuron, and so on. There is a vast array of ever-changing chemical-hormonal signals that guide each step and direct this process of migration. The DNA blueprints of these cells organize all of this; certain chemical signals are activated at precisely the right time in development to stimulate each developing cell to do the proper thing. Later, that chemical signal is turned off, supplanted by another appropriate chemical signal for the next step. As the neurons are moving outward from the germinal zone to their destination, they do not have physical impediments to this migration, as will be the case once the brain is fully developed and packed with cells. This entire process proceeds in countless steps, with wave after wave of new neurons moving to their correct location in the developing brain and then forming the appropriate synaptic connections. The sequence and timing of this process are obviously critical. This developing network of brain cells can only proceed if each component of the overall process occurs at precisely the right place and time in the sequence.

What does this have to do with cell transplantation for PD? If you understand the complexity of brain development, you can then appreciate the challenges to researchers wishing to restore cognitive circuits or rewire nondopaminergic motor control systems. The obstacles are those of time and space.

1. *Time.* The wiring of brain circuits is programmed early in our lives by a precise sequence of events, with each event triggering the next. These complex brain connections only occur when the process proceeds in the proper order and at the right time in brain development. To date, we have no sense of how to replicate this precisely programmed cascade of cellular events.

2. *Space.* Once the brain wiring is in place in the mature brain, there is no extra space. Neurons and glia are tightly packed together, along with the connections (axons and dendrites). Of the entire volume of the brain, perhaps only 15–20% is not occupied by some cellular element. Thus there are physical impediments to forming connections

(synapses) with other brain cells, except in the immediate vicinity. In the mature brain, if an axon were to grow, it would be blocked from extending very far by the surrounding cells and cellular elements.

What are the implications for cell transplantation? If new neurons were to be implanted into the adult brain, we currently have no means of inducing these cells to form the appropriate complex connections that occur in normal brain development. This would require a cascade of chemical signals, one after the other and in exactly the right location to make this happen. Moreover, there is no space in the adult brain for transplanted neurons to physically grow axons to distant targets. Implanted cells do indeed survive, form synaptic connections with the native neurons, and release neurotransmitters. However, these may not be the right connections or provide the right neurotransmitter for that particular location.

DO STEM CELLS HAVE THE CAPACITY TO RECONSTITUTE DEGENERATED COGNITIVE OR MOTOR CONTROL BRAIN CIRCUITS?

If brain organization develops in such a complex fashion, might stem cells be able to replicate this process? That begs the question: what are stem cells?

Stem cells are the most immature cells that have not yet taken on the defining characteristics of neurons, muscle cells, or kidney cells, among others. The excitement about stem cells for implantation is that they can reproduce themselves and hence proliferate in cell culture. They could thus provide an unlimited supply of cells for transplantation.

Stem cells may be obtained from a variety of sources. *Embryonic stems cells* come from a very early fertilized maternal egg (i.e., an early embryo). *Mesenchymal stem cells* are from connective tissue cell lines; adult bone marrow is a common source. *Induced pluripotent stem cells* can be developed in the laboratory with technology to transform adult cells into immature cells. With genetic engineering, it is possible to induce stem cells to become neurons (or other types of cells).

Stem cells could be used to replace degenerated dopamine neurons, as could early neural cells from aborted fetuses. However, reconstituting brain circuits to restore cognition is a fundamentally different matter. If we recognize the ultimate source of PD disability in the current era (dementia, levodopa-refractory imbalance, etc.), reconstitution of complex brain circuits with stem cells seems far beyond the capabilities of scientists. There are simply too many precisely timed steps in the development of the brain to do more than replace one cell type. Stem cells should theoretically restore a diseased liver, where hepatocytes are interchangeable. Unfortunately, stem cells cannot be engineered to rebuild the very complex circuitry of brain cognitive or motor networks.

The History of Cell Transplantation Therapy for PD

There has been considerable experience with cell transplantation directed at restoring dopamine function in PD patients. This has been ongoing for more than a quarter century. These treatment trials have included transplantation of adrenal cells, fetal brain cells, as well as pig (porcine) brain cells into the brains of people with PD.

ADRENAL–BRAIN TRANSPLANTATION

Adrenal–brain transplantation involves removing an adrenal gland from a PD patient, dissecting out the inner portion (adrenal medulla), and then transplanting that into the striatum of that same person. Since the adrenal medulla cells produce dopamine and related substances, this was expected to treat the dopamine deficit of PD. People have two adrenal glands, with each located on top of their two kidneys. People typically tolerate loss of one adrenal gland; the other could be taken for transplantation.

The first adrenal–brain transplantation surgeries were done in the mid-1980s. By the late 1980s, this procedure was being performed at many major medical centers in North America and Europe. Unfortunately, despite widespread optimism, it turned out to be a failure. Some patients may have partially benefited, but this might have been a placebo effect. The primary reason for the poor success became clear when several of the transplanted patients died of natural causes: brain examination revealed no surviving adrenal cells. Thus, it seemed that the surgery failed because the adrenal cells died. This surgery is no longer performed.

FETAL TRANSPLANTATION

Presumably, the old adrenal cells used in adrenal–brain transplantation were near the end of their normal life span; they could not withstand the rigors of transplantation surgery. Cells at the other end of the life spectrum are expected to be much more viable: fetal cells. To treat the dopamine deficiency state of PD, surgical research teams next focused on the midbrains of aborted human fetuses for implantation into the brain of people with PD. The dopaminergic substantia nigra neurons are located in the midbrain, which could be microscopically dissected soon after the abortion and implanted into the striatum of a PD patient. These fetuses were in the first trimester, and these immature cell lines were presumed to be viable and capable of forming mature dopaminergic neurons. Because the fetal midbrain is small and provides only limited numbers of cells, tissue from several fetuses was used for each PD patient.

By the mid-1990s a number of medical teams had implanted fetal midbrain tissue and reported improvement in parkinsonism. Encouraging reports of fetal brain implantation for PD were tempered by concerns that the results were not being objectively analyzed. Furthermore, placebo effects could have been playing a role, as was undoubtedly the case with adrenal-brain transplantation.

The efficacy of fetal transplantation was subsequently assessed in two independent, randomized, controlled, clinical trials funded by the U.S. federal government. Outcomes were tabulated by independent evaluators with measures to control for the placebo effects. In these trials, PD patients who volunteered were randomly assigned to one of two groups, receiving either the fetal cell implant or "sham" surgery. Patients were informed that they might not receive the actual fetal implant (i.e., sham surgery). Neither patients nor the clinicians evaluating the outcomes knew whether fetal tissue had been implanted in any given patient, controlling for possible placebo effects. Those who had the sham surgery had a hole drilled in their skull but received no implant. Those undergoing the actual surgery had midbrain tissue containing dopaminergic substantia nigra neurons from multiple fetuses implanted into their putamen. Immunosuppressive treatment was used in all of the patients in one of these two studies to minimize immunological rejection.

The aggregate outcomes of these two fetal transplantation trials were a bit discouraging. After 1 to 2 years, the groups of patients who had received the fetal implants had parkinsonism scores that were only modestly better than those of the sham surgery groups. In one study, it seemed that benefits were confined to people less than age 60 years. In the other study, benefits seemed to be among those who had milder parkinsonism at the start of the study. Even more discouraging was the development of dyskinesias (involuntary movements) in half of the patients in one study and 15% in the other; these persisted despite no medications. In several patients, further brain surgery was necessary to control these dyskinesias.

This lack of striking success was not due to poor implant survival. To the contrary, the implanted fetal midbrain tissue not only survived, but grew into mature-looking dopaminergic cells. This was apparent from special dopamine brain imaging studies (positron emission tomography, PET) as well as brain examination of patients who subsequently died.

Several PD patients who had received fetal implants died around a decade later. Brain examination revealed Lewy bodies not just in the expected brain regions but also in the transplanted tissue in most of these subjects. However, these Lewy neurodegenerative findings were not sufficient to explain the less than stellar outcomes.

This story has not yet reached the last chapter. Recently, two PD patients were reported to have had remarkable success following fetal midbrain transplantation. After 15–18 years post-transplant, these two patients had motor scores consistent with only mild parkinsonism, despite discontinuing all PD drugs. This outcome has rejuvenated interest in dopaminergic cell transplantation, launching a new PD surgical trial in Europe (the so-called TRANSEURO project).

PORCINE (PIG) TRANSPLANTATION

At the peak of enthusiasm for cell transplantation treatment of PD, concerns were raised about the availability of human fetal tissue. In the trials just described, brain tissue from several fetuses was used for implantation into each person with PD. To provide a more available source of brain tissue, fetal pig brain was suggested. Limited transplantation surgeries using porcine midbrain were done at that time. It appears that this strategy has now been abandoned as treatment for PD.

Stem Cells for Nurturing Neurons Rather Than Replacement

Direct replacement of diseased or dying neurons is not the only proposed benefit of stem cell transplantation. Notably, stem cells are known to be a source of neurotrophic hormones, such as brain-derived neurotrophic factor (BDNF) and glial cell line–derived neurotrophic factor (GDNF). They also may provide anti-inflammatory effects and may improve cell survival. They have been proposed to possibly promote clearance of aggregated alpha-synuclein.

Based on these general cell-nurturing mechanisms, mesenchymal stems cells have been used to treat another alpha-synuclein disorder, multiple system atrophy (MSA; see Chapter 6). This study was performed in a small cohort of Korean MSA patients, obtaining stem cells from the patients' own bone marrow. In contrast to the fetal cell implantation into brain, discussed earlier, these stem cells were infused outside the brain via a peripheral vein and artery. Moderate benefit was documented, compared to a control group of MSA patients. This study is now being repeated in the United States. Whether this strategy can be replicated and then subsequently expanded to PD treatment is unclear at this time.

Neurotrophic Factor Therapy

The promise of neurotrophic factors in treating neurodegenerative disease led to investigations of direct brain infusion of the neurotrophic hormone GDNF. GDNF is one of the most potent growth factors for enhancing survival and development of cultured dopaminergic neurons. Unlike BDNF, GDNF does not cross the blood-brain barrier and must be directly infused into the brain to reliably reach the brain target. Evidence from animal studies led to four small clinical GDNF trials involving PD patients.

The first GDNF trial was conducted about a dozen years ago and was negative: GDNF was infused into the cerebrospinal fluid of people with PD via *cannulas* (small tubes) implanted into the lateral ventricles. Recall that the lateral ventricles are slit-like reservoirs located in the center of our brains, containing cerebrospinal fluid (depicted in Figure 2.5 in Chapter 2). Given the negative outcome, concern was raised that the cannulas should have been implanted directly into the striatum. Thus, two subsequent uncontrolled trials (i.e., no placebo group) assessed GDNF directly infused into the putamen (striatum) through chronic indwelling cannulas. These two studies documented improved parkinsonism, as well as increased striatal dopamine signal with PET imaging. Unfortunately, these results could not be replicated in a double-blind, controlled trial, reported in 2006 (i.e., a trial with a control group and the treatment status unknown to the evaluators). Despite the negative clinical outcome, the GDNF group had increased putamen dopamine signal documented with PET imaging. A debate ensued as to whether this strategy should be further explored, although others concluded that the need for permanently implanted brain cannulas was a bit extreme.

OTHER MEANS OF GENERATING BRAIN GDNF: AEROBIC EXERCISE

People like quick fixes. The promise of benefit from brain infusion of GDNF convinced some with PD to allow cannulas to be implanted into their brains. There is an alternative strategy, however, for increasing brain GDNF that is safer, albeit more difficult: engaging in regular aerobic exercise. Multiple animal studies have documented exercise-induced increases in brain GDNF and BDNF. Rats or mice regularly running on treadmills or running wheels had significantly increased brain concentrations of both GDNF and BDNF. This was discussed in Chapters 9 and 31.

Gene Therapy

Theoretically, genetic programming might be used in a wide variety of ways to treat PD:

- Genes could be introduced directly into the brain to modify the function of the native brain cells. Thus neurons already in place could be genetically reprogrammed and transformed into dopaminergic cells or generate other neurotransmitters. This could be done with viruses carrying an appropriate genetic code. There are several viral candidates for this strategy, utilizing viruses known to be benign and not infectious.

- Stem cell lines grown in culture could be genetically modified. For example, these stem cells could be induced to make dopamine and form a certain type of synaptic connection. Once genetically programmed, they could be implanted into the brain.

- Living cells from the person with PD could be biopsied (e.g., bone marrow cells) and then genetically programmed; once genetically modified, they could then be implanted into the brain. Using one's own cells would obviously reduce any likelihood of immune system rejection.

The technology is in place for genetically programming cells. In fact, scientists have been rewriting the genetic codes of cells for many years through several standard techniques. The challenge, however, begins with deciphering the codes of not only the very complex mechanisms that create unique brain cells but also, importantly, the codes that program the unique interconnections between neurons. Translating such deciphered codes into practical therapeutic strategies seems even more challenging.

VIRAL TRANSMISSION OF GENES TO RESTORE BASAL GANGLIA FUNCTION IN PD PATIENTS

Gene transmission into the brain using viral vectors has been performed in people with PD. In one recent small study, three genes crucial for generating dopamine were packaged into a benign virus and injected into the putamen of people with PD. The 1-year outcome suggested modest benefit without substantial adverse effects. In one other study, reported a few years ago, the gene for the neurotransmitter GABA was infused into the subthalamic nucleus in fluctuating PD patients. It is known that subthalamic nucleus GABA neurotransmission diminishes when striatal dopamine is lost. Hence, enhancing GABA neurotransmission in that nucleus should treat the dopamine-deficiency symptoms of PD. In fact, that was documented, although the improvement in motor scores was not dramatically different from those of the control PD group.

Attacking a Possible Cause of PD: Alpha-Synuclein

We do not know the cause of PD, but current evidence suggests that alpha-synuclein may have a central role. As summarized in Chapter 8, circumstantial evidence implicates alpha-synuclein accumulation and aggregation as a primary inciting factor in PD. To reiterate, reasons for implicating alpha-synuclein as a causative factor include the following:

- Causative alpha-synuclein mutations were discovered in several rare families with Lewy body PD.

- Other rare PD families were found to have one to two extra alpha-synuclein genes as the cause (resulting in increased brain alpha-synuclein production).

- Lewy bodies and Lewy neurites are full of alpha-synuclein (although there are a variety of other proteins as well).

- The progression of PD parallels the progression of Lewy (alpha-synuclein) pathology in the brain.

Alpha-synuclein is normally found in all neurons, but appears to become problematic when it aggregates. Neurons have mechanisms for disposing of extra or aggregated alpha-synuclein, but evidence suggests that this may become overwhelmed when the Lewy process reaches certain critical proportions.

This begs the question of how alpha-synuclein accumulation, especially when aggregated, might be controlled. Studies in cultured cells and animals suggest several possible treatment avenues:

- Development of monoclonal antibodies targeting alpha-synuclein. Such monoclonal antibodies attach to only one unique target (e.g., alpha-synuclein). This initiates immune disposal of that targeted protein.

  (Note that specific monoclonal antibodies (e.g., rituximab) are approved therapies for other conditions, such as certain rheumatological disorders and blood cancers, such as lymphomas/leukemias.)

- Vaccination targeting alpha-synuclein. (A small clinical trial of alpha-synuclein vaccination in PD patients has recently been launched.)

- Enhancement of the alpha-synuclein degradation processes.

  (For example, glucocerebrosidase mutations are a prominent PD risk factor. Glucocerebrosidase is an important enzyme in lysosomes, which are cellular organelles involved with breaking down unwanted cellular products. Animal studies have suggested that genetic strategies for enhancing glucocerebrosidase activity attenuate alpha-synuclein accumulation.)

- Strategies for inhibiting the alpha-synuclein gene. (If the alpha-synuclein gene were blocked, alpha-synuclein would not be produced. A variety of medical conditions are caused by excessive production of specific protein products [e.g., Huntington disease], and countless researchers have focused on strategies for blocking responsible genes. Inhibiting the problematic gene has been possible in cell cultures but has not yet consistently translated into patient care. If a workable strategy is found for any one disorder, this should translate into others.)

This is not an exhaustive list of strategies for reducing alpha-synuclein aggregation. At present, alpha-synuclein seems to be the most appropriate therapeutic target for PD.

PART TWELVE

◆ ◆ ◆

Parkinson's Disease Information Services

35

$\blacklozenge \; \blacklozenge \; \blacklozenge$

Support and Advocacy
Groups and the Internet

Local Support Groups

Many communities have well-organized Parkinson's disease (PD) support groups that meet regularly. These meetings allow people with PD and their families to exchange information and share ideas for dealing with common problems. Frequently, guest speakers (doctors, nurses, therapists) are invited to discuss topics of interest. These groups additionally provide a social outlet and a chance to meet people in similar circumstances. If you are unaware of a PD support group in your community, check with your doctor's office, clinic, or hospital for information.

Not every local support group is appropriate for each person with PD. The mix of people differs from group to group. People generally feel most comfortable where they are similar in age and PD severity to the other members of the group. Some regions have special support groups tailored to specific segments of the PD community, such as young-onset PD. If your local group does not fit your needs, you always have the option of organizing your own support group.

National PD Advocacy Groups

Several national PD groups provide a variety of services, including dissemination of information, lobbying the government for research funding, as well as providing seed money for researchers starting new projects. The major national groups are listed at the end of this chapter, including website addresses. They encourage people to contact them.

The Michael J. Fox Foundation for Parkinson's Research focuses primarily on research directed at finding the cause of PD and better treatment for PD. The Parkinson's Action Network (PAN) is an organization specially focused on encouraging greater funding of PD research. The other national organizations listed here primarily function for the support and education of those with PD, although they also fund PD research.

The Internet

The Internet is a great source of information, but also misinformation. You must be discriminating. The websites for the national PD groups listed at the end of this chapter provide up-to-date information. Medical societies can also be good of information.

The Movement Disorder Society is a large international professional group open to all physicians and scientists with an interest in PD and other disorders of movement. They have a special website targeted to a lay audience: www.wemove.org. This website provides useful information about not only PD but also the Parkinson's-plus syndromes discussed in Chapter 6.

The U.S. National Institutes of Health (NIH) is also a reliable source. Their website includes specific information about Parkinson's disease: www.ninds.nih.gov/disorders/parkinsons_disease/parkinsons_disease.htm. The NIH website for all health issues is also worth viewing: www.nlm.nih.gov/medlineplus.

For those with a specific interest in genetic disorders, the NIH provides yet another rich source of information, albeit very detailed and nuanced. That is the Online Mendelian Inheritance in Man (OMIM) website: www.ncbi.nlm.nih.gov/omim. This addresses all heritable diseases and is regularly updated with the latest research discoveries. Although primarily targeted to clinicians and researchers, the OMIM website may be of interest to some with PD who have a specific interest in certain genes.

The cost of medications is important to many families, and relevant information is available online. As previously mentioned in Chapter 11, wholesale cost comparisons for most prescription drugs may be found at the U.S. government website: www.medicaid.gov. You will need to navigate through their website by first selecting "Prescription Drugs," then "Survey of Retail Drug Prices," then "Pharmacy Pricing," which then allows opening of the Excel spreadsheet of NADAC drug prices. Easier to navigate is the commercial website (mentioned in Chapter 11): www.goodrx.com. This provides comparative retail drug prices in local communities, searched by town or zip code.

National PD Advocacy Groups

American Parkinson's Disease Assoc., Inc.
135 Parkinson Ave.
Staten Island, NY 10305
Phone: (800) 223-2732 or (718) 981-8001
FAX: (718) 981-4399
E-mail: apda@apdaparkinson.org
Website: www.apdaparkinson.org

Davis Phinney Foundation
1722 14th Street, Suite 150
Boulder, CO 80302
Tel: 866-358-0285 303-733-3340
Fax: 303-733-3350
Email: info@davisphinneyfoundation.org
Website: www.davisphinneyfoundation.org

Michael J. Fox Foundation for Parkinson's Research
Grand Central Station
P.O. Box 4777
New York, NY 10163-4777
Phone: (800) 708-7644
Website: www.michaeljfox.org

National Parkinson Foundation, Inc.
200 SE 1st Street
Suite 800
Miami, Florida 33131
Toll-free Helpline: 1-800-4PD-INFO (473-4636)
Fax: (305) 537-9901
E-mail inquiries: contact@parkinson.org or helpline@parkinson.org.
Website: www.parkinson.org

Parkinson's Action Network (PAN)
1025 Vermont Ave. NW, Suite 1120
Washington, D.C. 20005
Phone: 800-850-4726 or (202) 638-4101
E-mail: info@parkinsonsaction.org
Website: www.parkinsonsaction.org

Parkinson's Disease Foundation
1359 Broadway, Suite 1509
New York, NY 10018
Phone: (800) 457-6676 or (212) 923-4700
FAX: (212) 923-4778
(Columbia Office: 710 West 168th St., NY, NY 10032)
E-mail: info@pdf.org
Website: www.pdf.org

<h1 align="center">♦ ♦ ♦</h1>

Glossary

Acetylcholine—A widespread neurotransmitter, relevant to PD, memory, bowel and bladder function.

Aerobic exercise—Physical exercise that, continued over weeks to months, tends to lead to fitness. It is assessed by physiologists via measurement of oxygen utilization efficiency during exercise. In simple terms, it is vigorous exercise that tends to induce sweating, shortness of breath, body heat, and tiredness.

Agonist—A drug that activates a specific receptor (e.g., dopamine agonists activate dopamine receptors).

Akathisia—Inner restlessness; unable to comfortably sit still.

Alpha-synuclein—A protein normally found in neurons and present in high concentrations in Lewy bodies. A genetic mutation is the basis for a rare inherited form of parkinsonism.

Amantadine—A drug used in the treatment of PD. Its primary role is in the treatment of levodopa-induced dyskinesias. It is a mild and partial blocker of glutamate.

Amino acids—The building blocks of protein, and also the class of biological chemicals that includes levodopa.

Amitriptyline—An antidepressant medication from the tricyclic class that is also used for other purposes, such as a sleep aid.

Antagonist—A drug that blocks a specific receptor (e.g., a dopamine antagonist blocks dopamine receptors).

Anticholinergic—Drugs that block acetylcholine receptors.

Apomorphine—A dopamine agonist available for injection under the skin (subcutaneous). It is used for a quick response when in a levodopa off-state.

Apraxia—The inability to smoothly program small motor movements into a larger, more complex movement, such as waving, or throwing a ball.

Aspiration—Inappropriate passage of food or liquid into the lungs.

Ataxia—Incoordination, as occurs in problems involving the cerebellum, as well as imbalance.

ATP (adenosine triphosphate)—A high energy substance manufactured by the mitochondria within cells, which is necessary for multiple metabolic processes

Autonomic nervous system—The internal nervous system that controls bladder, bowels, sweating, sexual function and blood pressure.

Axon—A wire-like extension from the neuron that transmits an electrical signal from the cell body to the terminal, where the neurotransmitter is released.

Basal ganglia—A term for the combination of striatum, globus pallidus and interconnected nuclei (including substantia nigra and subthalamic nucleus).

BDNF (brain-derived neurotrophic factor)—A specific molecule (protein) that potentially increases survival and development of neurons. It is present both in the brain and can be measured in the circulation.

Benserazide—A drug that is identical in its function to carbidopa. This drug is available in certain countries outside the United States, including Europe.

Benztropine (Cogentin)—An anticholinergic drug.

Beta-blockers—Drugs that block one type of adrenalin-like responses. These are used in the treatment of tremor, high blood pressure, certain heart conditions, and migraines.

Biphasic dyskinesias—Levodopa-induced dyskinesias that occur twice during the levodopa on-cycle, transiently at the beginning and again at the end. Also called the D-I-D response (dyskinesia-improvement-dyskinesia).

Blepharospasm—Dystonia of the eyes, manifest as involuntary eye closure.

Blood-brain barrier—The lining around the blood vessels of the brain that prevents undesirable substances within the bloodstream from entering the brain.

Bradykinesia—The slowness of movement that is typical of PD.

Bradyphrenia—Slowness of thought.

Brainstem—The lowest end of the brain that interfaces with the spinal cord. Tracts passing from higher brain centers to the spinal cord pass through the brainstem, and vice versa. The brainstem contains nuclei that control elementary functions, such as breathing and eye movements.

Bromocriptine (Parlodel)—A dopamine agonist drug from the ergot class, no longer used to treat Parkinson's disease.

Carbidopa—A drug that blocks the conversion of levodopa to dopamine in the circulation but not in the brain (it does not cross the blood brain barrier).

Catechol-O-methyltransferase (COMT)—One of the enzymes that breaks down levodopa and dopamine. Blocking this enzyme is a PD treatment strategy.

Caudate—This brain nucleus forms the front portion of the striatum.

Cerebellum—A brain structure located just above the brainstem. Damage to this area causes ataxia (incoordination, imbalance).

Chemoreceptive trigger zone—A small region in the brainstem that senses certain substances circulating in the bloodstream. When stimulated by one of these substances, nausea results. Since there is no blood-brain barrier at this site, circulating dopamine can stimulate this region and cause nausea.

Cholinergic—Neurons that release acetylcholine as the neurotransmitter.

Chorea—Involuntary movements characterized by their rapidly flowing, chaotic pattern. These are the primary movements caused by an excessive levodopa effect.

Choreiform—A descriptive term implying that the appearance is that of chorea.

Clonazepam (Klonopin)—A sedating medication from the benzodiazepine class that is used to treat REM sleep behavior disorder.

Clozapine (Clozaril)—A medication used to treat hallucinations and delusions. It is very effective, but has very significant side effects.

Coenzyme Q (Coenzyme Q_{10})—A substance that participates in the chemical reactions of mitochondria. Supplementation of coenzyme Q was initially thought beneficial for Parkinson's disease but failed in larger and more comprehensive clinical trials.

Colon—The large intestine where feces form.

COMT inhibitor—Drugs that block the enzyme, catechol-O-methyltransferase, thereby prolonging the action of levodopa.

Cortex—Outermost layers of the brain, which are most highly developed in humans. Complex human thought, language and behavior are conceived and programmed here.

Corticobasal degeneration—A neurodegenerative condition that has some resemblance to PD. The clinical picture is termed corticobasal syndrome.

Corticospinal—One of the primary brain and spinal cord systems involved with controlling movement. This is spared in PD.

CR (controlled-release)—The sustained-release form of carbidopa/levodopa (Sinemet CR). This is to be distinguished from a recently developed combination formulation of regular and sustained-release carbidopa/levodopa with the brand name Rytary.

CT scan—Computed tomography scan, which is used to image the brain.

Deep brain stimulation (DBS)—Therapy employing high frequency stimulation of a specific brain region through a device similar to a heart pacemaker.

Delusions—Beliefs that are inappropriate, patently false, and sometimes bizarre.

Dementia—Loss of intellectual abilities, usually due to a neurodegenerative disorder.

Dendrites—Short, wire-like processes on neurons that receive neurotransmitter signals from axon terminals.

Diaphoresis—Sweating.

Diastolic—A blood pressure parameter corresponding to the second number in blood pressure readings (such as "80" in the reading of "120/80").

Diffuse Lewy body disease (Lewy body dementia, dementia with Lewy bodies)—A condition in which the neurodegenerative changes, including Lewy bodies, are widespread, typically affecting both the substantia nigra (resulting in parkinsonism) and the cortex (resulting in dementia).

Diplopia—Double vision.

Diuretic—A water pill (increases urine output).

DNA—Deoxyribonucleic acid, which is the molecule used to write the genetic codes of living cells.

Dominant inheritance—The inheritance pattern in which a trait is passed from one generation to the next. Half of the offspring in any generation tend to display the trait passed from one parent (if it is fully expressed).

Donepezil (Aricept)—A medication that increases brain levels of acetylcholine, which is used to treat memory disorders.

Dopa decarboxylase—The enzyme that converts levodopa into dopamine.

Dopamine—The neurotransmitter that is deficient in PD.

Dopamine agonist—Synthetic drugs that behave like dopamine.

Dopaminergic—Adjective relating to neurons that release dopamine as their neurotransmitter.

Droxidopa (Northera)—A recently approved drug for treating orthostatic hypotension. It requires dopa decarboxylase to be converted to the active substances norepinephrine and epinephrine. Administered carbidopa blocks dopa decarboxylase.

Duodopa—Brand name for a recently approved gel formulation of carbidopa/levodopa administered into the small intestine via an implanted tube in the abdomen. Because it bypasses the stomach with delivery directly into the jejunum (where levodopa is absorbed into the circulation), the levodopa response is more consistent and sustained. It is used for treatment of levodopa fluctuations that cannot be adequately treated with adjustment of carbidopa/levodopa pills.

Dysarthria—Impaired precision of speech.

Dyskinesias—In the context of PD, these are involuntary movements provoked by medications, primarily levodopa. These are especially characterized by flowing, dancing movements (chorea) of the limbs, trunk, neck, or face

Dysphagia—Impaired swallowing.

Dyspnea—Shortness of breath.

Dystonia—A muscle contraction state resulting in an abnormal posture of a foot, toes, hand, etc. This is caused by abnormal motor programming within the central nervous system. Among those with PD, this is usually a parkinsonian symptom, rather than a medication side effect.

Dysuria—Painful urination.

Entacapone (Comtan)—A COMT inhibitor that prolongs the levodopa effect and is used to enhance the carbidopa/levodopa response.

Enzymes—Cellular molecules used to transform or modify specific biochemical substances. An example is dopa decarboxylase, which transforms levodopa into dopamine.

Ergot—A class of drugs that includes bromocriptine, pergolide and cabergoline. These have unique side effects not shared by other dopamine agonists. They are no longer used to treat Parkinson's disease.

Esophagus—The passageway from the mouth to the stomach.

Essential tremor—The most common cause of tremor, sometimes confused with PD. People with this condition experience no other neurological symptoms other than tremor.

Extrapyramidal—A term for the basal ganglia and its connections. The term originated to distinguish this from another movement control circuit, the pyramidal motor system.

Fluctuations—Variations in the levodopa response, with transitions between on- and off-states.

Fludrocortisone (Florinef)—A medication used to elevate the blood pressure, which works by causing the kidneys to excrete less sodium (salt).

Freezing—Transient paralysis of movement. In PD, this most often relates to walking, where the feet become stuck to the floor.

GDNF (glial cell line-derived neurotrophic factor)—A specific molecule (protein) that supports neuron survival and development, including dopaminergic neurons.

Gene—A DNA code for a specific protein.

Glia—The supporting cells of the nervous system. They perform a variety of metabolic and housekeeping tasks that are critical to neurons.

Globus pallidus—This nucleus is located between the striatum and thalamus. Most of the striatal output is to this nucleus, which in turn, has important projections to the thalamus.

Glutamate—A brain neurotransmitter.

Glutamate antagonist—Drugs that block the brain neurotransmitter, glutamate.

Hesitancy—Slowed, hard-to-start urination.

Homocysteine—A metabolite normally present in the bloodstream. Elevated concentrations are a risk factor for atherosclerosis and dementia.

Hypokinetic—The type of speech problem (dysarthria) found in PD.

Hypophonia—The soft voice of PD.

Hypotension—Low blood pressure.

Immediate-release—The regular formulation of a medication, distinguished from sustained-release products. Carbidopa/levodopa comes in two forms, immediate-release and sustained-release.

Lesioning—Surgically destroying a small area of brain tissue.

Levodopa—The amino acid that is the precursor to dopamine.

Levodopa treatment—This implies carbidopa/levodopa treatment. Plain levodopa without carbidopa is no longer used.

Lewy body—Round collections of amorphous material inside neurons in PD, including the substantia nigra. Aggregated alpha-synuclein is one important component, among many others.

Lewy body dementia—See diffuse Lewy body disease.

Lewy dots—Microscopic, small accumulations of alpha-synuclein and other products, representing part of the Lewy neurodegenerative process.

Lewy neurites—Accumulations of aggregated alpha-synuclein and many other substances in the dendrites and axons of neurons, seen microscopically with special tissue stains.

Long-duration levodopa response—A sustained effect from levodopa, which develops over about one week. If levodopa is discontinued, this benefit conversely dissipates over a week.

Madopar—The brand name for benserazide/levodopa, which is used in some European countries.

MAO-B inhibitor—Drugs that block one of the two major forms of monoamine oxidase (the B-form). This results in slightly higher brain dopamine levels. The primary drugs in this class are selegiline (Eldepryl; formerly, known as deprenyl) and rasagiline (Azilect).

Midodrine (ProAmatine)—An adrenalin-like drug that elevates blood pressure, but spares the heart.

Mirabegron (Myrbetriq)—A medication used to treat urinary urgency. Unlike the other bladder drugs used for that purpose, it does not block acetylcholine and hence does not have anticholinergic side effects. It tends to relax muscles in the bladder wall by activating beta-3 adrenergic receptors.

Mirtazepine (Remeron)—An antidepressant medication.

Mitochondria—Components of all cells that carry on critical oxidative chemical reactions that generate ATP.

Monoamine oxidase (MAO)—An enzyme that breaks down dopamine. Blocking it will enhance PD treatment. Blocking the B-form is well tolerated, whereas also inhibiting the A-form of MAO has the potential for serious side effects.

Motor—Term for movement and action; for example, brain circuits that program motor function.

MRI—Magnetic resonance imaging, which generates high-resolution views of the brain.

Multiple system atrophy (MSA)—A neurodegenerative disorder that may resemble PD.

Nadolol (Corgard)—A beta-blocking drug that does not cross the blood-brain-barrier, which is used to treat tremor.

Neurodegenerative—A class of disorders in which certain brain systems slowly die (degenerate); this includes conditions such as Parkinson's disease, Alzheimer's disease and Lou Gehrig's disease (ALS).

Neurogenic bladder—A malfunctioning bladder due to impaired nervous system control.

Neuroleptic—A class of medications used to treat psychosis (e.g., hallucinations, delusions). Most drugs in this class block dopamine receptors and may induce or exacerbate parkinsonism (except for quetiapine and clozapine).

Neuron—The primary brain cell, of which there are approximately 10 billion in the normal brain. Neurons contain a cell body with a nucleus and an axon extending from that cell body.

Neuropathology—The study of disease states within the nervous system, which might include visual inspection and microscopic evaluation of brain, spinal cord, and nerves, as well as laboratory measurements.

Neurotransmitter—The chemical released by nerve terminals used to signal the next neuron in the brain circuit.

Neurotrophic hormone—A class of chemicals found in the nervous system that enhance the growth and viability of neurons.

Nigrostriatal—The projection from the substantia nigra neuron to the striatum. Each nigrostriatal neuron has a cell body located within the substantia nigra, with an axon extending to the striatum.

Nocturia—Urination during the night.

Norepinephrine—A neurotransmitter, also called noradrenalin.

Normal pressure hydrocephalus (NPH)—A disorder of senior citizens in which the brain ventricles expand; this impairs the function of nearby brain circuits. The symptoms include a parkinsonian gait, urinary incontinence, and cognitive dysfunction.

Nortriptyline (Pamelor, Aventyl)—An antidepressant medication that is some-times used for other purposes, such as a sleep aid.

NSAIDs—Nonsteroidal anti-inflammatory drugs, such as ibuprofen, naproxen, plus a variety of prescription pain relievers.

Nuclei—Collections of neurons grouped together in a somewhat homogeneous brain structure.

Off—The state when levodopa is not working.

Olanzapine (Zyprexa)—A medication used to treat hallucinations and delusions. It may induce parkinsonism.

On—The state when levodopa is working and parkinsonian symptoms are relieved.

Opioid—A drug with narcotic properties.

Orthostatic—Standing, as in orthostatic hypotension, where the blood pressure is low when erect.

Osteoporosis—Weakening of bones. A related term, osteopenia, implies mild, early loss of bone integrity.

Oxybutynin (Ditropan)—An anticholinergic medication used to treat urinary urgency.

Pallidotomy—Surgically lesioning the pallidum to treat PD.

Pallidum—Another name for the globus pallidus, a target of one form of PD surgery.

Parcopa—A formulation of carbidopa/levodopa that dissolves in your mouth and is then swallowed. Water or other liquid is not necessary to take this pill.

Parkin—A component of the ubiquitin proteasome system. Mutations of the gene coding for parkin are responsible for many cases of parkinsonism starting before age 40 years.

Parkinsonism—Implies that the clinical appearance resembles Parkinson's disease; however, it may or may not be PD.

Pathological—Adjective, implying extreme, reaching the level of a disease state. In this text, this term has been used for the most severe compulsive behaviors pro-voked by dopamine agonist medications (e.g., gambling, sexual acts).

Pathology—The study of disease states within the body, which might include visual inspection, microscopic evaluation and laboratory measurement.

Pergolide (Permax)—An ergot dopamine agonist drug no longer used to treat Parkinson's disease.

Peristalsis—Contractions of the gut that move food products through gastrointestinal system during digestion.

PET scan—Positron emission tomography, a nuclear medicine scanning technique. With certain injected substances, dopaminergic neurons are imaged.

Placebo—A "sugar pill" used in clinical trials.

Polymorphisms—Normal variations of genes.

Postmortem—After death, such as a brain autopsy.

Pramipexole (Mirapex)—A dopamine agonist drug.

Praxis—Programming of smaller motor movements to make a more complex movement.

Progressive supranuclear palsy (PSP)—A neurodegenerative condition often mistaken for PD.

Propranolol (Inderal)—A beta-blocking drug sometimes used to treat tremor. It is also used to treat high blood pressure, certain heart disorders, and migraine.

Protein—A class of biological chemicals, composed of strings of amino acids.

Putamen—The back portion of the striatum. This region sustains greater loss of dopamine than the caudate in PD.

Quetiapine (Seroquel)—A medication used to treat hallucinations and delusions.

Rasagiline (Azilect)—An inhibitor of MAO-B, used to treat the symptoms of Parkinson's disease. Some clinicians believe it may slow the progression of Parkinson's disease but this is unproven.

Receptor—The region of the synapse that binds a specific neurotransmitter.

Recessive inheritance—Traits that occur within a generation but are not passed from one generation to the next (except in rare situations). The trait is expressed only when both genes of a pair are affected; that is, both the mother and father contribute an abnormal gene.

REM sleep behavior disorder—Acting out dreams during rapid eye movement (REM) sleep. Normally, the body should be limp during this dreaming stage of sleep, except for eye movements.

Restless legs syndrome—A creepy-crawly feeling in the legs when trying to sleep, associated with the urge to get up and walk to gain relief.

Rest tremor—The typical tremor of PD. When affecting the hands, it is present when they are not being used, such as in the lap, or at one's sides when walking.

Reuptake—The mechanism whereby neuron terminals control the duration and intensity of a neurotransmitter effect. The presynaptic terminal sucks up the neurotransmitter after release to prevent the effect from being excessive.

Rigidity—The increased tone of limbs seen in PD.

Ropinirole (Requip)—A dopamine agonist drug.

Rotigotine (Neupro)—A dopamine agonist drug that is administered as a skin patch. It has properties very similar to ropinirole.

Rytary—Brand name of a newly released drug, combining sustained-release and immediate-release carbidopa/levodopa.

Selegiline (deprenyl, Eldepryl)—An MAO-B inhibitor drug, which tends to enhance the levodopa effect.

Serotonin—A brain neurotransmitter, which may be deficient in some cases of depression.

Short-duration levodopa response—A one to six hour response that is time-locked to each levodopa dose.

Sinemet—The brand name for carbidopa/levodopa.

Sleep apnea—Impaired breathing during sleep.

SNRI (Serotonin-norepinephrine reuptake inhibitor)—A class of antidepressant medications, also used to treat chronic pain. Similar to SSRI drugs, they block reuptake of serotonin; however, they also block norepinephrine reuptake.

Spasticity—The clinical features of someone with damage to their corticospinal tracts. This variably causes increased deep tendon reflexes and limb tone, Babinski signs (extension rather than flexion of the great toe when the undersurface of the foot is scratched), as well as a specific pattern of weakness.

SPECT scan—Single photon emission computed tomography, which can be used to image brain dopamine systems when certain chemicals are injected.

Spinal cord—This, along with the brain make up the central nervous system. It is an elongated extension of the brain, extending downward from the brainstem. Tracts from the cortex and subcortex pass through the brainstem to the spinal cord, which is the final common pathway controlling movement. Conversely, sensory information (e.g., touch, pain) passes in the opposite direction via other tracts, up to the brain.

SSRI (selective serotonin reuptake inhibitor)—A class of antidepressant medications; the effects are mediated by blocking the reuptake of serotonin.

Stalevo—A combination drug containing entacapone, carbidopa, and levodopa.

Stem cell—A very immature cell with potential to differentiate into a wide variety of cells, including neurons.

Striatum—The brain region that receives the dopaminergic projections from the substantia nigra. The striatum is comprised of two components: putamen and caudate.

Subcortex—Brain centers located underneath the cortex, which tend to have more elementary functions than cortical circuits. The basal ganglia is subcortical.

Substantia nigra—Neurons containing a black pigment and located at the upper end of the brainstem, in the midbrain. This degenerates in PD.

Subthalamic nucleus—A nucleus located just beneath the thalamus, which is intimately connected with the striatum and globus pallidus. Strokes here cause involuntary movements. It is a target for neurosurgical treatment of PD.

Sustained-release (SR)—Formulating a medication to make it dissolve very slowly; hence, the effect is delayed and prolonged. Sinemet CR is a sustained release formulation of carbidopa/levodopa.

Synapse—The interface between a nerve terminal and a receptor. The terminal releases a specific neurotransmitter into the synaptic cleft, which then binds to the receptor.

Systolic—A blood pressure parameter corresponding to the upper number in blood pressure readings (such as "120" in the reading of "120/80").

Terminal—The end of the axon, which releases a neurotransmitter.

Thalamotomy—Lesioning the thalamus, primarily done to treat tremor.

Thalamus—A centrally located brain nucleus with widespread connections to the cortex. It receives extensive input from the globus pallidus, as well as from a variety of other brain regions.

Tolcapone (Tasmar)—A COMT inhibitor drug that enhances the levodopa response. Because of potential for life-threatening liver failure, it is now rarely prescribed.

Tolterodine (Detrol)—An anticholinergic medication used to treat urinary urgency.

Tracts—Collections of axons running together like a telephone cable.

Transporter—A component of cells that moves (transports) a chemical across a cell membrane. For example, the dopamine transporter is responsible for the reuptake of dopamine from the region of the synapse.

Trazodone (Desyrel)—An antidepressant medication often used as a sleep aid.

Tremor—A rhythmic (back and forth) movement.

Trospium (Sanctura)—An anticholinergic drug used to treat urinary urgency. This medication is unique among the anticholinergic bladder drugs in that it does not cross the blood-brain barrier; hence it has no potential to block cholinergic memory circuitry within the brain.

Tricyclic—A class of antidepressant medications.

Trihexyphenidyl (Artane)—An anticholinergic drug.

Trimethobenzamide (Tigan)—A medication used to treat nausea. This does not worsen parkinsonism, as do most of the other prescription nausea drugs.

Ubiquitin—A cellular molecule that is used to tag proteins destined for degradation.

Ubiquitin-proteasome system—A complex system within cells for disposing of unwanted or abnormal proteins.

UPDRS—Unified Parkinson's Disease Rating Scale, which is the PD scoring system used by clinicians for quantifying parkinsonism. A major component is the test battery that tabulates the PD motor examination. Each item on this motor subscale (e.g., facial masking, arm rigidity, bradykinesia, etc.) is scored from zero (normal) to 4 (maximum severity). The scores from all of the items are added to provide a single UPDRS value. Although this may be used in routine care, it is especially a clinical research tool.

Ureter—The conduit from the kidneys to the bladder.

Urethra—The conduit out from the bladder, through which urine externally passes.

Urgency—An enhanced sense that one must urinate.

Vertigo—One form of dizziness, characterized by a subjective sense that the room or person is spinning or moving.

Wearing-off—When the levodopa beneficial effect is declining, typically before the next dose.

Wilson's disease—A rare disorder of copper metabolism, with liver and neurological problems. Tremor and parkinsonism may occur in this condition.

Index

♦ ♦ ♦

Page numbers followed by t indicate a table on the designated page